G. Antes/F. Eggemann · Small Bowel Radiology

Günther Antes · Franz Eggemann

Small Bowel Radiology

Introduction and Atlas

Preface by Professor J. Lissner, M.D., Munich

With 276 figures

Springer-Verlag
Berlin Heidelberg New York
London Paris Tokyo

Günther Antes, M.D.
Chief Physician
Department of Radiology
Stadtkrankenhaus Kempten
Robert-Weixler-Str. 50
D-8960 Kempten

Franz Eggemann, M.D.
Senior Physician
Department of Diagnostic Radiology and Nuclear Medicine
Städtisches Krankenhaus München-Neuperlach
Oskar-Maria-Graf-Ring 51
D-8000 München 83

Cover illustration: Meckel's Diverticulum (see Fig. 5.6.-9)

ISBN-13: 978-3-642-82475-3 e-ISBN-13: 978-3-642-82473-9
DOI: 10.1007/978-3-642-82473-9

Library of Congress Cataloging in Publication Data

Antes, Günther, 1943–. Small bowel radiology.
Bibliography: p. Includes index.
1. Intestine, Small – Radiography – Atlases.
2. Intestine, Small – Diseases – Diagnosis – Atlases.
I. Eggemann, Franz, 1941–. II. Title.
[DNLM: 1. Intestine, Small – radiography – atlases.
WI 17 A627s]
RC804.R6A58 1987 616.3′407572 87-28784

Product Liability: The publisher can give no guarantee for information about drug dosage and application thereof contained in this book. In every individual case the respective user must check its accuracy by consulting other pharmaceutical literature.
The use of registered names, trademarks, etc. in this publication does not imply, even in the absence of a specific statement, that such names are exempt from the relevant protective laws and regulations and therefore free for general use.

Softcover reprint of the hardcover 1st edition 1988

Reproduction of figures: Karl Porupski GmbH & Co. KG, Stuttgart

2329/3321-543210

Contents

Preface

In this book, Dr. Antes and Dr. Eggemann have communicated their vast experience in the complicated field of radiology of the small bowel. In my opinion, this is a highly valuable and successful study and I would like to congratulate the authors on this most worthwhile, comprehensive presentation.

Dr. Antes worked at our institution for many years and I am happy to comment on his great personal commitment. Observing Dr. Eggemann's scientific activity at close range, I am aware of both his subtle examination technique and admirable results.

It only remains for me to wish this well-approved book the success it really deserves.

J. Lissner, Munich

Acknowledgements

We would like to thank Professor Dr. J. Lissner of the Department of Radiology, University Hospital, Munich-Großhadern, and Dr. U. Schulz, Chief Physician, Department of Diagnostic Radiology and Nuclear Medicine, Municipal Hospital, Munich-Neuperlach, for their unlimited support, concerning our work. Our gratitude extends to all colleagues from the Radiological Departments of the hospitals at Munich-Großhadern, Munich-Neuperlach and Kempten for their enthusiasm and also to Professor Dr. H.J. Clemens from the Springer Publishing Company for the organization of this book.

Last but not least, we would like to thank our families for sacrificing their time during our work on the manuscript.

G. Antes, Kempten *F. Eggemann, Munich*

1 Introduction

Since the small bowel except the duodenum and terminal ileum is largely inaccessible during endoscopic examination, radiology of the small bowel attains special significance as a diagnostic method. Owing to the length and position of this organ, good images are difficult to obtain. Furthermore, the considerable variation of transit time, unpredictable response of the contrast medium, and superimposition with the filled loops make small bowel radiology difficult. As a result, few radiologists specialize in this field. With the exception of Crohn's disease, disorders of the small bowel are relatively rare. Thus, not many clinicians and radiologists are interested in the small intestine.

The follow-through method according to Pansdorf (1937) is still the most frequently employed roentgenological investigation of the small bowel. In most cases, "no significant abnormality detected" is a very convenient phrase for the diagnostician. Only the most careful follow-through investigations can obtain good diagnostic results (Golden 1959; Marshak and Lindner 1976). Early attempts by Einhorn (1926), Pribram and Kleiber (1927) and especially Pesquera (1929) were made to improve small bowel radiology by selective intubation of the duodenum. In the following years, attempts were made to optimize small bowel enema (*enteroclysis*) and to accelerate the passage. In 1939, Gershon-Cohen and Shay already obtained good images of the small bowel in single and double contrast. In 1943, Schatzki advocated larger quantities of dilute contrast medium. Previously, the major problems in enteroclysis were inadequate equipment and difficulties with intubation. In 1951, however, Lura reported over 300 successful investigations. Further improvements in small bowel intubation technique were described by Scott-Harden et al. (1961), Pygott et al. (1960), Gianturco (1967) and Bilbao et al. (1967).

Sellink, however, was really responsible for the widespread recognition of enteroclysis (1971, 1974, 1976). In spite of the increasing popularity of this method, the necessity for substituting this apparently viable method for the peroral examination is still equivocal (Rabe et al. 1981; Fried et al. 1981; Maglinte et al. 1982; Ott et al. 1985). Comparisons of both methods, however, (Fleckenstein and Pedersen 1975; Sanders and Ho 1976; Ekberg 1977; Vallance 1980) have confirmed the superiority of enteroclysis. It achieves a high accuracy (Antes and Lissner 1983).

Sellink, with his *Radiological Atlas of Common Diseases of the Small Bowel* (1976) created a standard reference for radiology of the small bowel. This book contains a vast amount of information concerning investigational technique and radiological-clinical correlations. He prefers the enteroclysis with a barium suspension of low specific weight which, however, does not obtain successful results in every case. For this reason, like previous authors, Sellink tried to obtain double contrast images of the small intestine. He used *water* or *air* for achieving a better transparency. Geiter and Fuchs (1977) popularized the double contrast method in Germany using water. Trickey et al. (1963) and later Gmünder and Wirth (1970) introduced methylcellulose as a negative contrast medium for double contrast. Herlinger (1978) described a modification of these methods. He found out that methylcellulose has a better stabilizing effect on the barium suspension than water. This method, which we have adopted, yields better morphological images of the small bowel.

Herlinger (1978, 1979), however, does not report on motility disturbances. Generally in literature there is little information concerning this subject. Sellink, on the other hand, brought it to attention which inspired us to concern ourselves with these functional changes and to develop a method which may include motility disorders as well as morphological changes during one examination (Antes and Lissner 1981). It consists of a combination of single and double contrast and thus unites the advantages of both methods in the same investigation.

A detailed examination of the duodenum has been omitted, since this is task of the double contrast study of the stomach. Enteroclysis, however, may demonstrate gross changes in the duodenum. Standardization of method obtains films which allow a reinterpretation by others. The investigations can always be reproduced.

This book compiles the results of more than 5000 investigations of the small intestine in double contrast since 1977. Examination with barium and methylcellulose has been performed since 1979. In our opinion, this method produces optimal diagnoses of the small bowel. Furthermore, we are convinced that the most suitable method and best radiographs alone do not produce an accurate diagnosis. Of paramount importance are adequate knowledge of small bowel diseases and continuous clinical correlation. An optimal result also requires an experienced investigator.

We have selected the most interesting and most instructive cases, whereby considerable importance was attached to the clinical findings. Every diagnosis has been confirmed by histology, laboratory tests and follow-up observations. The first section of this book discusses *investigational technique, indications* and *fundamental roentgenological interpretation.* The second part is an *atlas* in which small bowel diseases are subdivided into groups and illustrated with examples. Special attention is focussed on motility disorders. A systematic organization makes an intersection of pathological entities inevitable (e.g. obstruction by tumor or Crohn's disease). We have tried to overcome this problem by referring to other chapters. Our experience in infants and children is limited. Enteroclysis, however, is of growing importance in this area, too.

As far as further progress in enteroclysis and clarification of small bowel diseases are concerned, we keep an open mind about other imaging procedures (CT, sonography, angiography, and MRI). We have referred to these methods as far as possible.

2 Examination Technique

2.1 Patient Preparation

Emptying of the large bowel is a prerequisite for optimal investigation of the small bowel (Sellink and Rosenbusch 1981). Adequate preparation is therefore important, particularly in patients suffering from chronic constipation. A filled cecum inhibits the contrast medium passage, thus prolonging the investigation. Furthermore, in the assessment of the ileocecal region, more contrast medium has to be introduced if the bowel contents have to be washed out of the cecum. This can lead to artifacts in this region which may be misinterpreted for inflammatory lesions, tumors or worms (Figs. 2.9.-1 and 2). A filled cecum also inhibits the assessment of the distal ileum, especially if the cecum is situated low in the pelvis.

The following procedure is recommended:

One day before the examination:
a) Food: a light breakfast; clear soup for lunch and then liquids only. Amount of fluid for the rest of the day: 2.5–3 liters. No milk or milk products.
b) Purgation: in the early afternoon e.g. with Prepacol® or X-Prep®.

Day of investigation: The patient is given nothing to eat and the bladder should not be emptied!

The filled bladder lifts the small bowel loops out of the pelvis minor, allowing better accessibility for the investigator.

The above procedure may be modified for patients with diarrhea. In such cases, preparation would include fluids only. In extreme cases of constipation, more intensive cleansing methods may be necessary. Drugs which have a peristaltic inhibitory effect, e.g. sedatives, antipsychotic drugs, strong pain killers and spasmolytics, should be discontinued, if possible, several days before.

2.2 Instruments

Tubes: Special tubes for enteroclysis, e.g. Bilbao-Dotter tube, Nicholas tube, are supplied by various companies (Cook Co., Nicholas Ltd). The roentgen opaque tube should be 125–150 cm long, the distal end of which may be open or closed. For guiding the tube, a guide wire of the same length is provided. The set may be used again. It is a good idea to coat the wire with silicone or olive oil. After several applications, the plastic tubes become hard and shrink. The discrepancy between the tube and wire makes application difficult. This problem may be overcome by placing the tube in warm water and stretching it to the required length. At present we use the small bowel tube of Nicholas Ltd (Nicholas Small Bowel Tube)[1] (Fig. 2.4.-1). This tube is only 2.8 mm in diameter and is provided with a double mandrel (spiral mandrel with steel core), which simplifies the intubation considerably. The transnasal intubation is well-tolerated, retching is rare. The gastral passage is much easier to perform than with other special tubes. Fluoroscopy time can be reduced, too (Antes and Eggemann 1987).

[1] Nicholas Small Bowel Tube, Art. Nr. 810; Nicholas Ltd, D-6231 Sulzbach, Germany

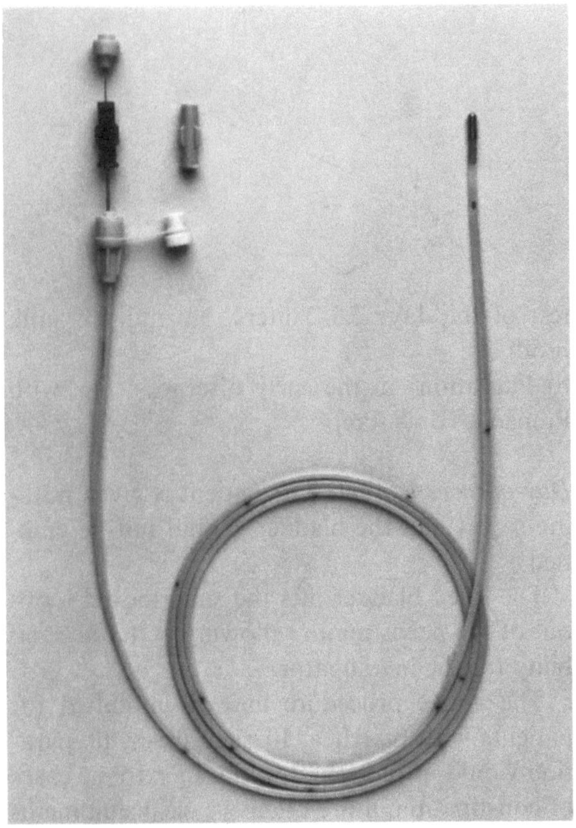

Fig. 2.4.-1. Intubation. Nicholas Small Bowel Tube with double mandrel (spiral mandrel with steel core)

Injection/pumping: There are various methods of instilling the contrast medium. A steady flow rate is important. The simplest method is to administer the barium from a container as in the colon contrast enema (see chapter 2.7) and the more viscous methylcellulose by injection (e.g. by means of a bladder syringe).

The application of an electric pump has proved to be best. We work with a roller pump[2] which facilitates the investigation procedure. Thus, the small bowel enema can be easily performed by one person (Trüber and Fuchs 1981). Prior to investigation, it is important to check that the connection to the duodenal tube is compatible.

[2] Fresenius Ltd, Borkenberg 14, D-6370 Oberursel/Ts. 1, Germany

2.3 Contrast Medium and Preparation

Barium: The barium suspension should be of low viscosity and free of bubbles. According to Sellink the specific gravity should be 1.2–1.3 corresponding to the patient's weight (Miller and Sellink 1979; Sellink and Rosenbusch 1981). With our method, however, the specific gravity of 1.3 is independent of the patient's weight and is adequate in every case.

Barium preparation: one part barium to two parts water (e.g. 300 ml Micropaque® fluid[3] and 600 ml tap water). This quantity is recommended, even if there is a surplus, as it is important to have enough contrast medium available for special cases (e.g. obstructions).

Methylcellulose: Tylose®[4] e.g. may be used. The 0.5% aqueous solution can be prepared either shortly before the investigation or on the day before.

10 g methylcellulose is stirred into 200 ml of hot water. This stock solution is then diluted with 1800 ml tap water.

For measuring purposes, a drugs cup may be marked to indicate the appropriate amount.

[3] Micropaque® fluid, Nicholas Ltd, Sulzbach, Germany

[4] Tylose MH 300 "Kalle", Caesar und Loretz Co., Hilden, Germany

This avoids having to measure each time. Before application, brisk stirring should smooth out any clumps which may be present in the methylcellulose solution. The temperatures of both barium and methylcellulose solutions should roughly correspond to room temperature (20° C) in order not to chill the patient too much.

2.4 Intubation

Peroral or transnasal intubation is possible. Transnasal intubation has certain advantages (Maglinte et al. 1986). We recommend a local anesthetic with lidocaine gel or spray. Swallowing and gastric transit is best accomplished in standing position without fluoroscopy. If the patient starts coughing, the investigator will know that the tube is going into the bronchial system. On reaching the cardia, the rest of the passage is controlled by fluoroscopy until the duodenum is approached. Particularly in stocky patients with transverse stomachs, the tube may touch the left gastric wall and coil up into a dorsal cascade of the fundus (Fig. 2.4.-2). By turning the guide wire, slightly bending its tip and pressing in the left epigastric region against the gastric fundus with the lead-gloved hand – with the patient in standing position or lying on the right side – the tube may be directed into the antrum (Fig. 2.4.-3). Care should be taken to avoid abrupt pushing against the wall of the stomach or coiling in the fundus since both may cause retching or vomiting. The same goes for the antrum whilst the tube is being directed into the pylorus canal. This often happens in slim patients with marked ptotic, "fishhook" stomachs. To direct the tube away from the stomach wall, the guide wire should be drawn back a little to allow the soft tip of the tube to be mobile. In ptotic stomachs, transit through the pylorus can be facilitated by pressing with the hand against the antrum from caudal, thereby lifting and stretching it. As soon as the duodenum is reached, the tube in most cases glides easily as far as the ligament of Treitz. There is no need for positioning the catheter distal to this region. When the tube has entered the duodenum, the guide wire should not be pushed over the level of the pylorus. The catheter is eased forward, holding the guide wire taut. If there is a sharp bend in the lower duodenal flexure, the tube usually has to remain there, since it is impossible to maneuver it farther. Gastric reflux may be avoided by positioning the patient on the left side or elevating the examination table. Should problems arise, the position of the catheter may be determined by introducing a small test dosage of contrast medium.

A coiling of the tube in the stomach should be avoided since the pressure of the flowing contrast medium will produce a spring effect, causing the tip of the tube to lever itself out of the duodenum or causing nausea. It is better for two people to perform the positioning of the tube; one can operate the fluoroscope and direct the tube by palpation whilst the other pushes and directs the catheter. The radiographer should not be alarmed if the tube coils above the diaphragm. This indicates a large intrathoracic hernia. Intubation may proceed when the loop is straightened (Fig. 2.4.-5).

Positioning of the tube will probably take some time before the radiographer becomes experienced. He or she will then be able to perform the operation more quickly.

Radiation exposure can be kept to a minimum by using proper collimation. If the patient is informed about the purpose of duodenal intubation well in advance, cooperation may be guaranteed which is certainly an advantage in control examinations.

In difficult circumstances, the tube may be introduced by means of a gastroscope. The introduction of the Nicholas tubes, however, has facilitated the intubation.

Drugs (e.g. Metoclopramide, Diazepam) are not necessary.

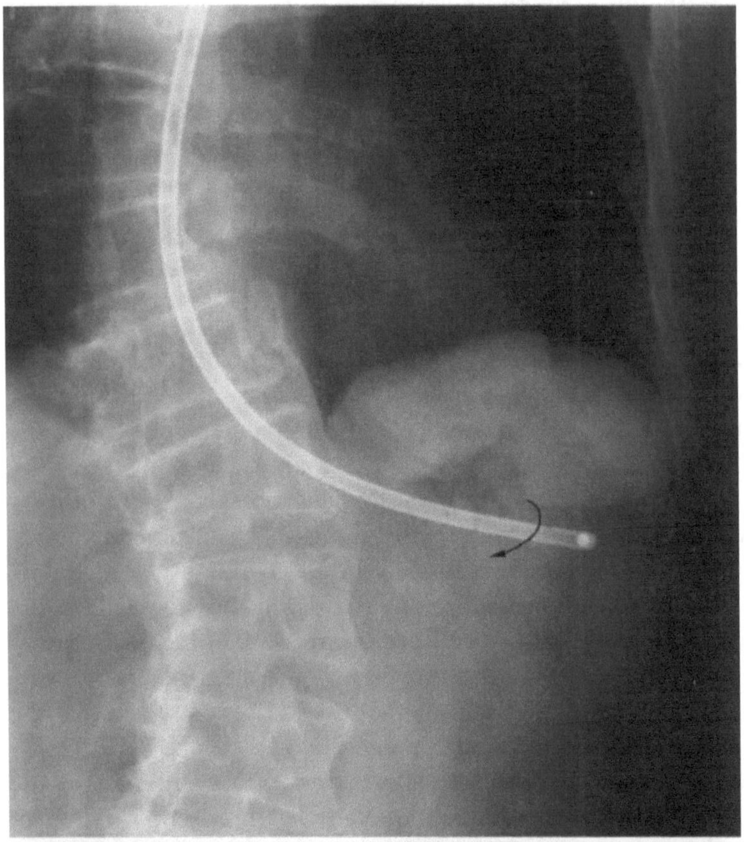

Fig. 2.4.-2. Intubation. On entering the stomach, the tube usually proceeds left and pushes against the stomach wall

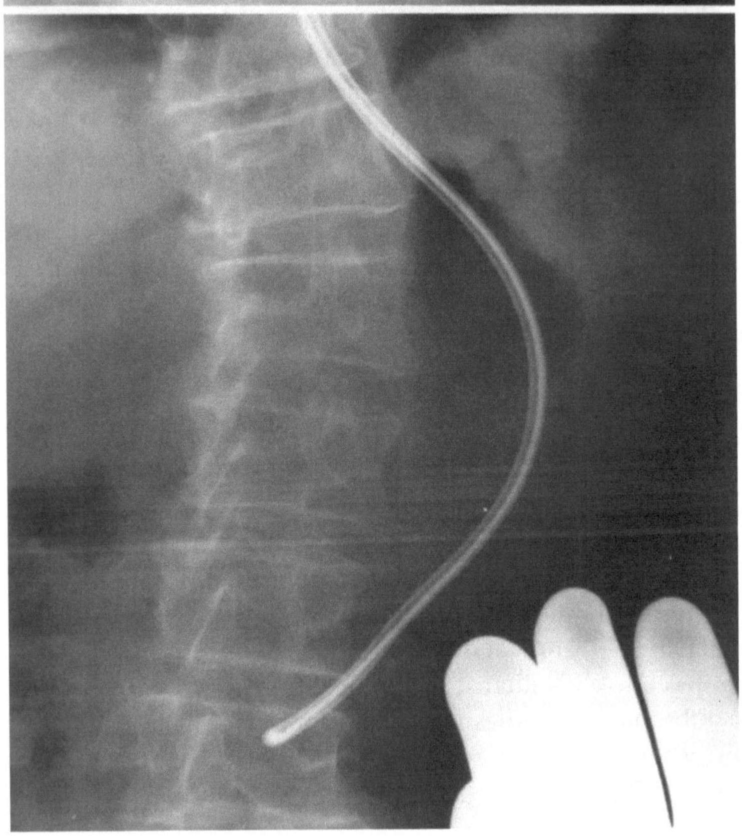

Fig. 2.4.-3. Intubation. The tube may be directed into the antrum by turning the guide wire, gently flexing the tip and pressing in the left epigastric region with the lead-gloved hand

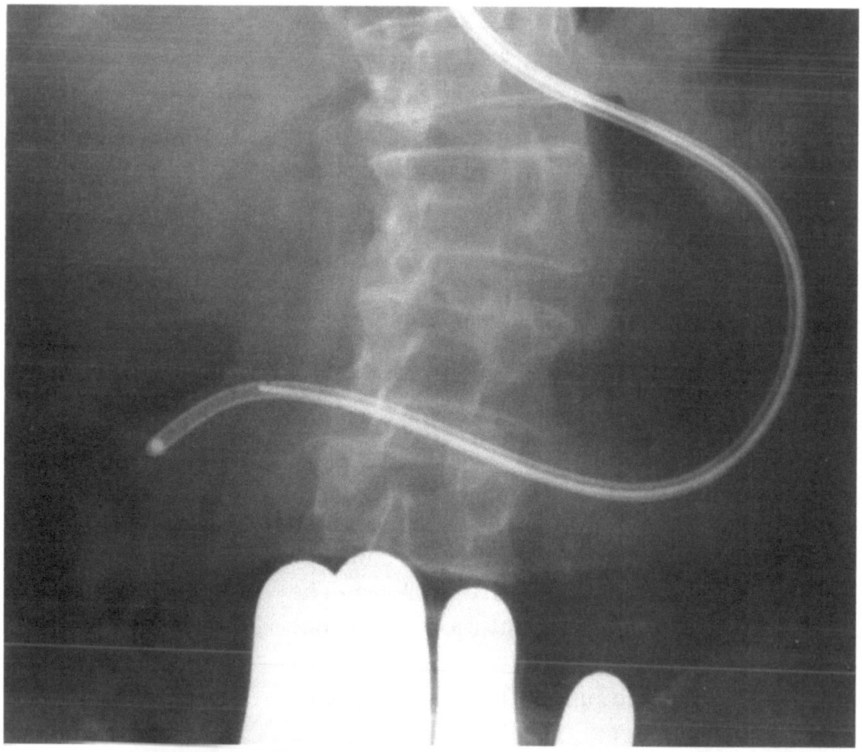

Fig. 2.4.-4. Intubation. Transit of the tube through the pylorus into the duodenum can be facilitated by pressing against the antrum from caudal. The tip of the catheter should remain flexible. The tube usually glides in the duodenum down to the ligament of Treitz

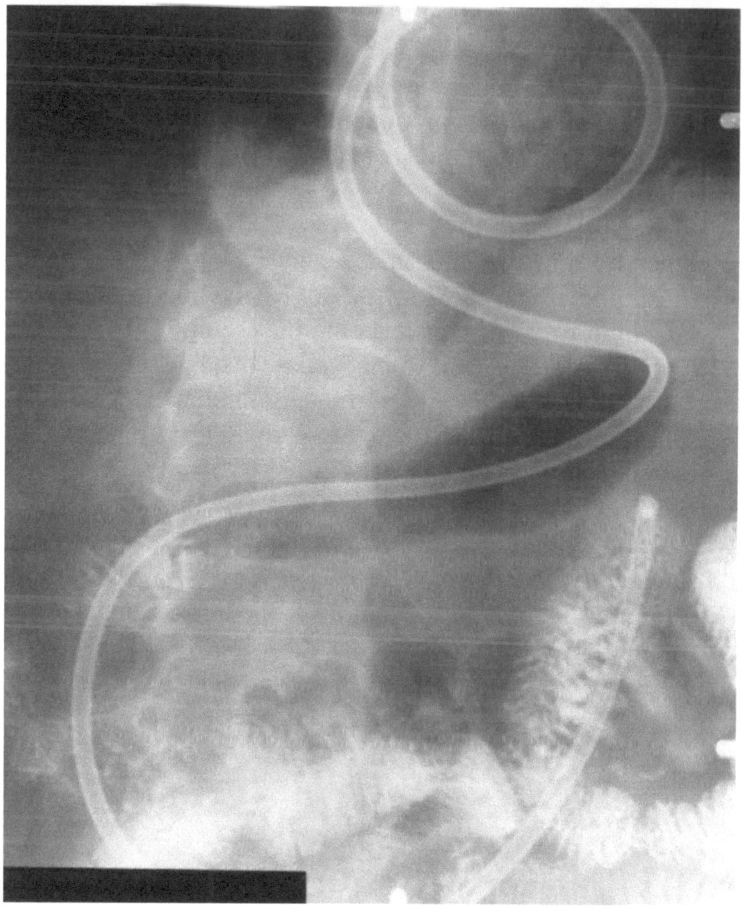

Fig. 2.4.-5. Intubation. The tube curls up into a large intrathoracic hernia. The loop should be straightened before administering the contrast medium

2.5 X-ray Equipment and Filming

The examination is carried out under fluoroscopy. A final film taken on the Bucky table may complete the investigation. The tube voltage depends considerably on the weight of the patient and the transparency of the bowel loops in double contrast. The voltage varies between 125 kV in obese patients and 90 kV in slim patients. The m As should be adjusted likewise.

2.6 Flow Rate of Contrast Medium

It has been shown that a 75 ml/min flow rate of barium solution produces optimal results (Sellink and Rosenbusch 1981). This infusion rate is certainly one of the most important factors for a successful enteroclysis. Its significance has not been appreciated well enough concerning the detection of motility disturbances. The exact determination for the infusion rate is not altogether simple. There are two possibilities:
1. Use of an electric pump (Trüber and Fuchs 1981; Abu-Yousef et al. 1983).
2. Empirical determination of the level of barium in the container. This can be adjusted if the barium suspension is too slow or flows too quickly. 300 ml of barium poured into a container and infused in 4 min is equivalent to 75 ml/min flow rate.

A higher flow rate results in a reactive hypoperistalsis and an increase in the amount of contrast medium necessary for reaching the cecum. A lower infusion rate leads to inadequate distension of the bowel lumen, which hinders the detection of motility disturbances. Some cases necessitate deviation from this standard rate.

A reduction of flow rate to 50 ml/min or less is necessary in the following cases:
- position of the tube in the middle of the duodenum and possible reflux;
- significant hypoperistalsis in the upper jejunum (e.g. with pseudoobstruction or drug-induced). From our experience, the application of 20–30 ml of metoclopramide into the tube or 10 mg i.v. recommended by Sellink (1981) does not always accelerate the flow and is rarely necessary;
- reflux caused by obstruction;
- in babies and children. Here our experience is limited. If the child is cooperative, intubation and further examination procedure do not pose any great difficulty. The investigation ensues likewise as in adults. If a child is sedated, a resulting hypoperistalsis must be anticipated. If there is gastric reflux in the infant, the flow rate should be reduced or another tube introduced into the stomach to remove refluxed fluid (Miller and Sellink 1979; Sellink and Rosenbusch 1981). In normal cases, we have not observed the early flocculation in babies, mentioned by Sellink.

An increase in flow rate to 100–150 ml/min is necessary in the following cases:
- considerable hypermotility, as in *intestinal hurry,* collagen diseases or carcinoid. Increase ensures adequate distension of the bowel lumen;
- inadequate filling of the proximal jejunum for different reasons (e.g. lumen dilatation in celiac disease).

The flow rate should be adjusted if any of the above mentioned situations evolve after filling of the upper jejunal loops.

2.7 Examination Procedure

The investigation is biphasic: the *barium phase* and the *methylcellulose phase*.

Barium Phase

The purpose is to assess the small bowel peristalsis and to detect motility disturbances. Maintaining constant examination conditions (infusion of contrast medium through the duodenal tube with a determined flow rate), the small bowel is subjected to a kind of "test". Its peristaltic reaction is documented on radiographs.

Normal peristalsis: After 300 ml of barium (75 ml/min) most of the jejunum is filled and roughly one third of the recorded loops show contractions (Fig. 2.7.-1).

Hyperperistalsis: After 300 ml of barium (75 ml/min) the contrast medium has reached the ileum and two thirds or more of the depicted loops show contractions. The term *intestinal hurry* is used if the cecum is reached after 300 ml (Fig. 2.7.-2).

Hypoperistalsis: After 300 ml of barium (75 ml/min) only a few proximal jejunal loops are filled showing only rare or no contractions. The loops are more or less dilated. Gastric reflux may occur (Fig. 2.7.-3).

Pendular or nonpropulsive peristalsis: This is hyperperistalsis (without propulsion). It is best assessed under fluoroscopy. Segmental contractions seen on the film may be a clue for this type of peristalsis (Fig. 5.2.-19).

Methylcellulose Phase

This allows for double contrast imaging and better detection of morphological changes, as well as for the assessment of mucosal coating. In normal mucosa, the coating remains intact for up to 20–40 min (Fig. 2.7.-4). Poor mucosal coating and early flocculation shortly after administration of methylcellulose which cannot be restored by repeated doses of barium and methylcellulose, are assessed as *nonspecific enteritis or mucosal irritation* (Fig. 2.7.-5).

Technical Procedure

Barium phase: A container hooked up at the appropriate level is filled with 300 ml of barium suspension. The level has first to be established in order to obtain the desired flow rate of 75 ml/min. It also depends on the type of tube/container connection. 300 ml barium should be instilled in 4 min. Here an electric pump is useful. After 300 ml of barium a fluoroscopically guided survey film is made for the assessment of intestinal motility. The subjective observation at fluoroscopy plays a secondary role. Pathological features seen during intermittent fluoroscopy (e.g. partial stenosis, alteration of folds) should be recorded on spot films.

Methylcellulose phase: The methylcellulose should be administered with the last drops of barium to ensure optimal mucosal coating and further propel the barium bolus. The aqueous methylcellulose solution is instilled into the tube either by means of injection by syringe or by a pump since its high viscosity prevents spontaneous flow. In order to avoid delay, everything should be prepared in advance. In particular, the connection system should be checked for compatibility.

Duodenum and jejunum first appear in double contrast and are recorded. As the investigation proceeds, again under intermittent fluoroscopy, the transit of the barium bolus is observed from the terminal ileum to the cecum. This ileocecal transit is recorded in a spot film. Thus, the terminal ileum can be identified and localized every time, even in the case of superimposition by less translucent small bowel loops or by a filled, ptotic colon later on.

The amount of methylcellulose depends on the desired transradiation. When adequate dou-

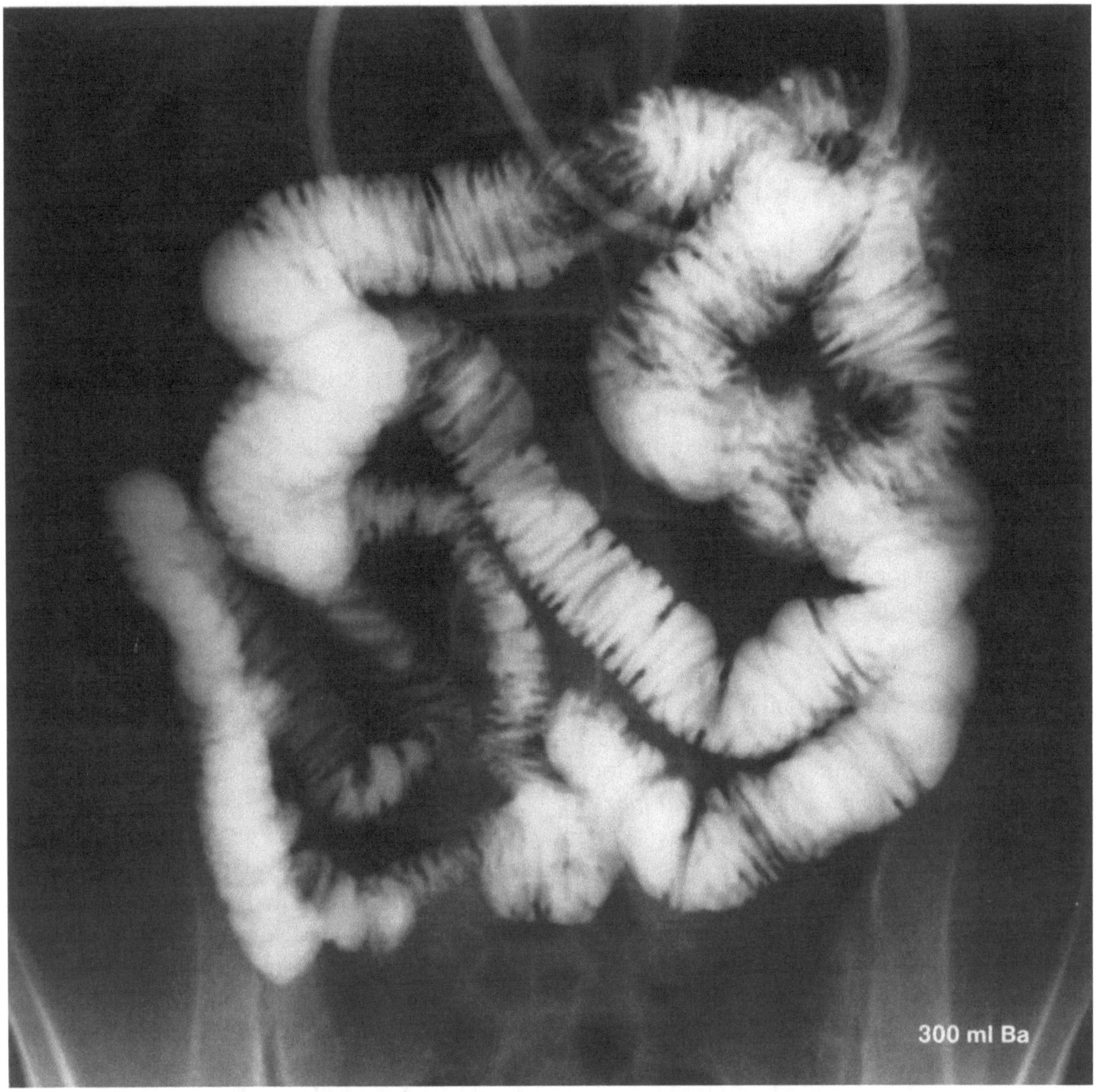

Fig. 2.7.-1. Barium phase with normal peristalsis. Most of the jejunum is filled, about $^1/_3$ of the imaged loops are contracted

ble contrast is obtained, survey and spot films are produced to record pathological processes under particular consideration of the terminal ileum and the ileocecal junction. As required, these are made in varying degrees of transparency, under graded compression, and in varied contractory and filling conditions.

If premature rinsing in the upper jejunum or poor mucosal coating or flocculation occur, a further dose of barium (e.g. 50 ml) should be administered. A normal mucosa can then keep good coating with a further dose of methylcellulose. If poor mucosal coating persists, there is evidence of a *nonspecific enteritis or mucosal irritation* which should be documented.

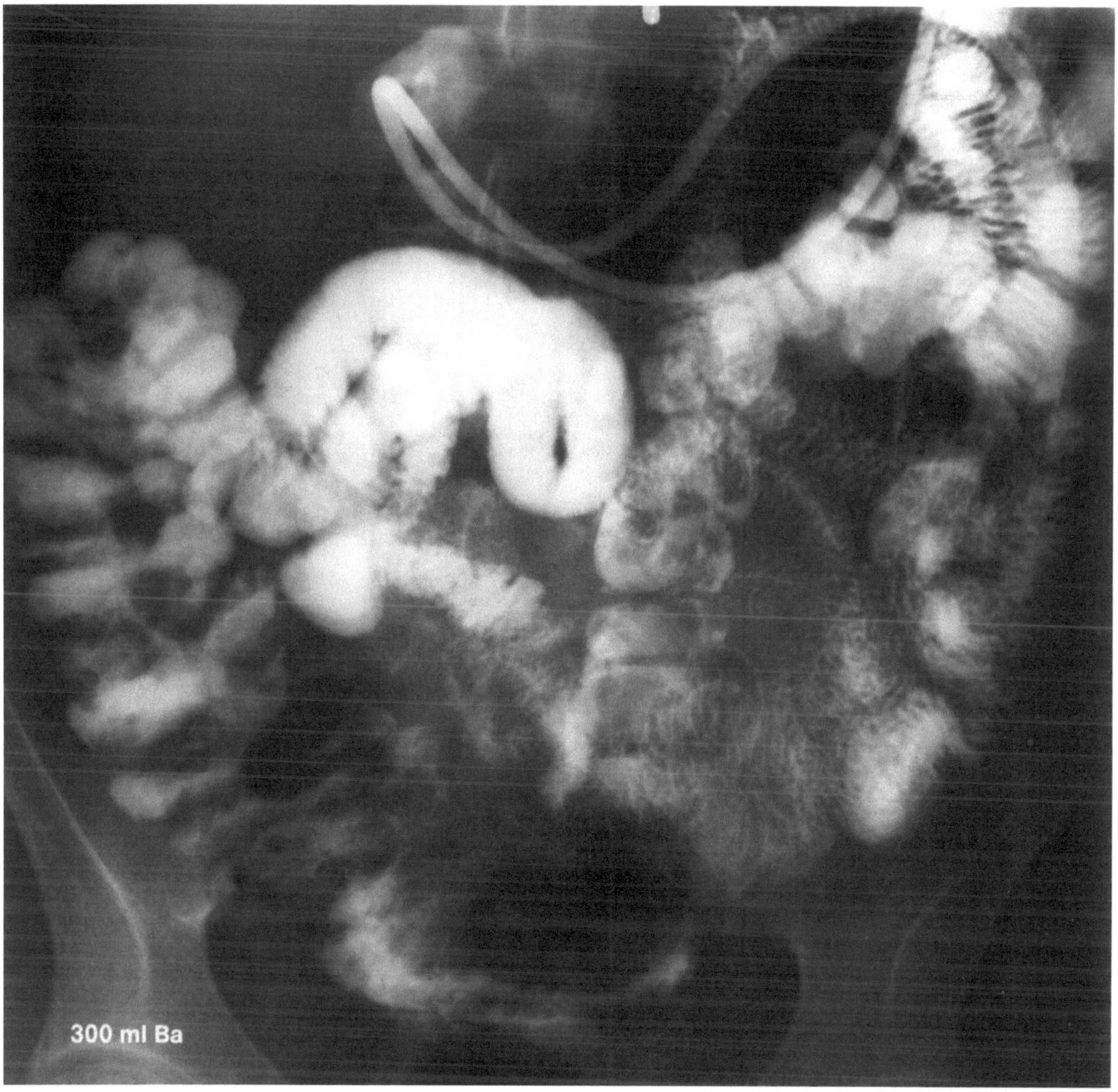

Fig. 2.7.-2. Barium phase with hyperperistalsis (*intestinal hurry*). The colon is reached after only 300 ml of barium. Almost every loop is contracted

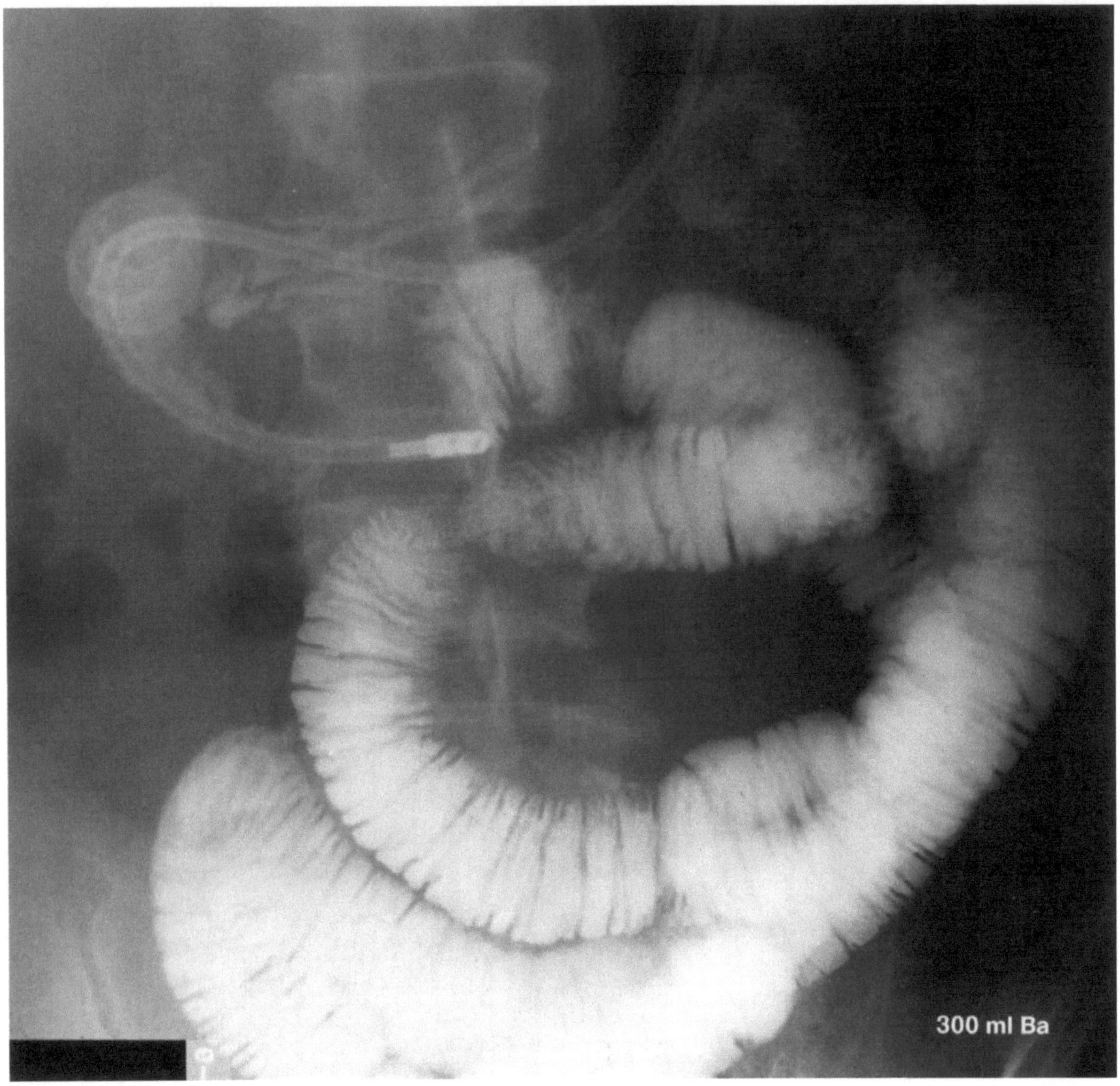

Fig. 2.7.-3. Barium phase with hypoperistalsis. After 300 ml of barium, only some of the upper dilated jejunal loops are filled. Only a few isolated contractions may be seen. Gastric reflux

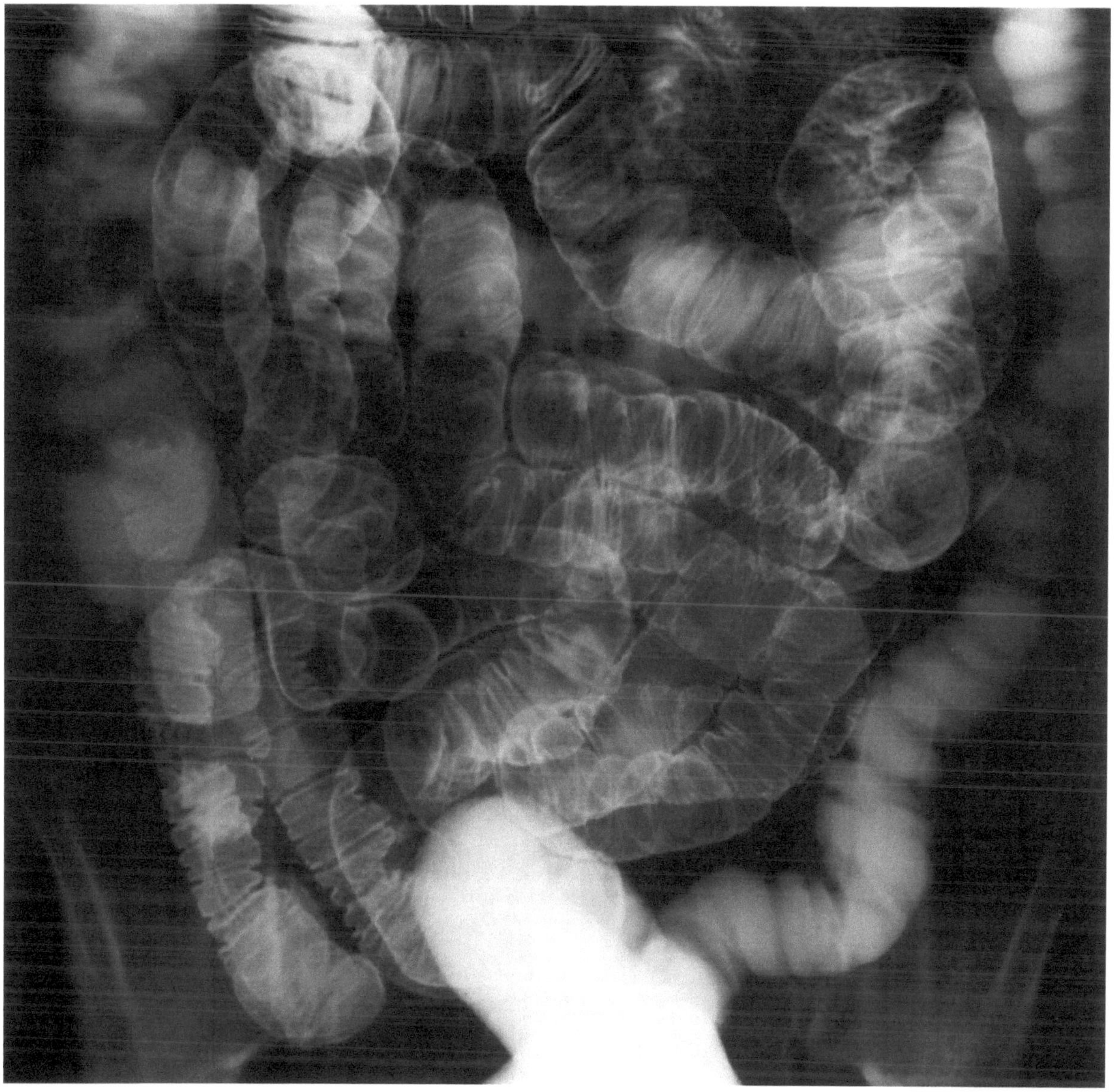

Fig. 2.7.-4. Double contrast of the small bowel in the methylcellulose phase. A good mucosal coating is usually maintained for 20–40 min

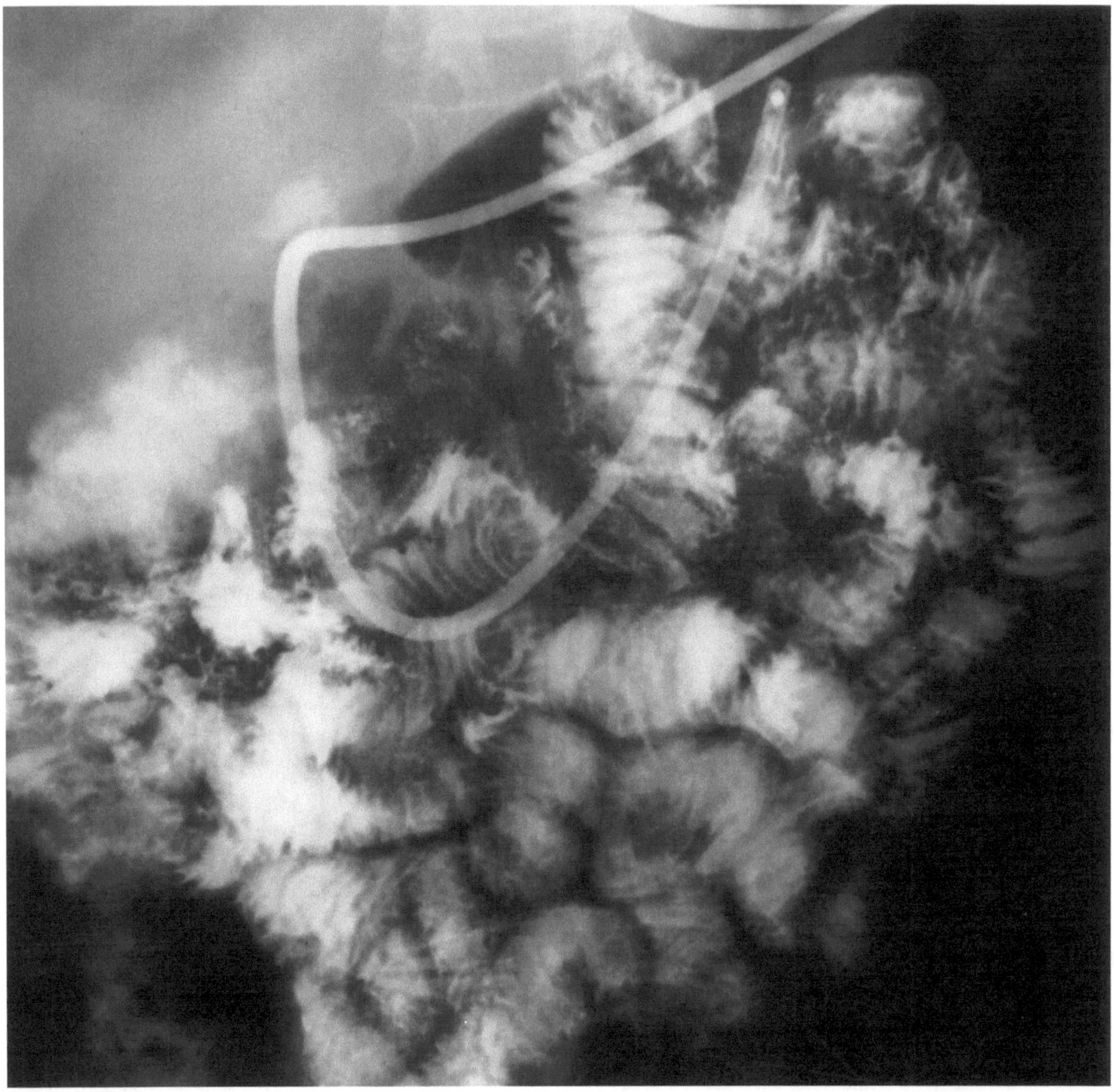

Fig. 2.7.-5. Nonspecific enteritis or mucosal irritation. During the investigation there is already early flocculation of the contrast medium and poor mucosal coating. Repeated doses of barium and methylcellulose have no effect. In addition, there is thickening of the folds and intestinal wall as well as hyperperistalsis (in this case nonpropulsive peristalsis). Patient suffers from malabsorption and insulin-dependent diabetes with diabetic and alcoholic polyneuropathy

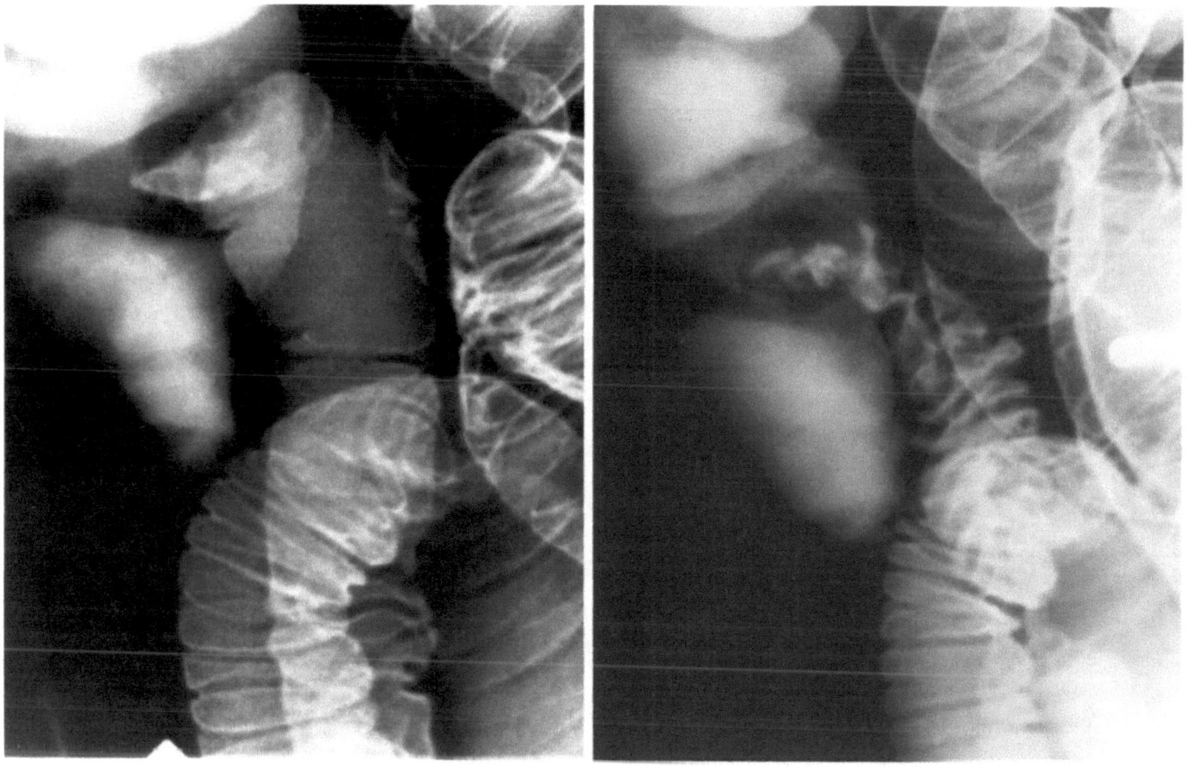

a b

Fig. 2.7.-6a and b. Terminal ileum in double contrast. Distended (**a**) and contracted (**b**)

Documentation

The radiological documentation during the small bowel investigation should be so detailed that the examination can be reinterpreted by others. In general, the following radiographs are adequate (the format depends on the type of x-ray equipment).

Barium phase:
1 survey film (see Fig. 2.7.-1).

Methylcellulose phase:
- proximal jejunum and duodenum in double contrast;
- terminal ileum in barium monocontrast;
- terminal ileum in double contrast and in stages of varying contraction (Fig. 2.7.-6);
- spot films under graded compression, varied transparency and varied contractions and filling conditions of the remaining small bowel;
- survey film in double contrast (Fig. 2.7.-7).

Careful palpation of the bowel loops under fluoroscopy is mandatory. Generally, 2–3 survey radiographs and 5 spot films suffice. The duodenal tube is not removed until the radiographs have been developed and assessed!

Radiation Exposure

Radiation exposure during enteroclysis is about the same as during small bowel follow-through examination (Vogel and Löhr 1978; Salomonowitz et al. 1980). Reports about higher values of exposure during enteroclysis (Ott et al. 1985) should be carefully considered in the light of the execution of the examination. The positioning of the tube under fluoroscopy may account for a higher skin dose. By means of limited fluo-

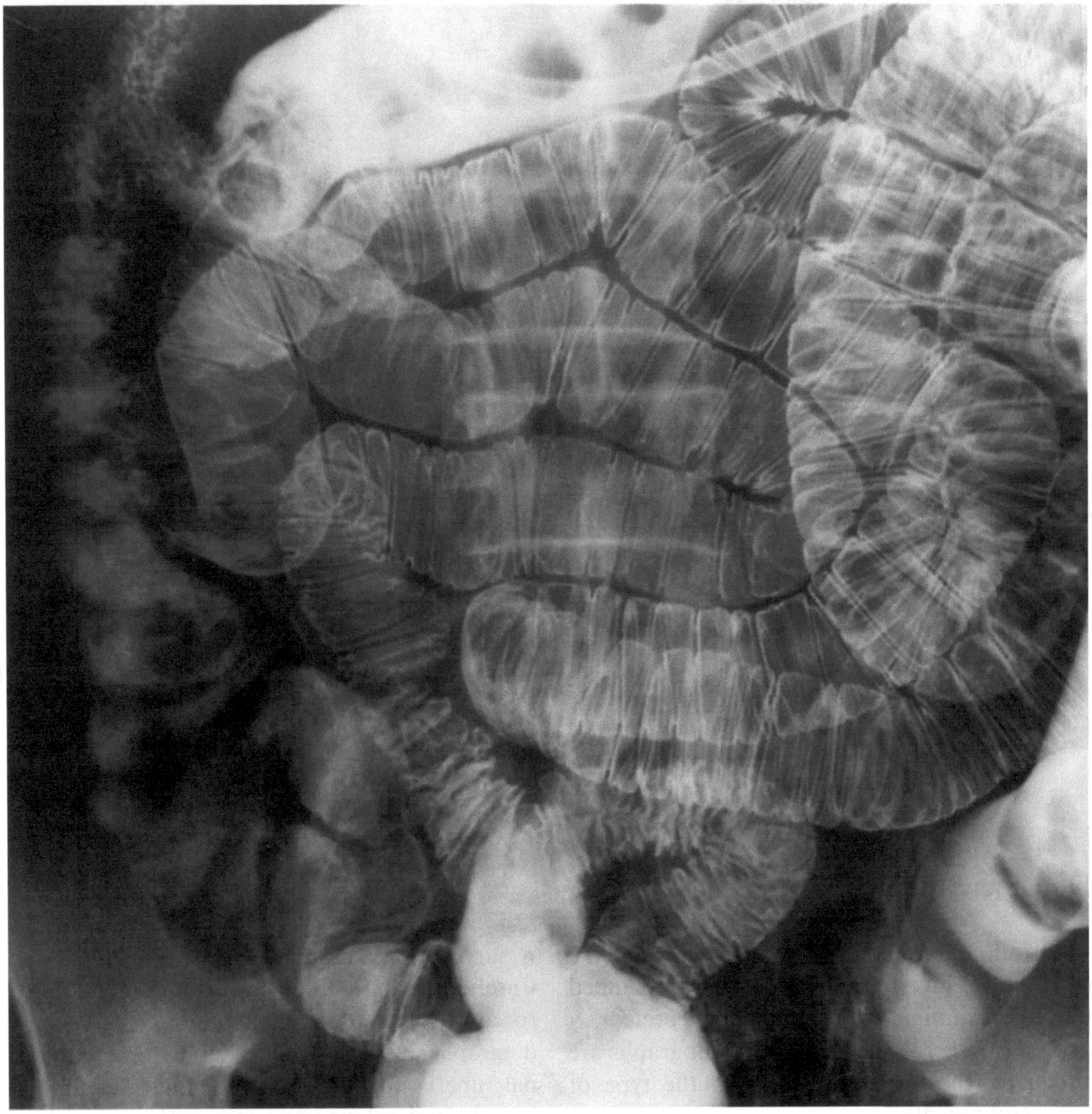

Fig. 2.7.-7. Final survey radiograph in double contrast

roscopy using good collimation, the gonadal dose in males can be maintained at an almost negligible amount. The ovarian dose is roughly similar to that of a barium enema of the colon. Experience with intubation and standardization of investigation will reduce radiation exposure.

2.8 Special Information

Although the aim is to standardize the examination procedure, individual cases require different approaches. This may become apparent before or shortly after commencement of the investigation when the radiologist has elicited the complaints from the patient in advance. This is particularly important for the examination procedure.

- Drug history should be evaluated.
- The duodenum should be included in the examination and assessed accordingly. The filming ensues either within the normal examination procedure or towards the end of the investigation when the tube is withdrawn into the upper duodenum, whereby additional contrast medium is administered.
- The filling and distension of the rectum may produce a defecation urge, which usually subsides quickly. The patient should be informed about this.
- Early filling of the rectum before the terminal ileum appears is suggestive of an ileorectal fistula, even if fluid is not seen directly. One should bear in mind that the aqueous contrast medium sometimes gushes into the rectum after entering the ascending colon, leaving the rest of the colon uncoated. This should not be misinterpreted for early filling of the rectum.
- Superimposition of the filled rectum and sigmoid can impede the assessment of the ileum in the pelvis. In such cases, the patient should be sent to the toilet to empty the large bowel. The small bowel loops then become free from overshadowing.

- *Inclusion of the colon for assessment*
  When the contrast medium has entered the well-purged colon, an assessment of the colon may ensue or in special cases be attempted with rectal air insufflation in drug-induced hypotonia (e.g. Crohn's disease) (Fig. 2.8.-1).

- *Desired transradiation*
  In double contrast examinations of the stomach and colon, superficial lesions can sometimes be better detected by working with a barium "puddle". Since this maneuver is not possible in the investigation of the small bowel, the barium concentration for the mucosal coating should be adequately thick. A transradiation which is too strong is not always suitable for the detection of lesions. A "milky" mucosal coating is often better (Fig. 2.8.-2a, b).
- If severe reflux is unavoidable during the examination, it is advisable to empty the stomach by means of an additional tube.
- Gastric reflux, especially while the catheter is being drawn, may cause vomiting. A suitable basin should be available.

- *Application of drugs*
  Spasmolytic drugs, e.g. butylscopolamine, glucagon, or peristalsis stimulating drugs, e.g. metoclopramide, are seldom necessary. The administration of metoclopramide in hypoperistalsis and likewise of butylscopolamine or glucagon is mentioned earlier in connection with the assessment of the colon. The application of a spasmolytic drug in advanced hyperperistalsis to improve the filling of the bowel in the methylcellulose phase and for better detection and presentation of morphological bowel alterations is not necessary in our opinion.

- *Small bowel obstructions*
  In suspected fibrous bands, subileus condition or obstruction, the barium bolus should be carefully monitored by intensive fluoroscopy, since short stenoses are difficult to detect and may later be concealed in double contrast by overlying loops (Fig. 2.8.-3a, b). The same goes for detection of Meckel's diverticula. In mechanical obstruction, depending on the severity, duration and localization, initially there is normal or increased peristalsis in the proximal jejunum. Distally, the bowel becomes dilated and hypoperistaltic.

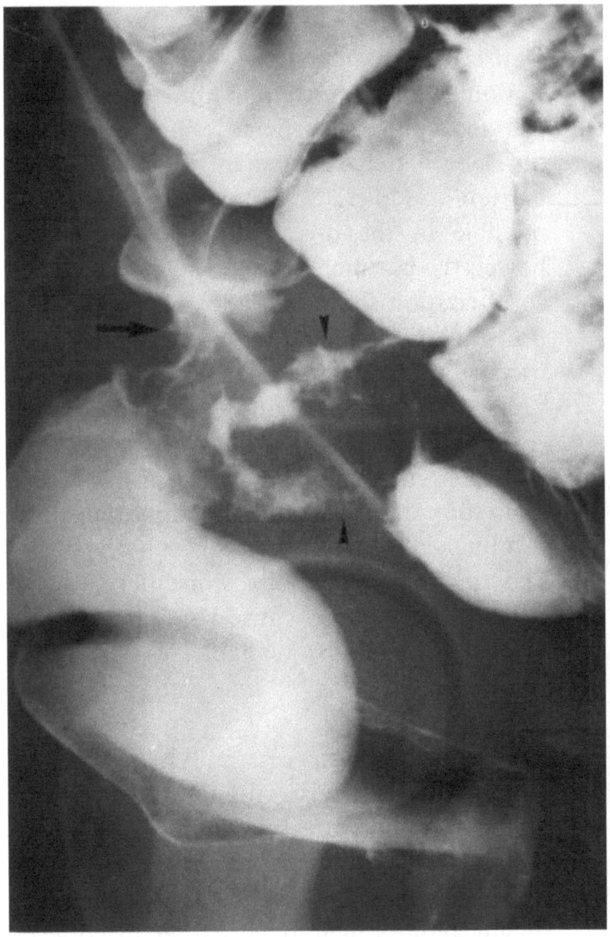

Fig. 2.8.-1. Colonoscopic insuperable stenosis at the rectosigmoidal junction. Enteroclysis, combined with rectal air insufflation in hypotonia, detects Crohn's disease in the terminal ileum (►), as well as an obvious stenosis due to Crohn's disease at the rectosigmoidal junction (→)

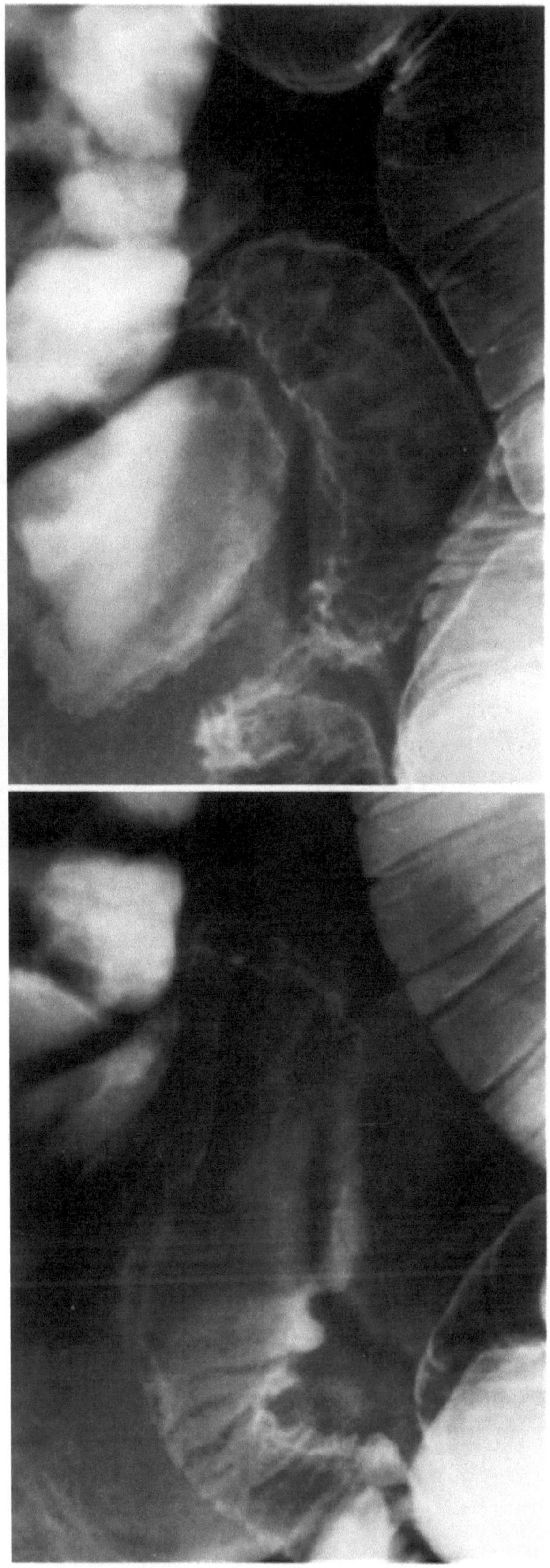

a

b

Fig. 2.8.-2a and b. Distinct lymphofollicular hyperplasia in the terminal ileum. Easily recognizable with "milky" mucosal coating (**a**), but unrecognizable if too much methylcellulose has flushed the mucosa (**b**)

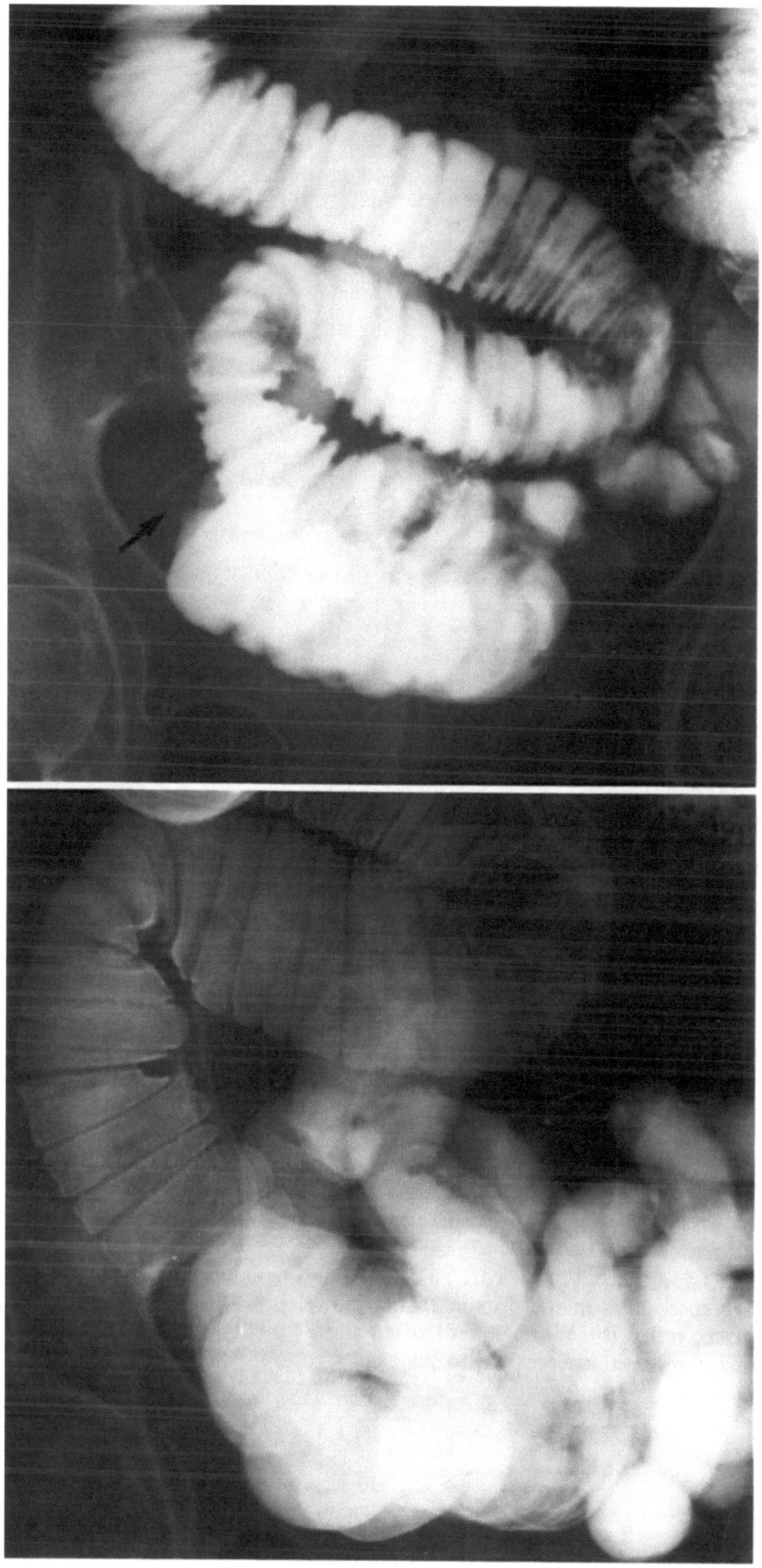

a

b

Fig. 2.8.-3a and b. Severe, short stenosis (→) by a post-ischemic scar at the jejunum/ileum junction (**a**). This was only detectable by following the barium bolus. In the methylcellulose phase, the stenosis is not visible due to overlying distal ileal loops (**b**). Prestenotic dilatation. A previous follow-through examination because of subileus symptoms was negative

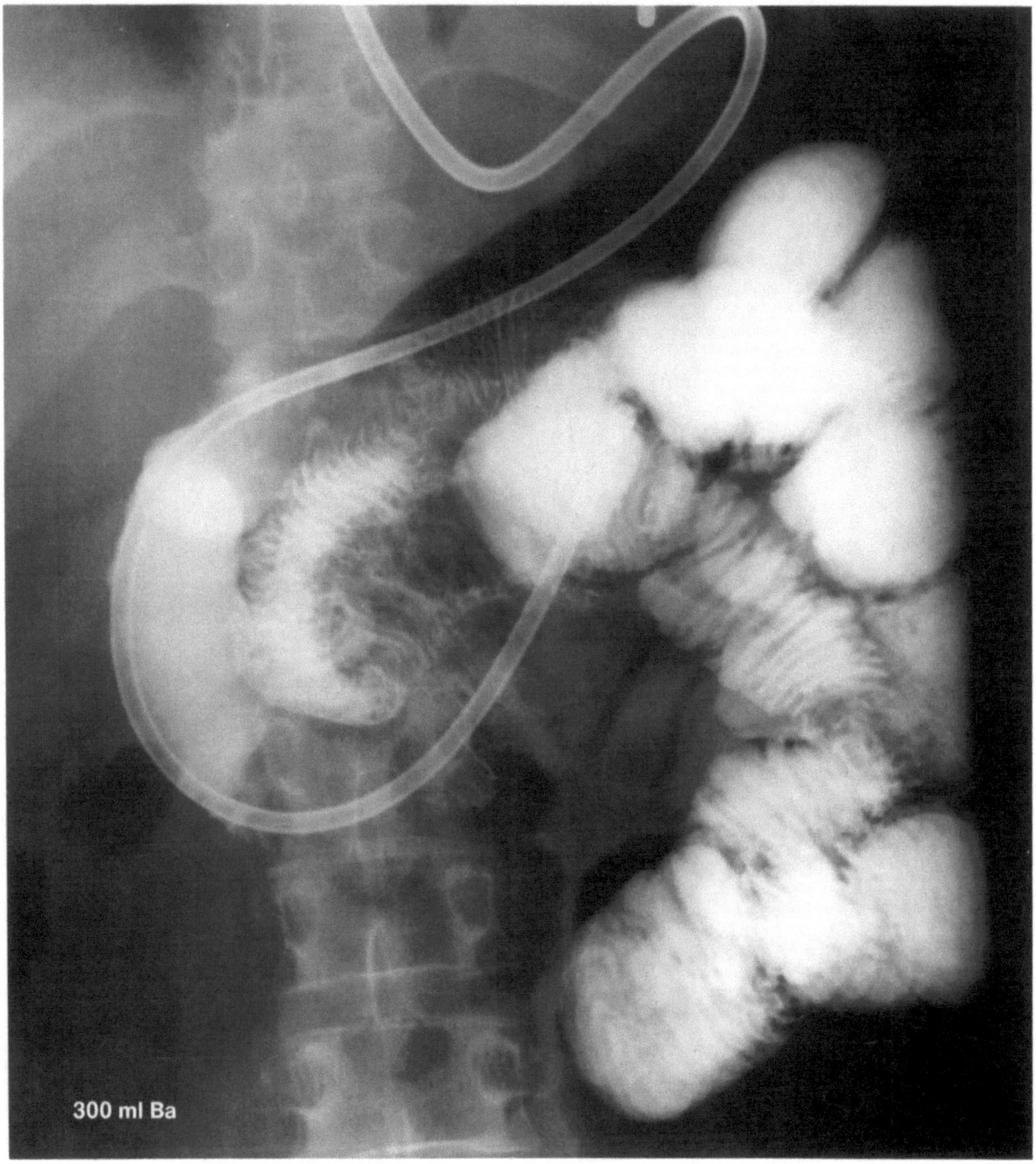

a

Fig. 2.8.-4a to c. Patient with subileus symptoms and chronic diarrhea. In the barium phase, there is initial hyperperistalsis in the proximal small bowel (**a**). Distally loss of peristalsis and increasing dilatation and gastric reflux (**b**). With 900 ml barium and 2 l methylcellulose, after 45 min and $2^1/_2$ h, an extremely dilated small bowel (**b**) emerges due to stenosing Crohn's disease (**c**)

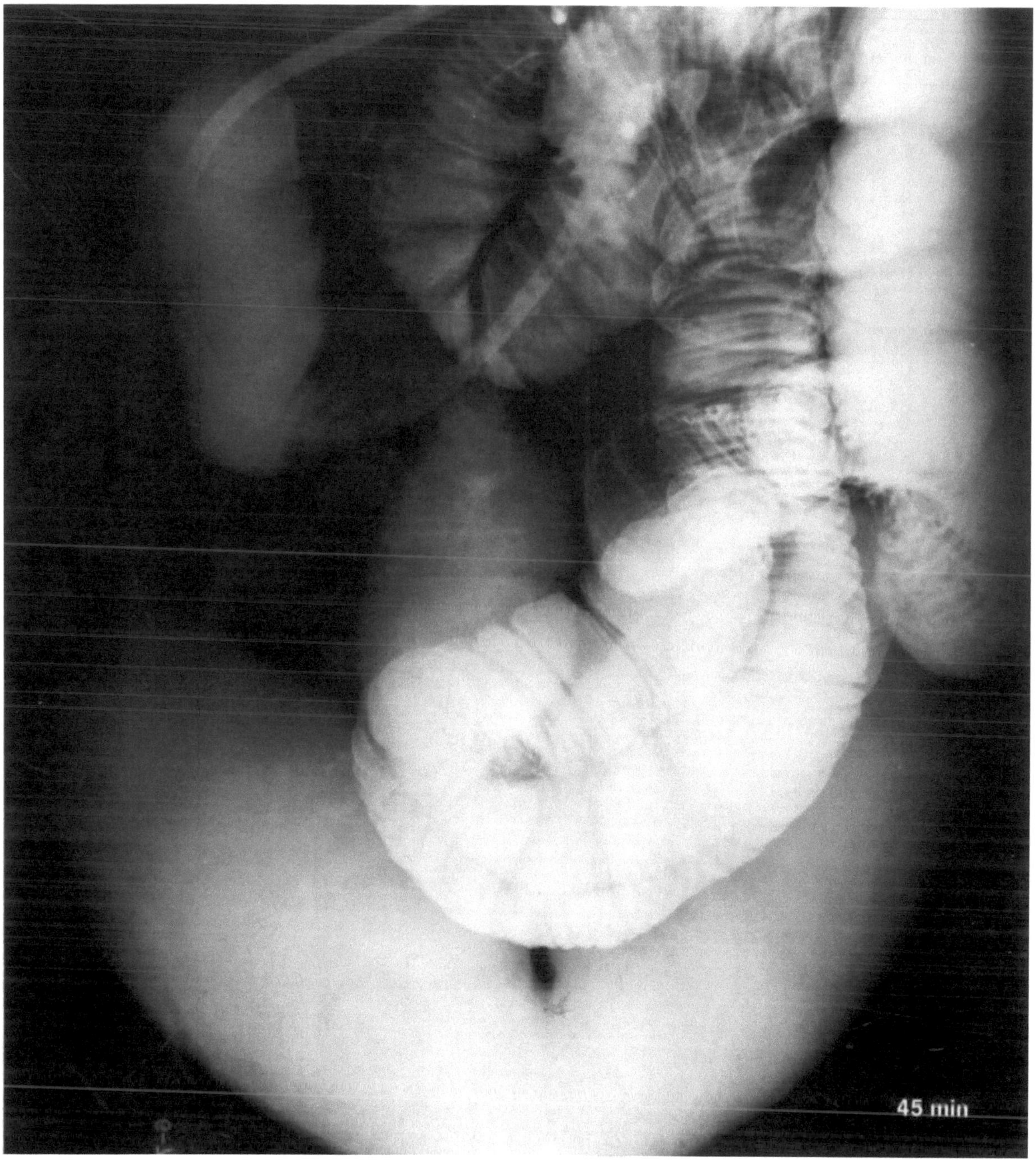

Fig. 2.8.-4b

If this is observed during the methylcellulose phase, sufficient barium must be added to ensure a good contrast. The barium is diluted by the increased fluid in the bowel.

Sometimes, large amounts of barium (e.g. 900 ml) and methylcellulose (e.g. 1.5–2 liters) are necessary (Miller and Sellink 1979). At any rate, adequate contrast as far as the ileocecal junction is necessary (Fig. 2.8.-4a to c). If the required amount of contrast medium

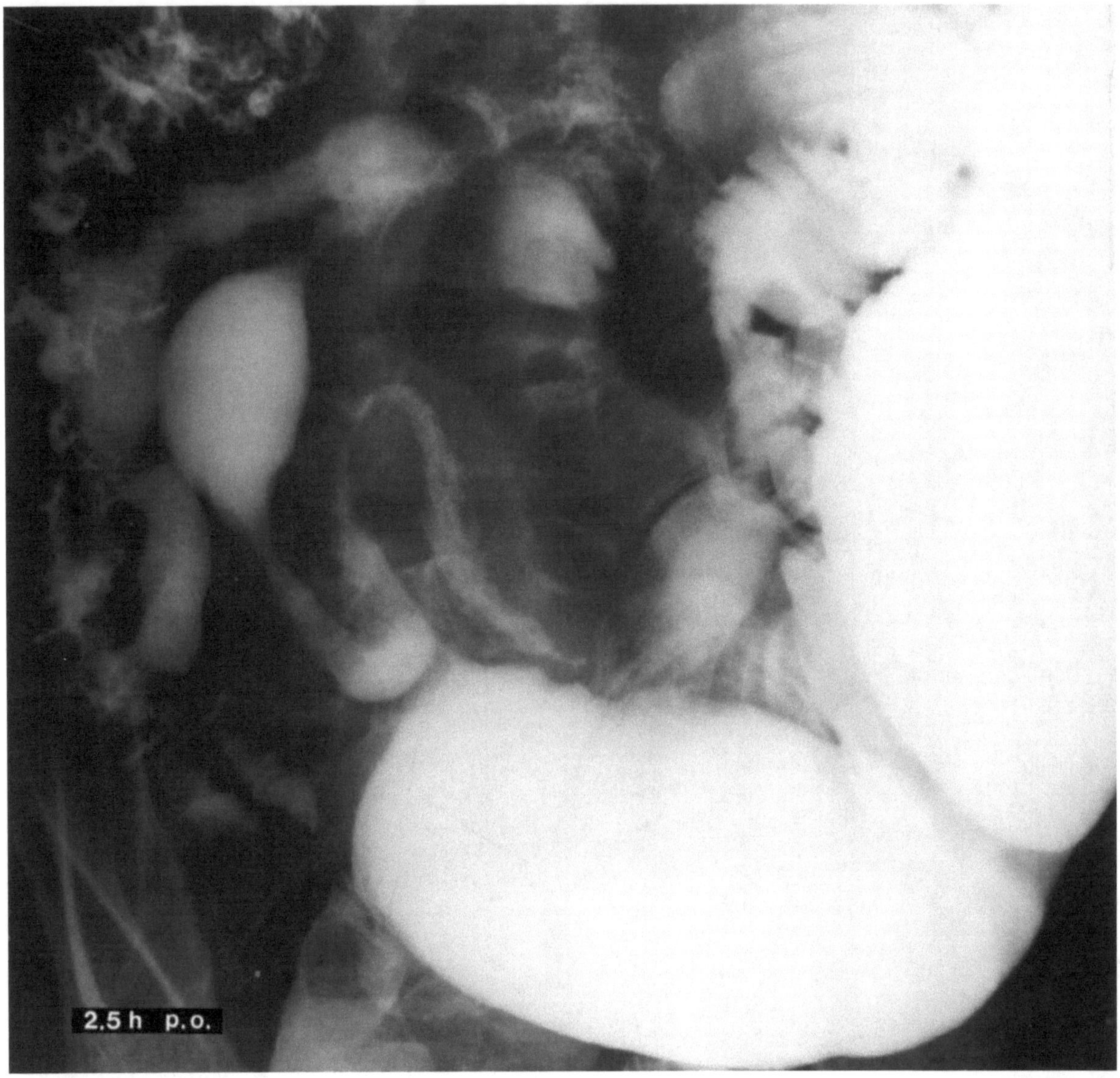

Fig. 2.8.-4c

is administered, the duodenal tube can be withdrawn and intermittent fluoroscopy is indicated for a longer period of time. If this is disregarded, etiology of an obstruction may be overlooked (Fig. 2.8.-5a to c).

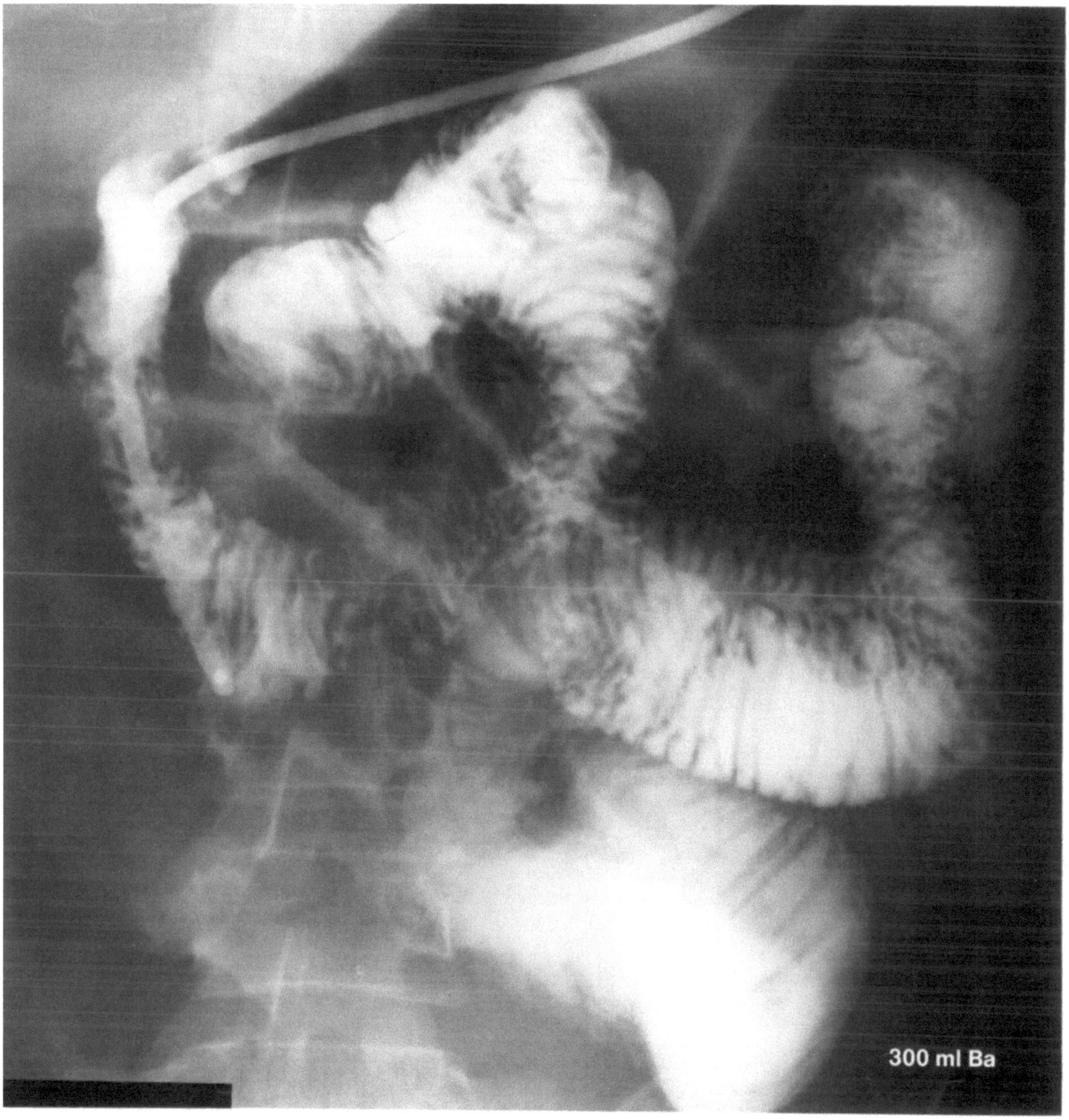

a

Fig. 2.8.-5a to c. Faulty investigation in a patient with subileus symptoms and diarrhea. In the barium phase, there is a slight hyperperistalsis with increasing bowel dilatation and loss of peristalsis distally (signs of a small bowel obstruction) (**a**). Due to an inadequate amount of barium and methylcellulose, it is difficult to obtain satisfactory contrast of the dilated and fluid-filled distal small bowel. A diagnosis was not possible (**b**). The retrograde filling of the terminal ileum via the colonoscopy yielded a stenosing Crohn's disease with a marked prestenotic dilatation (**c**)

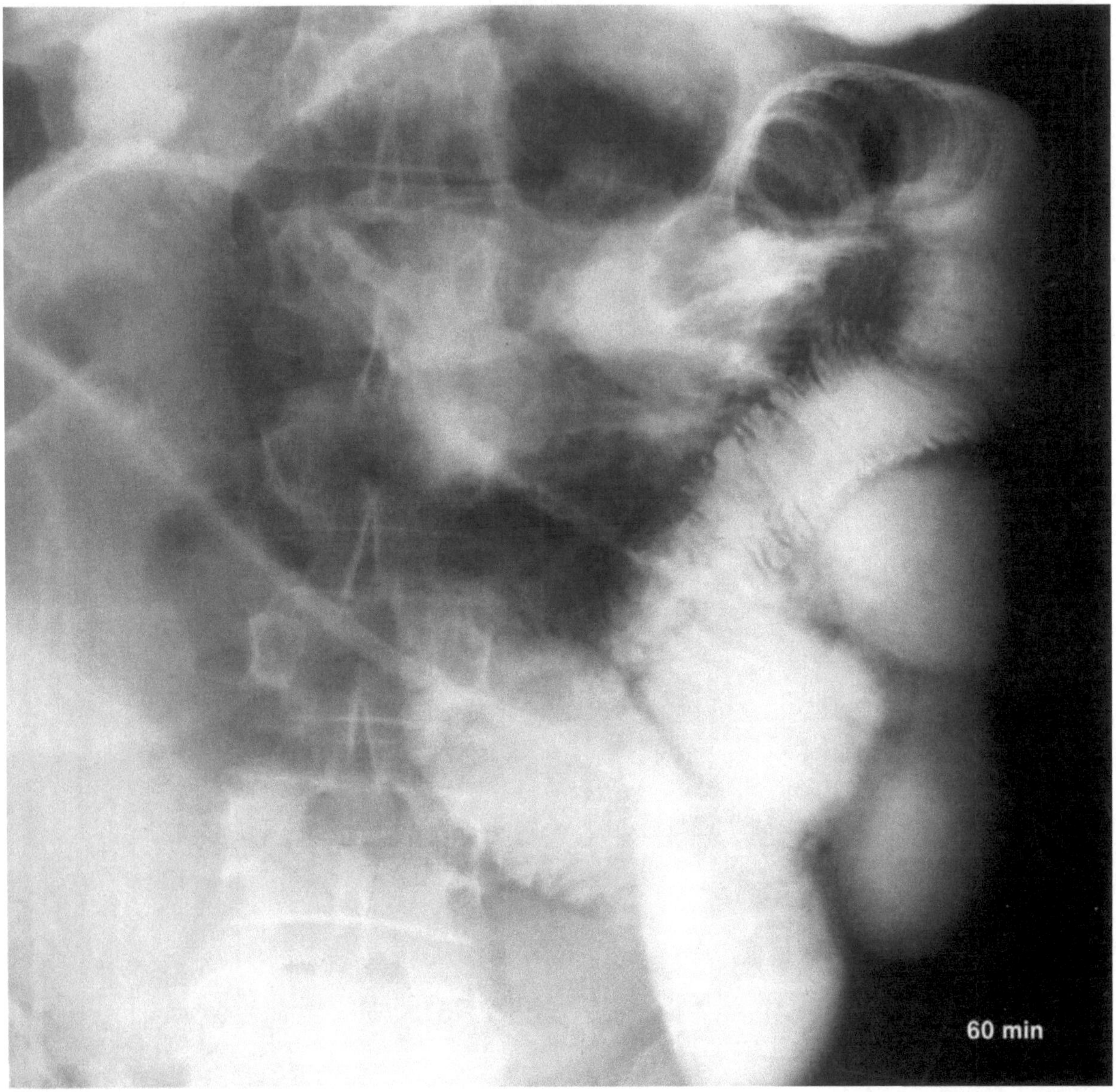

Fig. 2.8.-5b

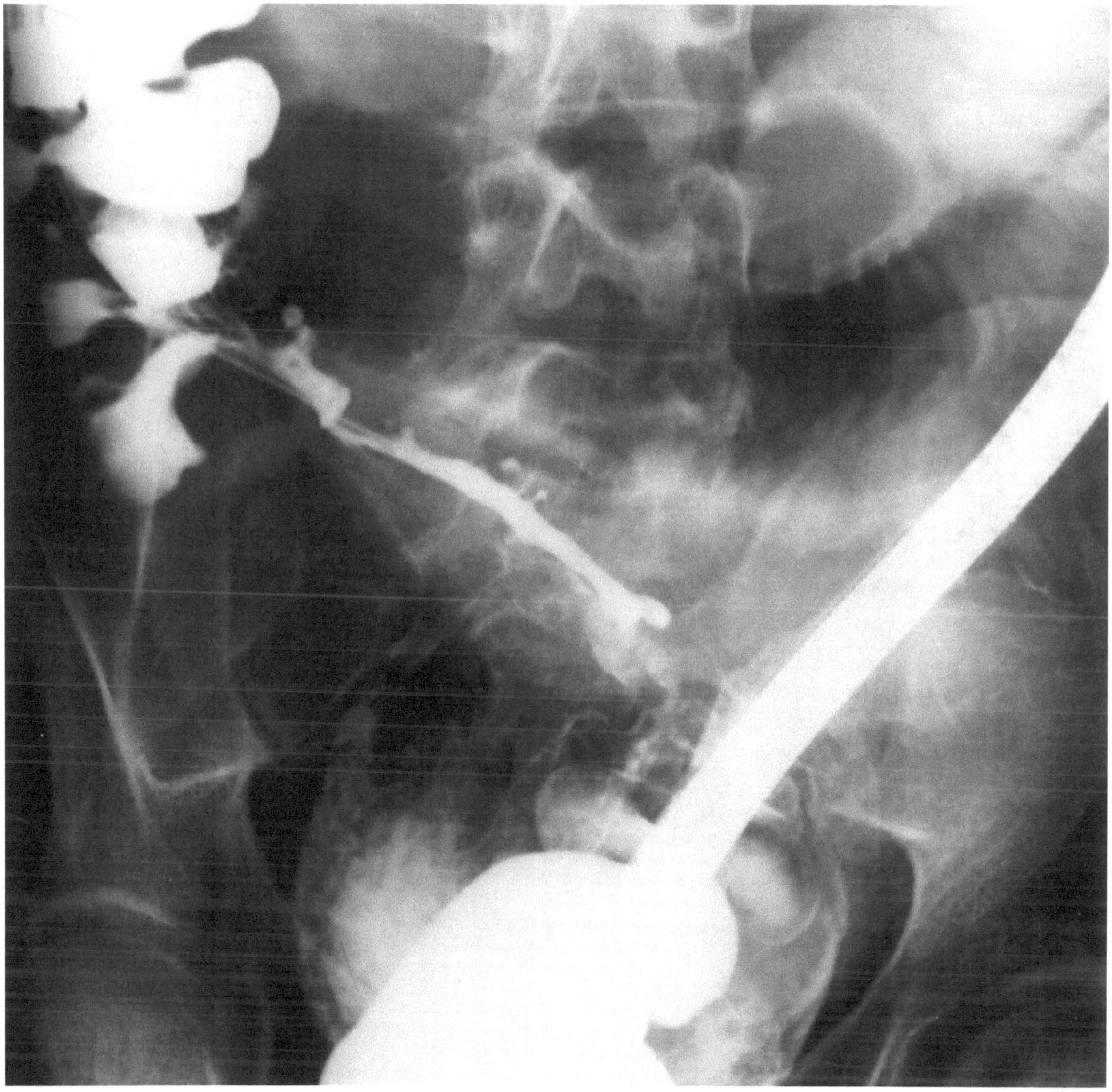

Fig. 2.8.-5c

Please observe: In the case of subileus and ileus, an enteroclysis may be carried out only if

- obstruction of the large bowel is excluded,
- there are no acute surgical indications,
- there is no severe congestive heart failure with ileus.

Concerning small bowel obstructions, there are no contraindications for enteroclysis, since the barium does not thicken in the small bowel, as is the case in large bowel obstructions. The resorbed fluid in the small bowel gets largely resecreted.

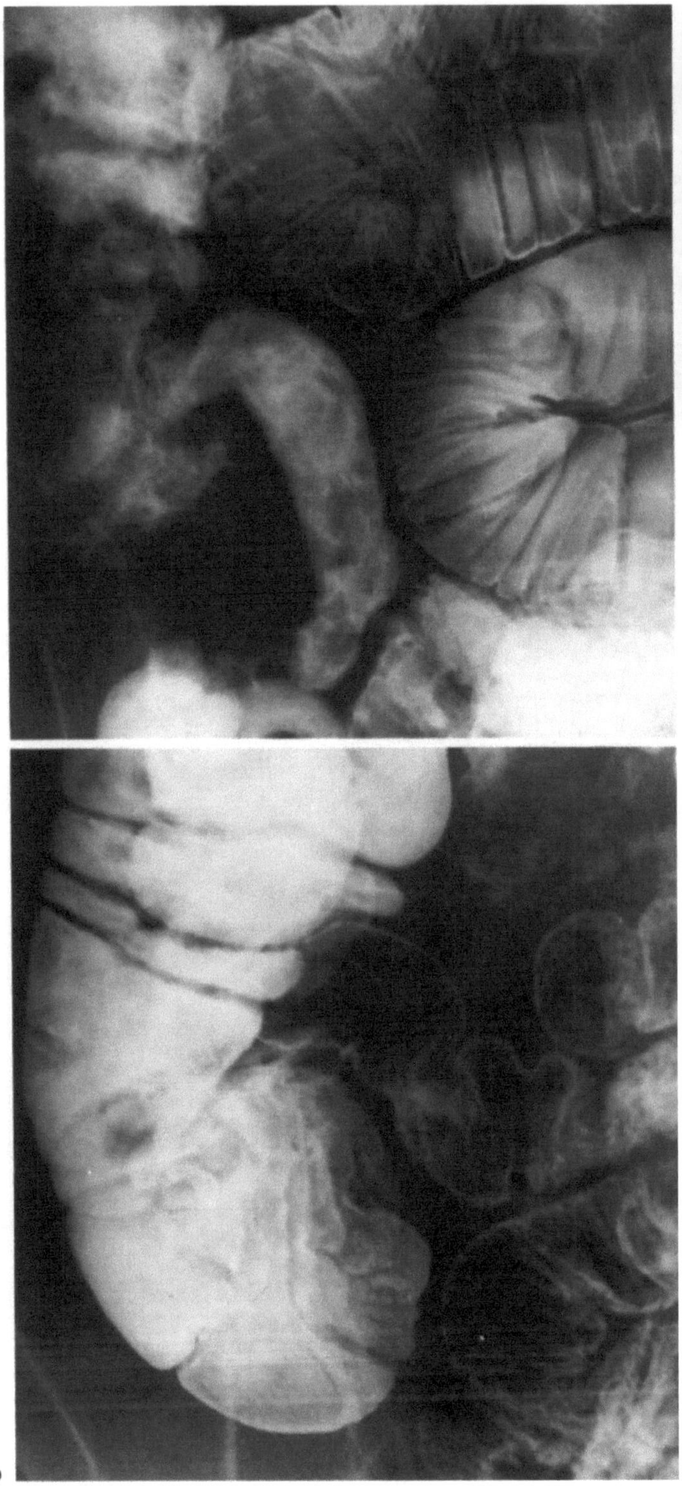

a

b

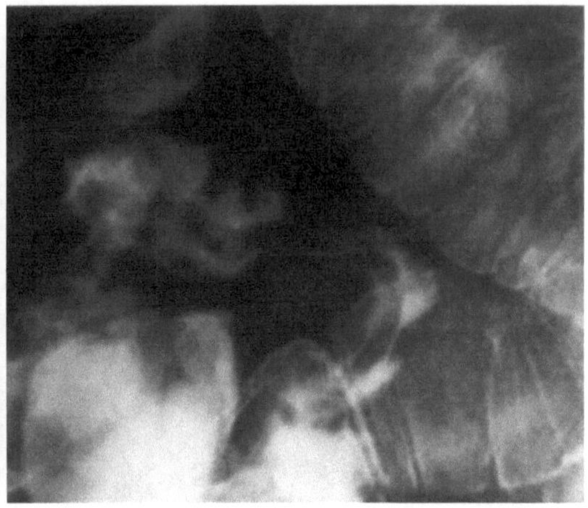

Fig. 2.9.-2. "Worm artifacts" due to residual food (vegetable fibers?)

Fig. 2.9.-1 a and b. Artifacts. Food remains in the terminal ileum and residual stool in the cecum, imitating Crohn's disease. The patient was suffering from chronic constipation and the bowel was not purged prior to investigation (**a**). On rinsing the bowel, no abnormality was detected in the ileum and the cecum (**b**)

Fig. 2.9.-3a and b. Artifact due to air bubbles and mucus during the first passage through the terminal ileum (**a**). No pathological findings after rinsing and optimal coating (**b**)

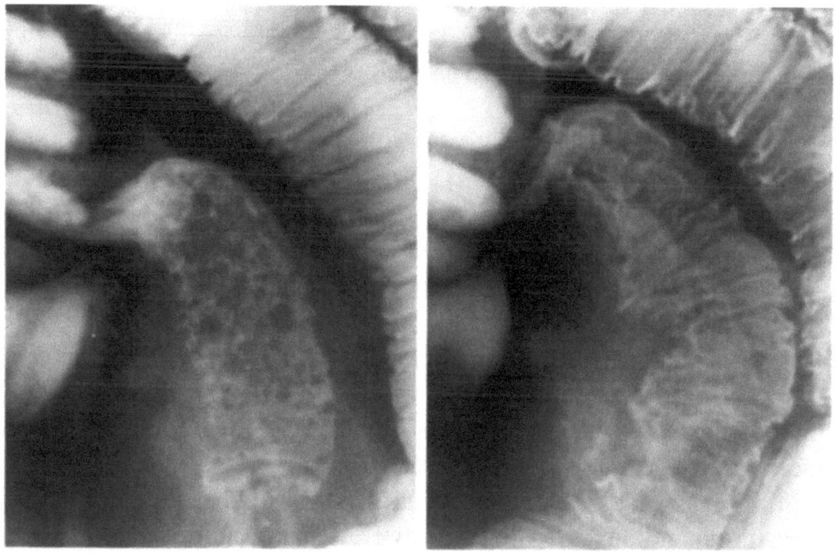

a b

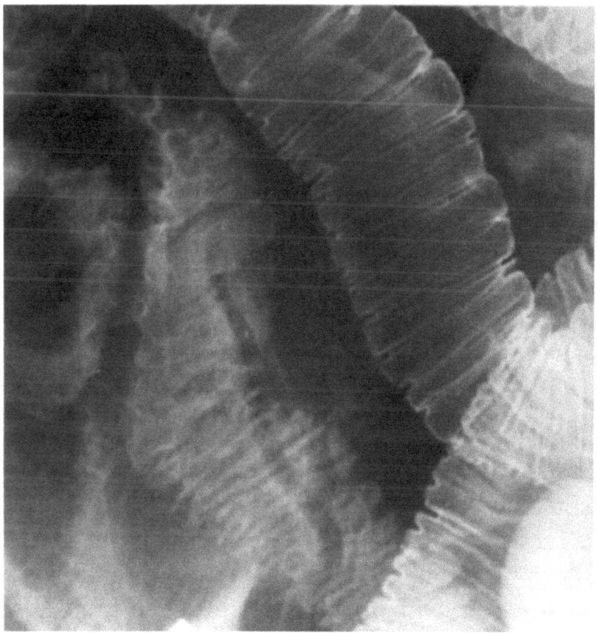

Fig. 2.9.-4. "Worm artifact" by superimposition of the ileosacral joint and the translucent terminal ileum

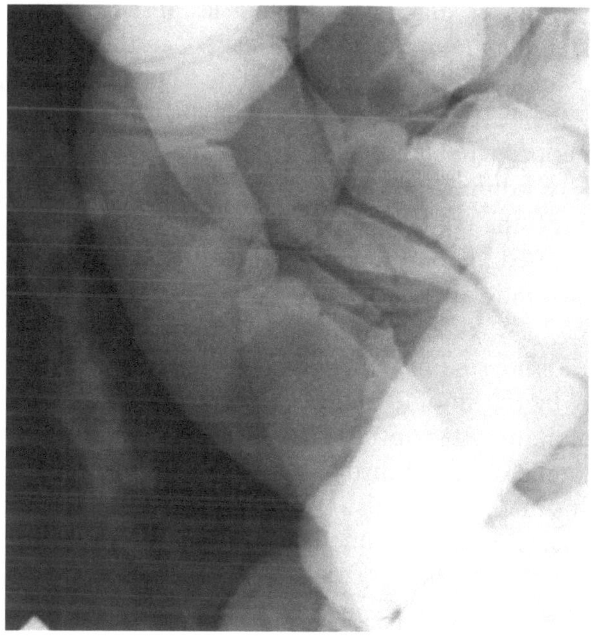

Fig. 2.9.-5. "Kissing artifact" due to trapped air bubbles

2.9 Artifacts

Artifacts may be caused by air bubbles, mucus and undigested intestinal contents, particularly when spot films are made, before the bowel lumen is sufficiently rinsed through with contrast medium. Other causes include superimposition or displacement by other structures, as e.g. air in the colon, vessels or calcified lymph nodes, residual contrast medium or bony structures. (Figs. 2.9.-1 to 2.9.-5).

2.10 Other Examination Techniques

• *Small bowel follow-through examination*
The advantage of this method is that it is easily performed. There are, however, various methods (Pansdorf 1937; Treichel 1981). Because fluoroscopy and documentation ensue only casually and regionally, the appropriate moment for detecting localized changes is jeopardized. Due to considerable physiological variations of the small bowel transit between 15 min and 5 h, the duration of the examination cannot be predicted (Geiter and Fuchs 1977). Motility disturbances cannot be assessed adequately. The fractionating function of the pylorus results in insufficient filling and distension of the bowel lumen. This makes diagnosis of small lesions, fibrous bands or minor stenoses difficult. Another disadvantage is that the barium-filled bowel loops in the pelvis often form an unpenetrable and unapproachable lump.

By administration of peristalsis stimulating drugs, the contrast medium transit may be accelerated (Thompson and Amberg 1978; Efsing and Lindroth 1980).

• *Reflux small bowel examination* (Miller 1965)
As in the double contrast examination of the colon, double contrast of the distal small bowel may be obtained through rectal air insufflation. This method appeals to patients who are apprehensive about the duodenal tubes. In cases of resection in the ileocecal junction, this method is useful for checking the anastomosis. However, a double contrast barium enema with retrograde filling of the small bowel seems to be better.

• *Enteroclysis in barium monocontrast*
This method has been preferred and perfected by Sellink (1976). As with the follow-through, however, when the ileum is overfilled, satisfactory assessment cannot be made. In such cases, an antero- or retrograde air insufflation is recommended for obtaining double contrast. Our method includes both single and double contrast examination in the same investigation.

• *Enteroclysis with barium and air*
This double contrast method of the small bowel also produces good results (Ekberg 1977; Salomonowitz et al. 1983; Bautz and Schindler 1983). It is not comparable with the examination of the stomach or colon. Difficulties in interpretation or orientation ensue because of excessive density differences and the multitude of intercepting lines of the valvulae conniventes (Herlinger 1979). Air and barium cannot be manipulated as in the investigation of the stomach and colon by change of position. Further disadvantages of this method are meteorism and stimulation of the peristalsis by air.

• *Enteroclysis with barium and water*
This method can produce good small bowel radiographs. But water washes the barium rapidly from the mucosa and excessive dilution with water leads to disintegration of the barium suspension which makes a regular interpretation impossible. As a result of this experience, Sellink has abandoned this double contrast method and advises against it (personal communication).

• *Water-soluble contrast medium*
The small bowel follow-through examination using water-soluble contrast medium is unsatisfactory in most cases and should be avoided as far as possible. Surgeons often want this type of examination for the exclusion of small bowel obstruction. Only in cases of advanced stenoses in the proximal small bowel a diagnostic report can be made. Often this method is inadequate for satisfactory interpretation in a subileus condition. If there is an indication for an investigation with water-soluble contrast medium (e.g. suspected obstruction in the small bowel and/or the colon), the tube already resting in the stomach should be farther advanced into the duodenum and an enteroclysma with undiluted water-soluble contrast medium should be carried out (e.g. Gastrografin®[5]). The proximal small bowel is easier to assess than the distal part. This is due to the dilution of the contrast medium by

[5] Gastrografin®, Schering Ltd, Berlin, Germany

retained fluid in the bowel. The modern nonionic water-soluble contrast media are better than the conventional ionic contrast media (Cohen 1982; Kaufmann and Langer 1985). Presently, the high costs limit the routine use. The nonionic contrast media, however, should be preferred in babies and infants.

- *Colonoscopic small bowel enema*

Frimberger et al. (1983) report on this method in connection with colonoscopy. Experience with this method is, however, limited. This examination will be spared for special cases only.

3 Indications

The indications for enteroclysis ensue from the clinical questions. The place of small bowel investigation in the diagnostic work-up varies. In suspected Crohn's disease, this investigation has priority. Otherwise, when all other examinations have proved negative – laboratory tests, ultrasound, CT, double contrast investigation of stomach and colon – it is last in the series.

Table 3.-1. Indications for enteroclysis

1. Unexplained abdominal complaints
2. Unexplained diarrhea
3. Malabsorption
4. Gastrointestinal bleeding
5. Suspected tumors
6. Fever of unknown origin
7. Postoperative condition
8. Recurrent fistulae
9. Small bowel obstruction

4 Basic Signs and Interpretation

4.1 Normal Findings and Variations

The length of a normal small bowel varies between 4–12 m (Hirsch et al. 1956; Underhill 1955). The difference is related to individual variations, racial differences, varied muscle tone and the problem in determining the length intra vitam.

In people with an abundance of mesenteric fat, the small bowel loops are separated from each other in the abdomen (Fig. 4.1.-1). In slim people, the loops are crowded together in the small pelvis (Fig. 4.1.-2).

It is difficult to determine the exact junction between jejunum and ileum. This junction is roughly situated in the middle of the entire length. The distribution of the valvulae conniventes varies considerably. They are more numerous in the jejunum than in the ileum. Rarification of folds in the ileum, however, is considered to be normal (Fig. 4.1.-3). In adolescents, particularly, there are numerous folds. The folds run circularly and are perpendicular to the longitudinal axis of the intestine. Sometimes, in the middle of the small bowel, there is a triangular arrangement of folds.

The fold pattern of the duodenum is different from that of a normal small bowel. There is a netlike arrangement of folds in this region. In ideal double contrast, the intestinal villi of the mucosa are recognizable (Fig. 4.1.-4).

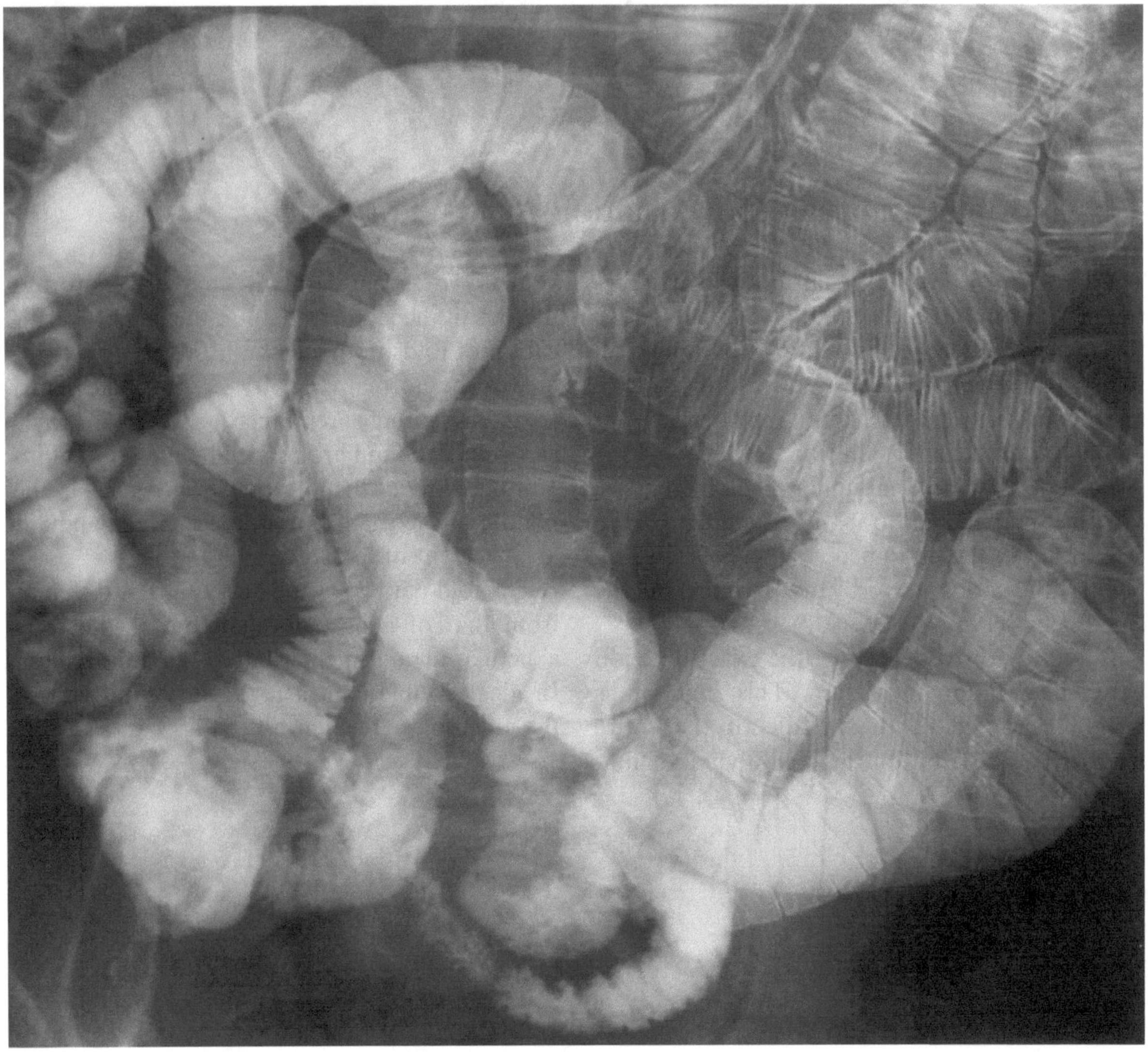

Fig. 4.1.-1. Normal small bowel in a patient with abundant mesenteric fat. The loops are well-separated from each other

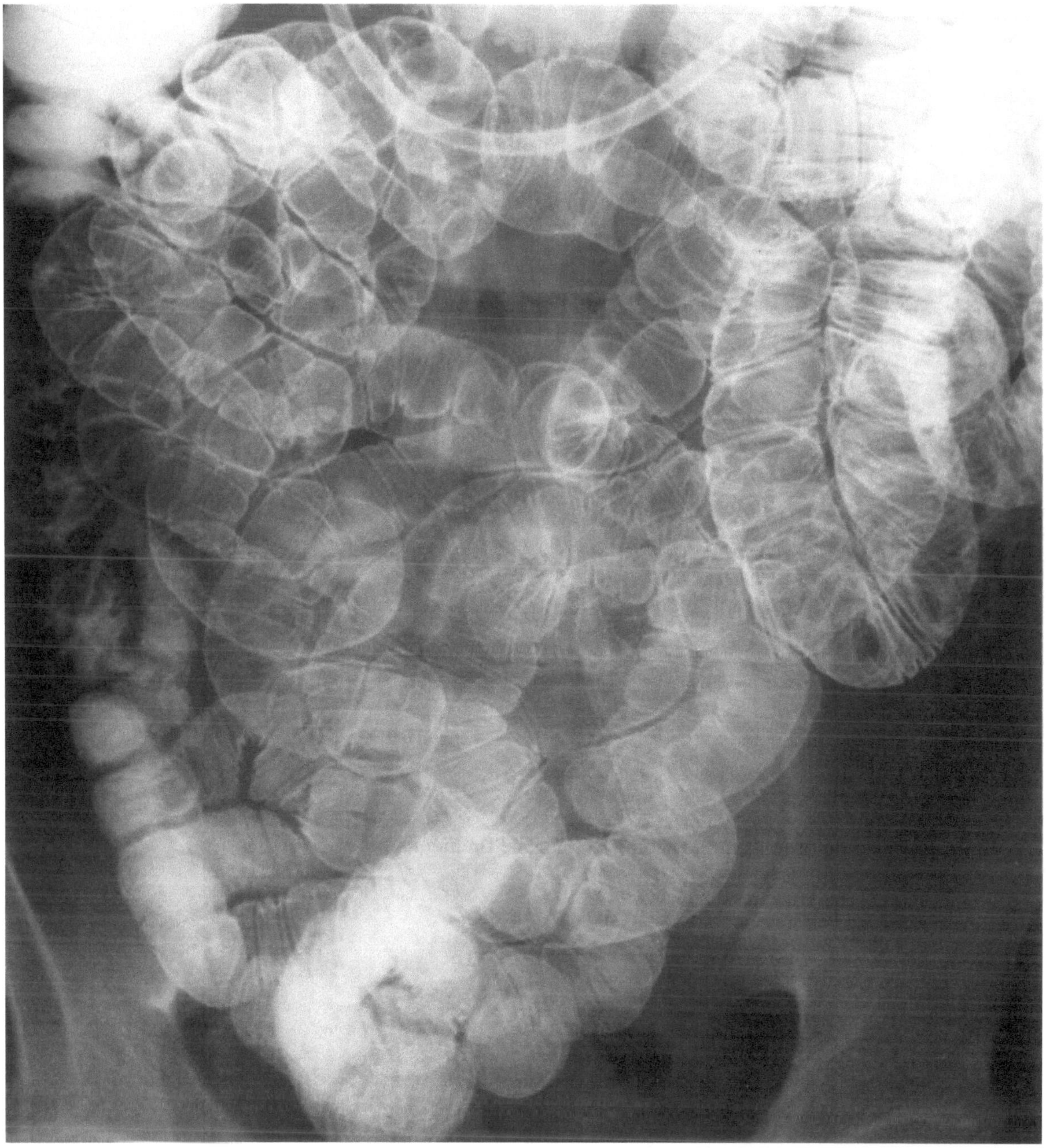

Fig. 4.1.-2. Normal small bowel in a slim person. The ileal loops are crowded together in the small pelvis

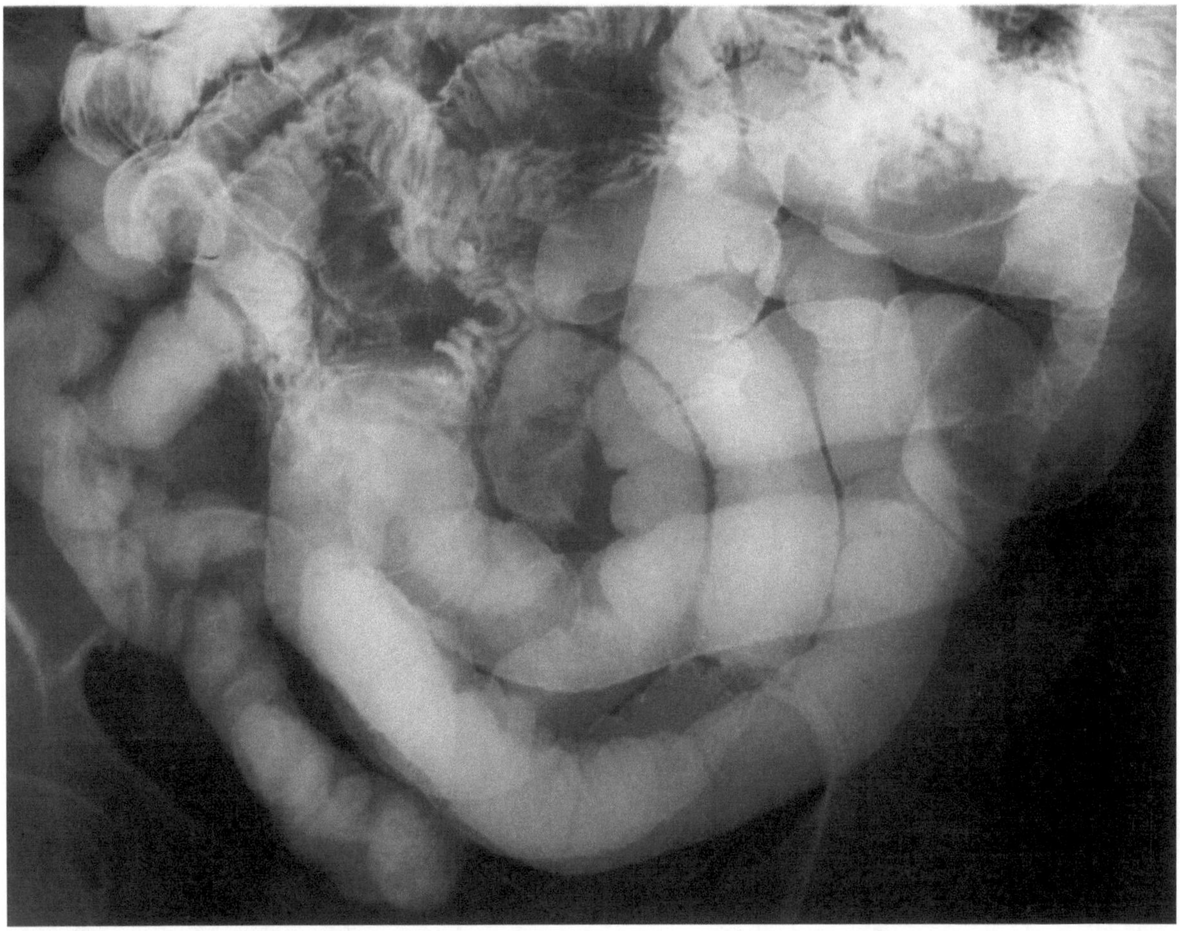

Fig. 4.1.-3. Rarification of folds in the ileum, as a normal finding in an elderly patient

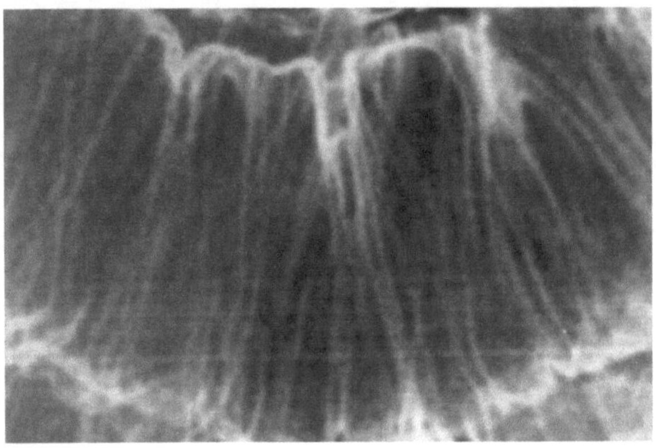

Fig. 4.1.-4. Normal fine relief (intestinal villi) of the small bowel mucosa

4.2 Small Bowel Folds and Wall Thickness

4.2.1 Small Bowel Folds (normal/abnormal)

In order to assess the folds, the small bowel has to be adequately distended. The thickness of normal folds is 1.7–2 mm in the jejunum, 1.4–1.7 mm in the ileum and does not vary with the lumen diameter (Herlinger 1979; Fig. 4.2.-1). A fold thickness of more than 2.5 mm is considered to be abnormal. There are no instances of folds which are "too thin".

In a well-distended bowel, normal folds – seen in profile – have rounded corners (Fig. 4.2.-1). Thickened folds seen in profile, may show an omega-like contour (Fig. 4.2.-2→). The fold height in the jejunum and the ileum varies considerably and is therefore of little diagnostic value. The fold arrangement is relatively regular throughout large sections of the intestine and there are no significant fluctuations.

An irregular arrangement of folds may be observed in inflammatory infiltrations (Figs. 4.2.-2 and 3), in chronic radiation enteritis (Fig. 4.2.-4), in lymphedema, in adhesions (Fig. 4.2.-5) or in tumor infiltrations and peritoneal carcinomatosis (Fig. 4.2.-6) as well as in scleroderma (Fig. 4.2.-7) and amyloidosis (see Fig. 5.4.-15, p. 157). Simultaneously, there is an abnormal configuration, thickness and height of the folds. Thick folds without deformation are caused by edema of varying origins (e.g. deficiency or loss of protein, Fig. 4.2.-8).

The average number of folds in a normal proximal jejunum is 4.88/2.5 cm (=1 inch) and varies between 3–7/2.5 cm. In the ileum there are usually 2–4 folds/2.5 cm, on average 3.15/2.5 cm (Herlinger and Maglinte 1986).

A rarification of folds in the duodenum and jejunum ("colonization") is very suspicious of adult celiac disease. A compensatory increase of folds ("jejunization") of the ileum may be observed (Figs. 5.4.-10 to 13, pp. 148–155).

4.2.2 Wall Thickness (normal/abnormal)

The wall of the small bowel measures between 1–1.5 mm in 75% of the normal population, 1.6–2 mm in 12.5% and under 1 mm in another 12.5%. A wall thickness of more than 2 mm must be regarded as abnormal (Herlinger 1979).

Fig. 4.2.-1. Normal jejunal folds. Circular arrangement of folds. Fold thickness is less than 2 mm. Rounded corners are shown in profile

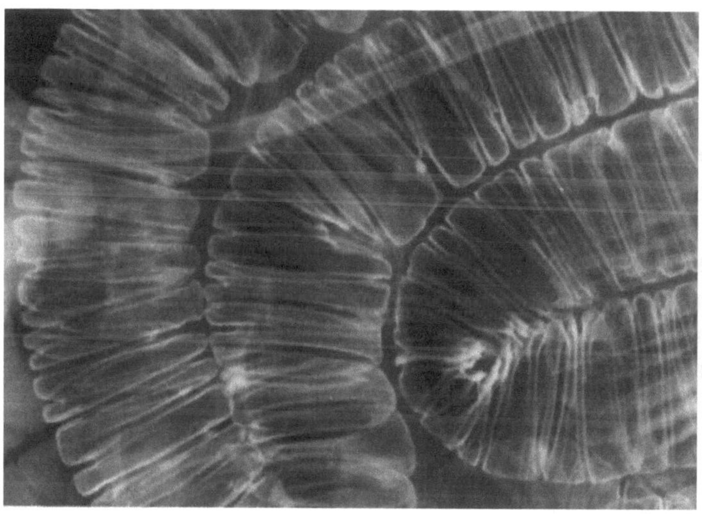

Fig. 4.2.-2. Irregular, thickened folds with omega-like configuration (→) due to inflammatory infiltration in eosinophilic enteritis

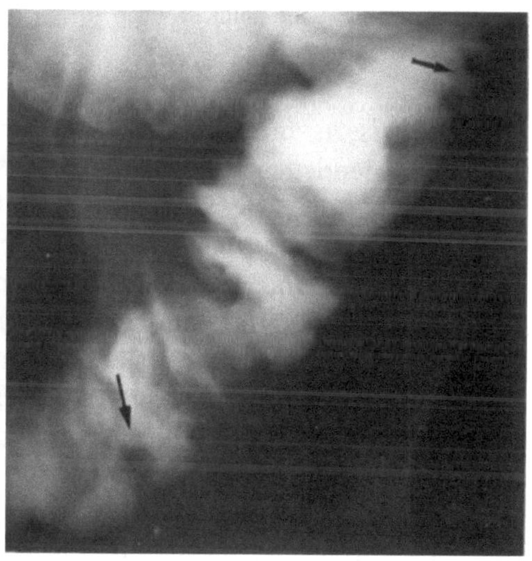

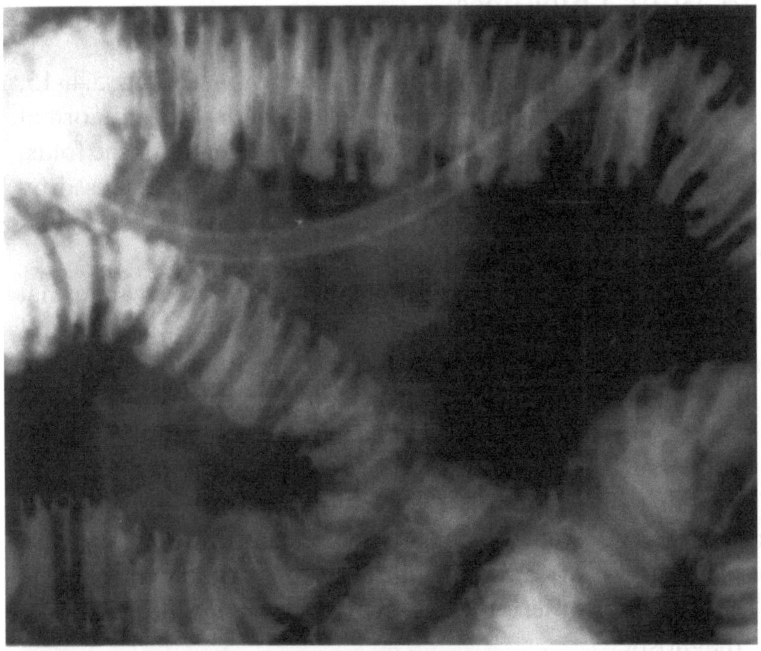

Fig. 4.2.-3. Irregular, thickened folds in the entire small bowel in Whipple's disease

Fig. 4.2.-4. Irregular, thickened folds with narrowing of the lumen in chronic radiation enteritis

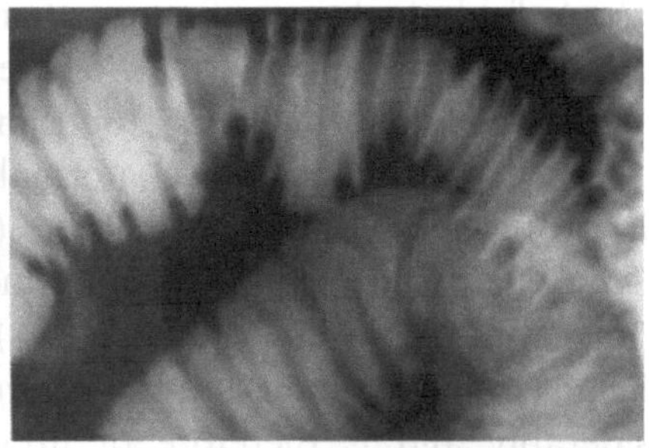

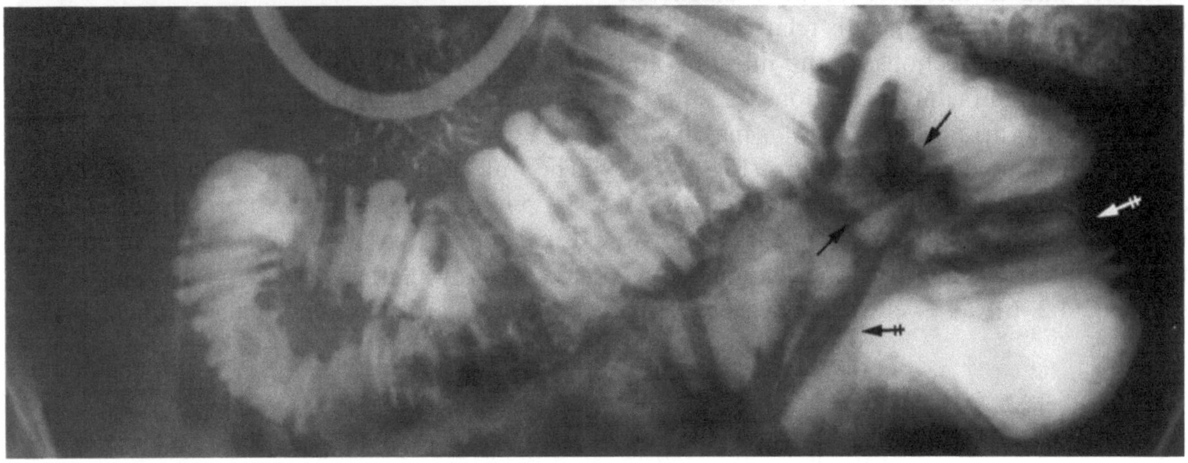

Fig. 4.2.-5. Thickened folds (→) because of marked postoperative adhesions (↠). The adhesions themselves may imitate thickened folds

The thickness is measured in a region where two well-distended bowel segments are seen to be strictly parallel over at least 4 cm. It is assumed that both serosal surfaces are in close contact. The distance between the two mucosal surfaces represents the combined thickness of the two bowel walls. This distance should not exceed 3–4 mm (Fig. 4.2.-9). Pathological processes, which result in thickening of the folds, usually result also in a thickening of the intestinal wall. Crohn's disease is the most frequent cause of intestinal wall thickening (Fig. 4.2.-9→).

4.3 Surface Changes

Surface changes are the most important manifestation of small bowel disease besides the alterations of folds and the mucosal coating. They may be observed in the mucosa and/or in the deeper layers of the intestinal wall. The changes are characteristic of certain small bowel diseases. In some of these cases, however, a picture typical of one disease may be imitated by other disorders. Surface changes are often combined with fold alterations and thickening of the wall.

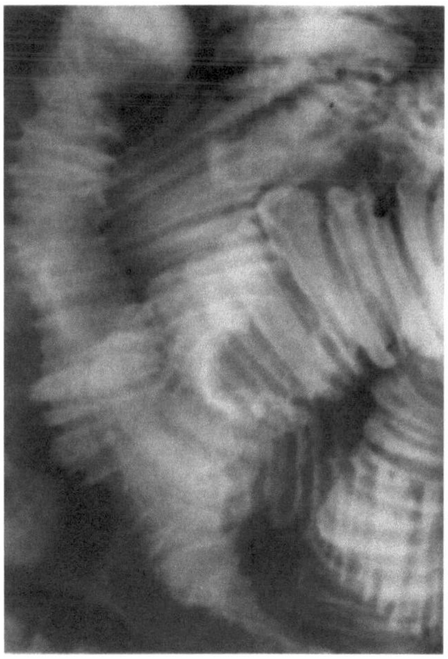

Fig. 4.2.-6. Thickened, irregular folds due to peritoneal carcinomatosis

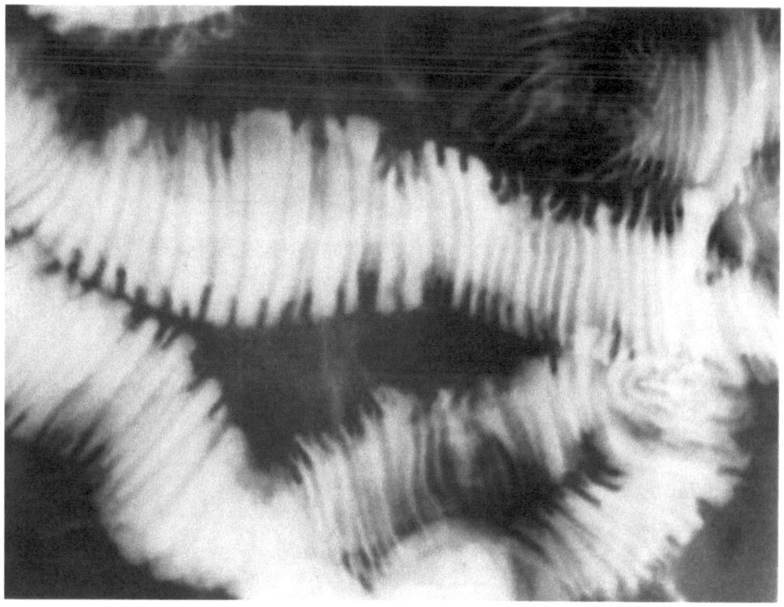

Fig. 4.2.-7. Irregular distribution of folds with segments of crowding folds with normal thickness and dilated segments in systemic sclerosis (scleroderma). So-called "hide-bound" sign

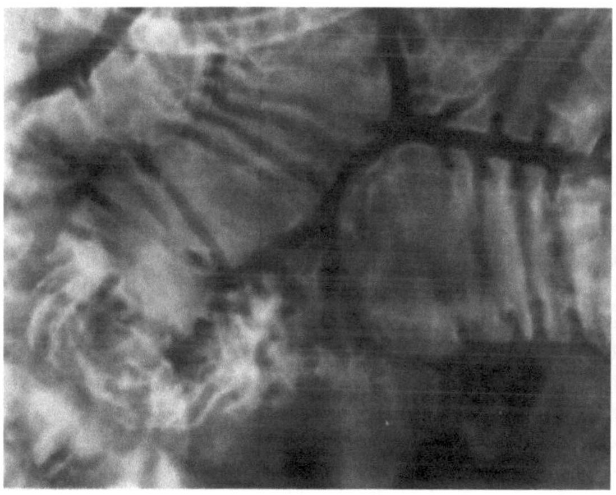

Fig. 4.2.-8. Omega-like thickening of folds and wall thickening in a patient with protein deficiency edema due to chronic pancreatitis

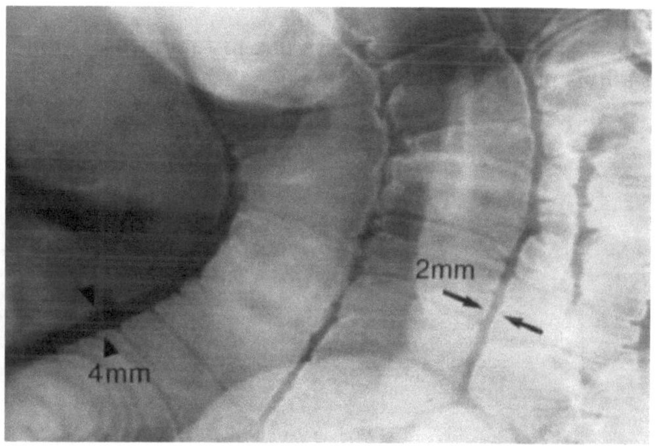

Fig. 4.2. 9. Crohn's disease. The distance between the healthy intestinal segment measures 2 mm (→), whereas the distance between the normal and diseased segment is 4 mm (►). This is due to inflammatory wall infiltration

4.3.1 Mucosal Thickening

Thickening of the mucosa in the distal terminal ileum, mainly at the mesenteric border (convex border), can be caused by enlarged Peyer's patches (Fig. 4.3.-1). A thickened, irregular mucosa in the terminal ileum is a manifestation of an inflammatory infiltration (Fig. 4.3.-2).

The differentiation from early Crohn's disease may be impossible. In such cases, histology, too, is often not diagnostic.

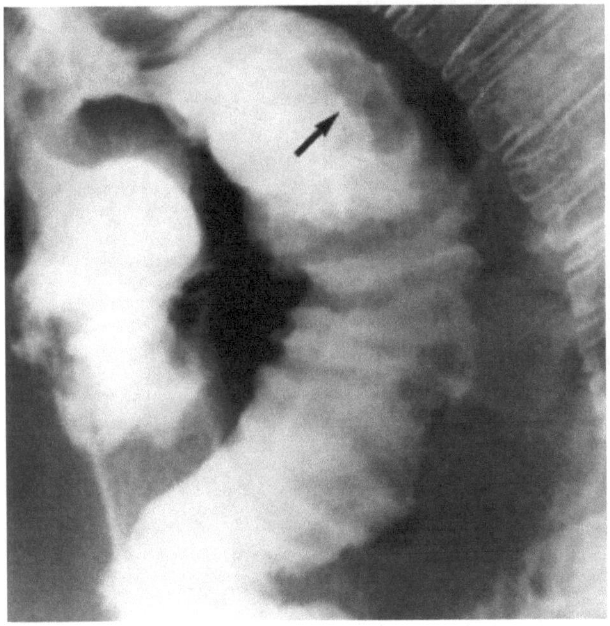

Fig. 4.3.-1. Prominent longitudinal fold and nodular surface changes in the terminal ileum due to Peyer's patches (→) on the mesenteric border. This may be a coincidental finding without significance or sometimes a manifestation of a nonspecific ileitis

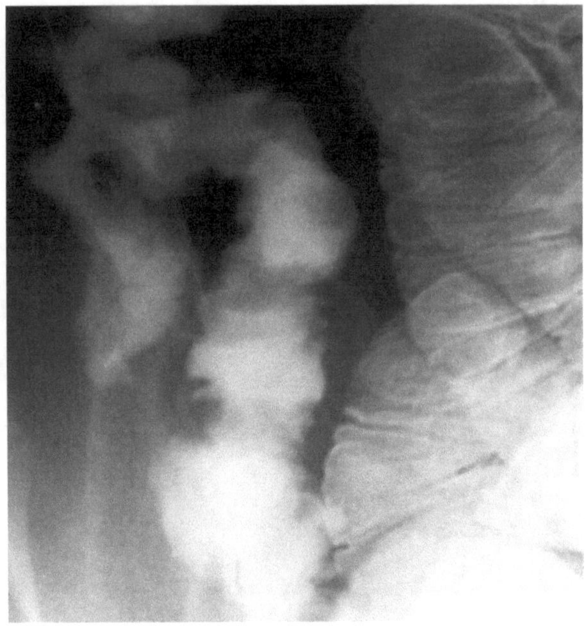

Fig. 4.3.-2. Significantly enlarged mucosal folds in the terminal ileum with thickening of the wall due to inflammatory infiltration in a nonspecific terminal ileitis

Fig. 4.3.-3. Cobblestone pattern due to submucosal infiltrations in Crohn's disease

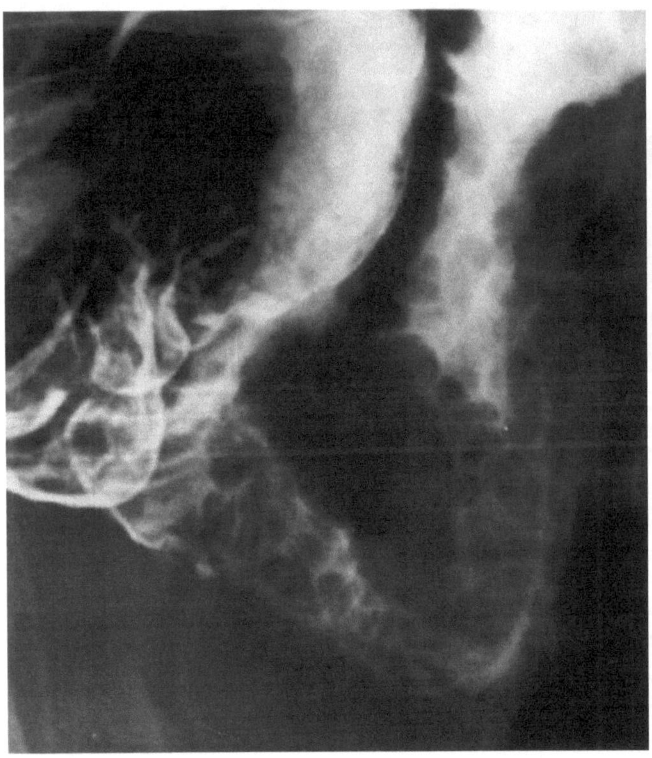

Fig. 4.3.-4. Flat, nodular surface changes due to granulomas in Crohn's disease (pseudopolyps)

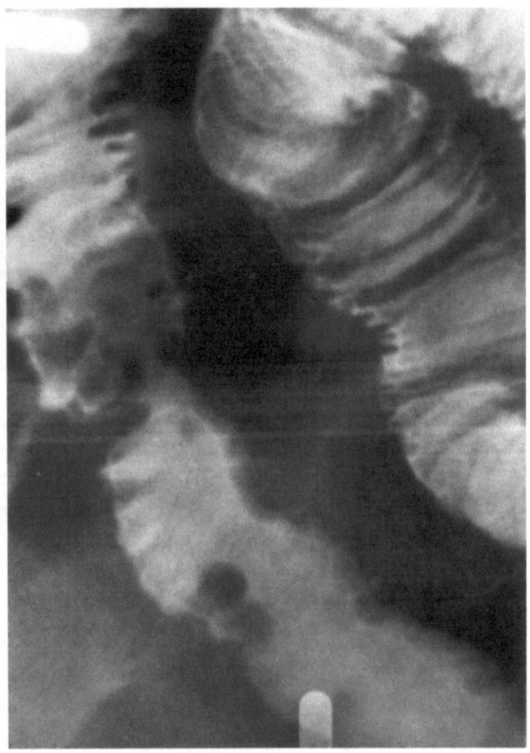

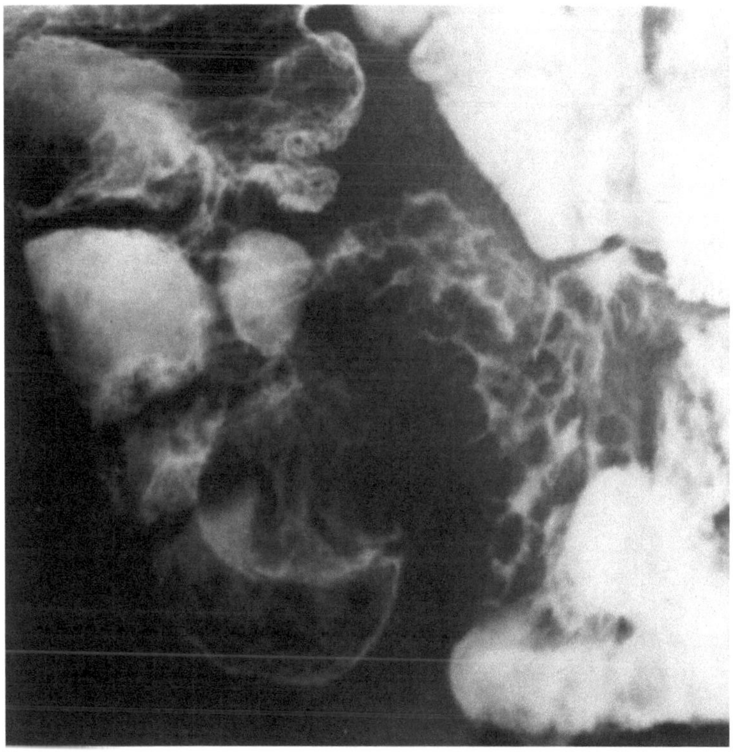

Fig. 4.3.-5. Irregular, cobblestone pattern in the terminal ileum with fissures due to granulomatous infiltrations in intestinal tuberculosis

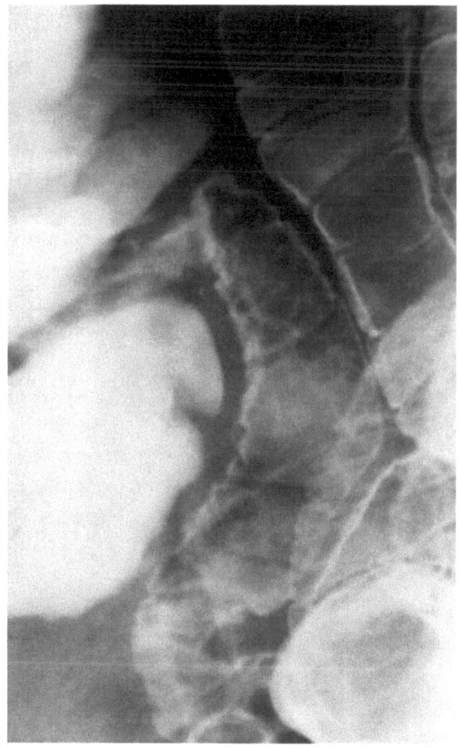

Fig. 4.3.-6. Small, uniform, flat elevations in the terminal ileum due to lymphofollicular hyperplasia. No thickening of the wall

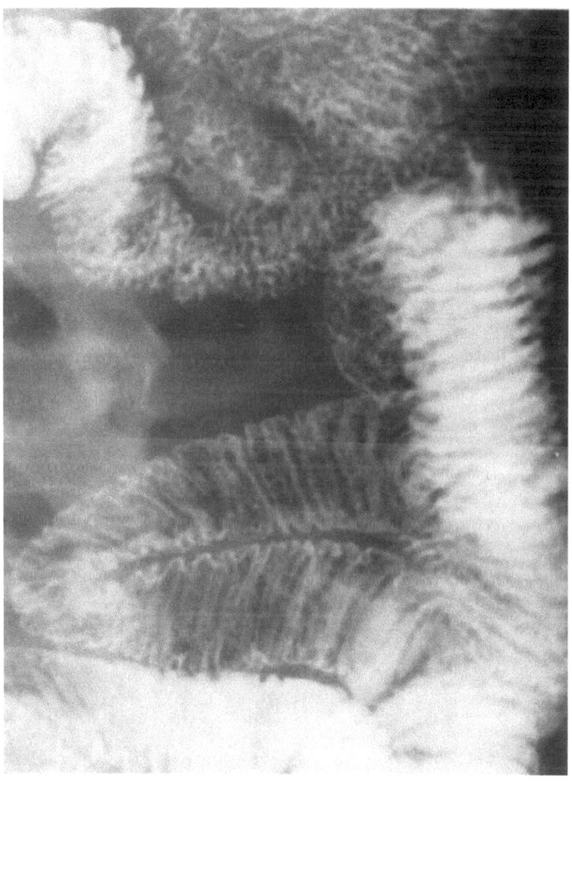

Fig. 4.3.-7. Tiny, regular nodules due to lymphofollicular hyperplasia, recognized only in a well-distended bowel. Not visible in the contracting segments and in monocontrast

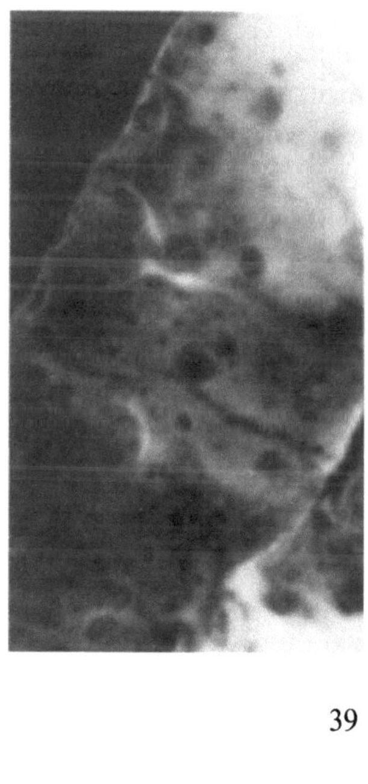

Fig. 4.3.-8. Irregular, small- to medium-sized nodular elevations in the ileum due to infiltrations in high grade non-Hodgkin lymphoma

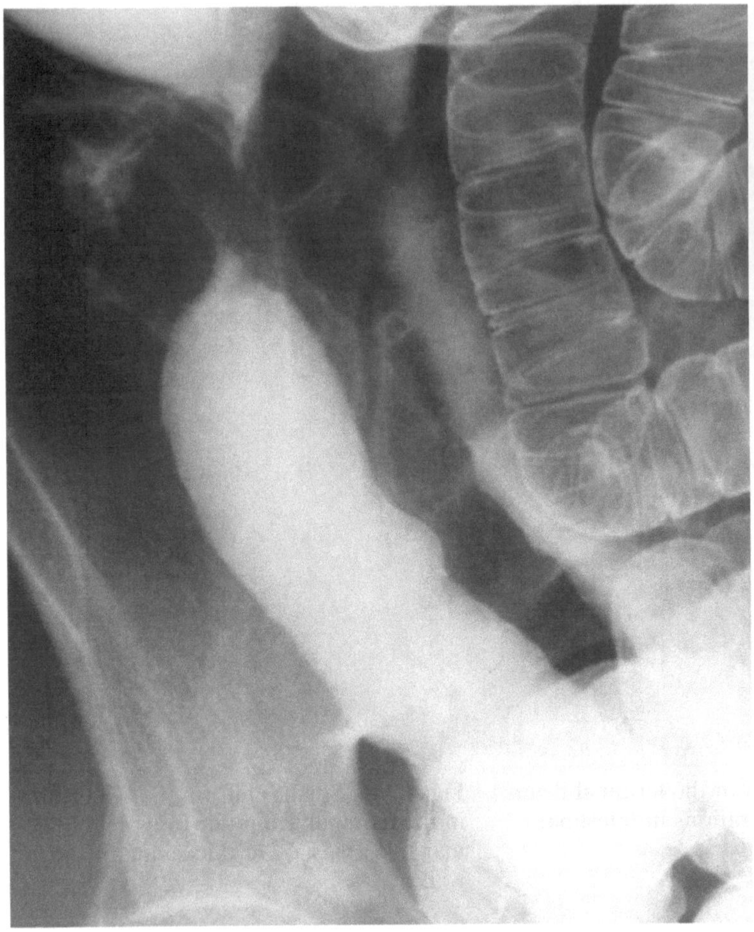

Fig. 4.3.-9. Loss of folds and smooth surface because of mucosal atrophy in Crohn's disease in remission

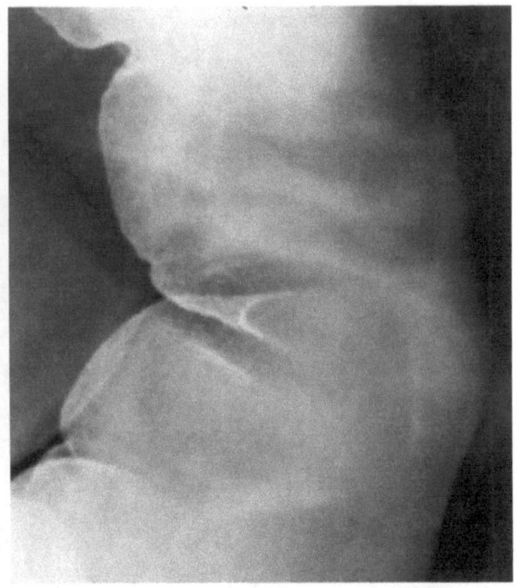

Fig. 4.3.-10. Complete loss of folds and lumen dilatation ("colonization"). Fine reticular pattern with small mesh size ("mosaic pattern") due to atrophy of the mucosal villi. Separation of the dilated and elongated mucosal crypts in adult celiac disease

Fig. 4.3.-11. Smooth intestinal surface through loss of folds and atrophy of the mucosal surface in chronic radiation enteritis (see Fig. 5.2.-14, p. 92)

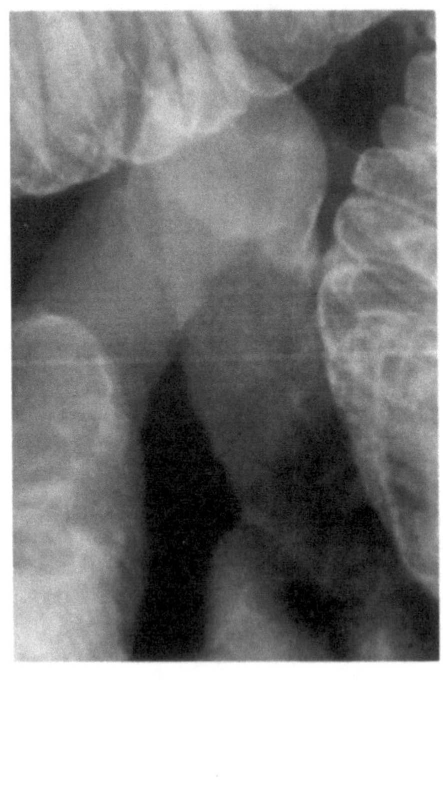

4.3.2 Polypoid Changes

The typical picture is a result of inflammatory infiltrates in Crohn's disease (cobblestoning and pseudopolyps). These infiltrates may be of different size and configuration. Tuberculosis can also produce similar changes (Fig. 4.3.-5).

Nodular changes of varying size and configuration on the intestinal surface may be caused by lymphofollicular hyperplasia of varied origin, nodular lymphoma infiltrations or so-called lipogranulomas (containing PAS-positive material) in Whipple's disease (Figs. 4.3.-6 to 8).

Attention: Lymph follicles can be simulated by orthograde viewing of the folds in an incompletely distended bowel.

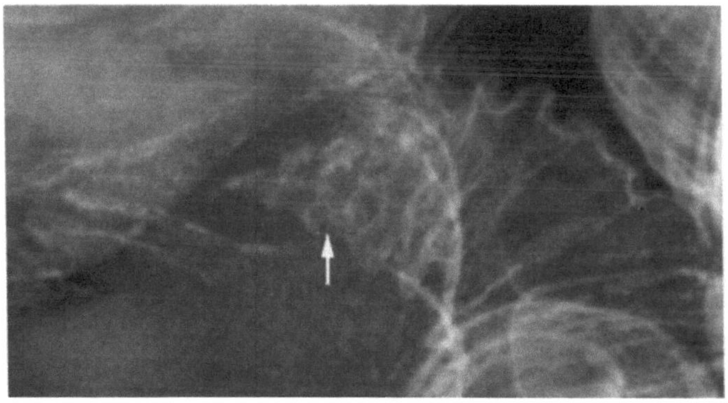

Fig. 4.3.-12. Aphthous ulcerations. Small, flat elevations with scattered central ulcerations in the terminal ileum close to the ileocecal valve (→). They represent the earliest roentgen features of Crohn's disease

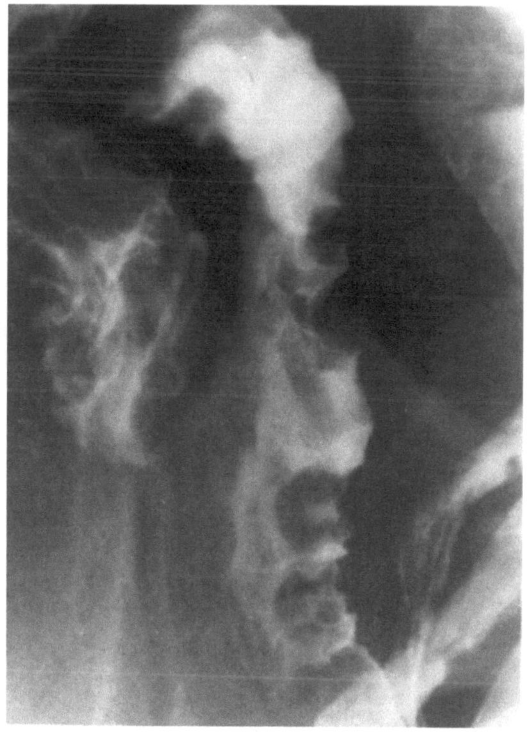

Fig. 4.3.-13. Polypoid thickening of the wall with superficial ulcerations (large aphthous ulcerations) in nonspecific terminal ileitis

4.3.3 Smooth Surface

A smooth bowel surface with loss of folds is observed in Crohn's disease, mainly in the stage of remission or slight clinical activity (Fig. 4.3.-9). With advanced celiac disease, there is a smooth surface with loss of folds and lumen dilatation. The villous atrophy and elongated crypts simulate areae gastricae in atrophic gastritis (Fig. 4.3.-10).

Amyloidosis (Fig. 5.4.-16, p. 158), chronic radiation enteritis (Fig. 4.3.-11) and chronic abuse of laxatives may produce atrophy of the folds with smooth surface as well.

4.3.4 Ulcerations

Aphthoid ulcerations are characteristic of the early form of Crohn's disease (Fig. 4.3.-12). Other inflammatory diseases of the small intestine rarely produce aphthae (Fig. 4.3.-13). Superficial mucosal ulcerations are difficult to image. Even under optimal conditions, the small defects are sometimes inadequately filled. Other signs, such as surrounding mucosal swelling, impaired mucosal coating, local hyperperistalsis and mural alterations are suggestive of inflammatory change. Ulcerations, which deeply penetrate the walls, are better portrayed, particularly in profile.

4.3.5 Fistulae

These usually develop in Crohn's disease when deep wall ulcerations spread in a tract-like fashion. They extend to adjacent organs. The most frequent types are enteroenteral or enterocutaneous fistulae (Figs. 5.1.-25 to 28, pp. 70–72). The fistular tracts are sometimes so thin that they might escape detection. Indirect signs of a fistula are e.g. early filling of the rectum or other parts of the colon before the ileocecal junction is reached, or the appearance of the contrast medium on the skin surface.

The increased amounts of contrast medium during enteroclysis produce good images of fine

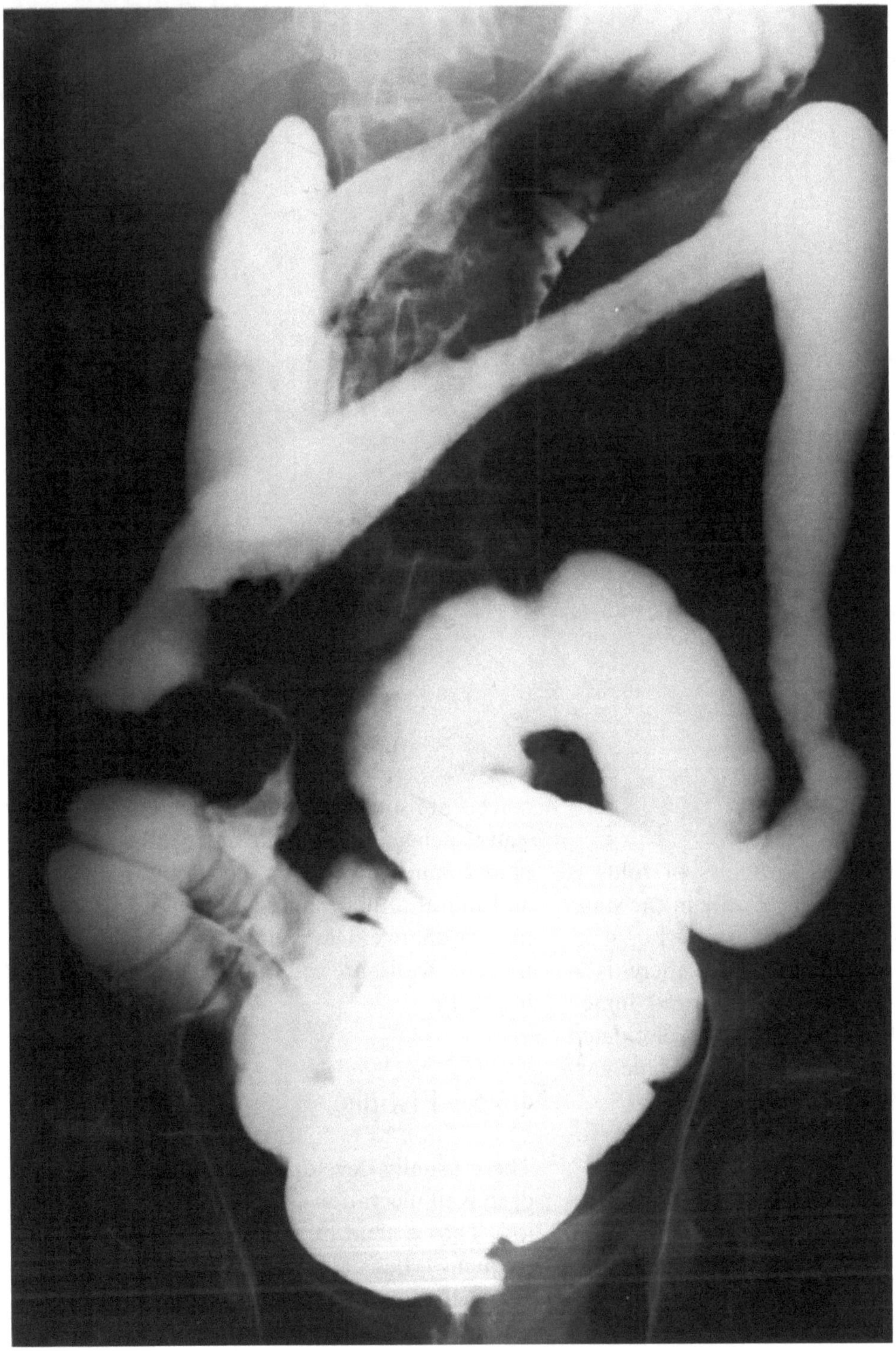

Fig. 4.3.-14. Retrograde filling of the stomach through a fistula between the terminal ileum/colon and the stomach in Crohn's disease. Retrograde filling of the fistula was only possible with a barium enema (check-valve mechanism). The patient suffered no malresorption or diarrhea

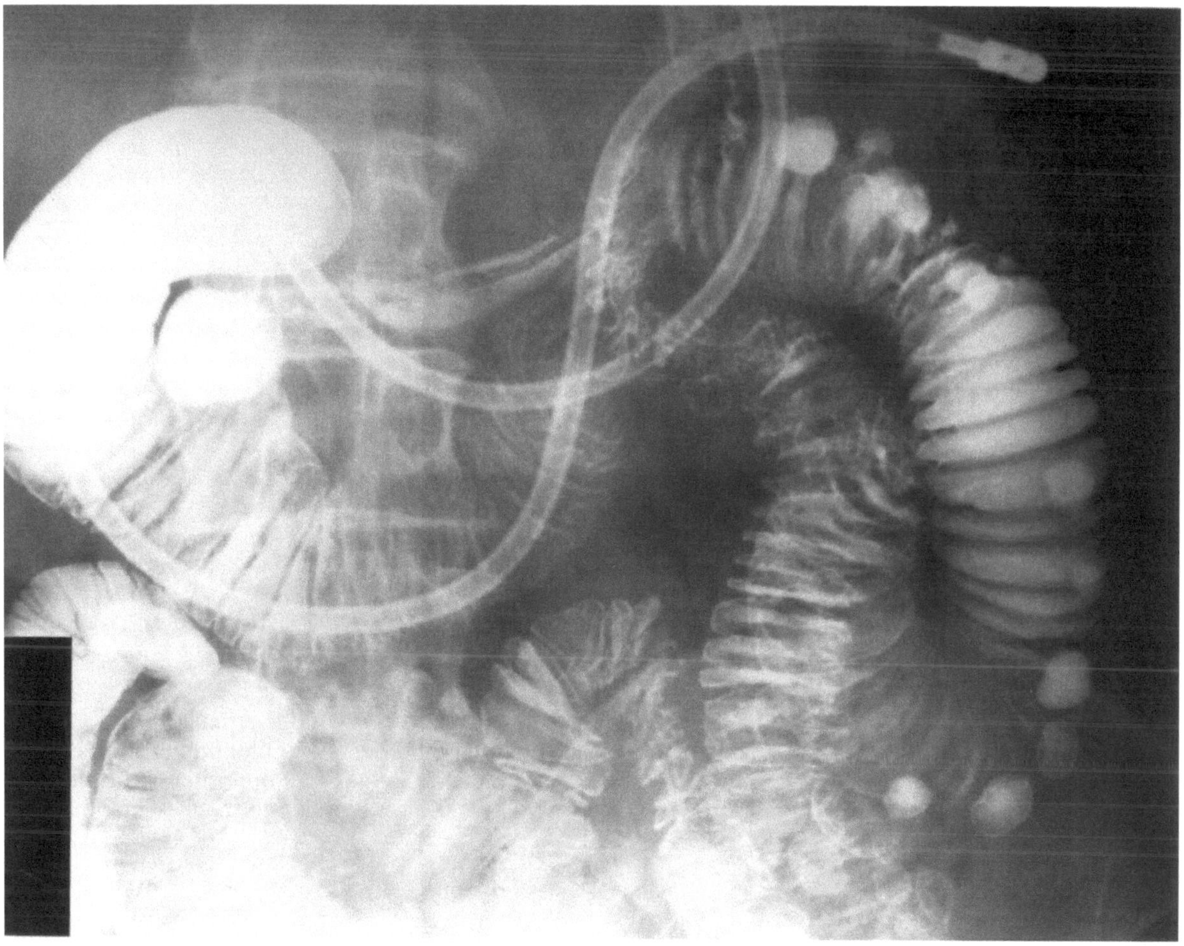

Fig. 4.3.-15. Numerous jejunal and duodenal diverticula localized partly on the mesenteric and partly on the antimesenteric border of the bowel

fistular tracts and so-called fox-earth fistulae. It has to be noted that only antegrade-filled fistulae, i.e. those which are to be filled from the small intestine into the large bowel, are probably functionally effective. On the other hand, fistulae which can be filled retrograde from the colon during barium enema are mostly functionally ineffective. In this case of a fistula, antegrade filling is inhibited because of a kind of valve mechanism (Fig. 4.3.-14).

4.3.6 Diverticula

Diverticula may be congenital, e.g. Meckel's diverticulum. Most small bowel diverticula are acquired. Diverticula on the antimesenteric border are most likely to be congenital whereas those on the mesenteric border are acquired (Fig. 4.3.-15; Meyers 1976). Absolute differentiation between the two types is, however, not always possible. Smaller contractile diverticula may escape detection if the contrast medium bolus is not carefully pursued. This is also true for Meckel's diverticulum.

Diverticula-like changes are observed in Crohn's disease. These are due to increase of

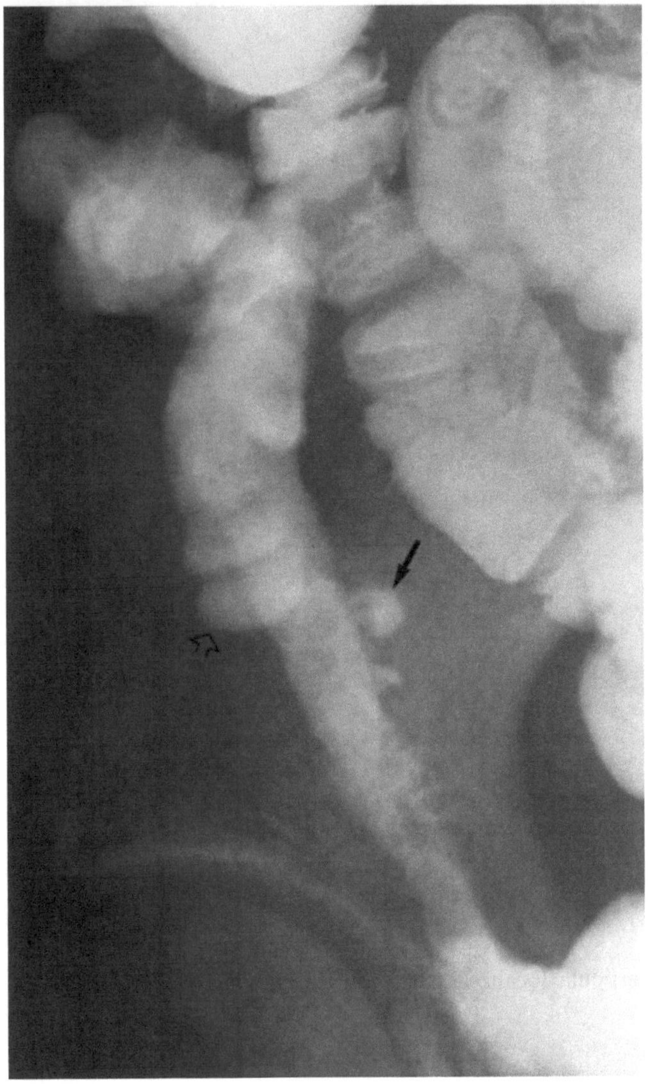

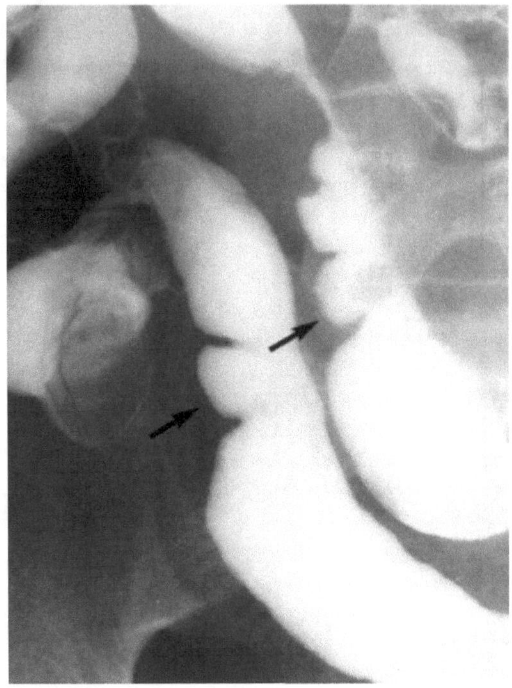

Fig. 4.3.-17. Pseudodiverticula on the antimes enteric border (→). Due to puckering of the intact intestinal wall opposite the fibrotically healed ulceration along the mesenteric border

Fig. 4.3.-16. False diverticula (→) on the mes enteric border in Crohn's disease. Pseudodiverticula on the antimesenteric side (⇒)

Fig. 4.3.-18. Broad-based diverticular sacculation, due to segmental intestinal infiltration in scleroderma

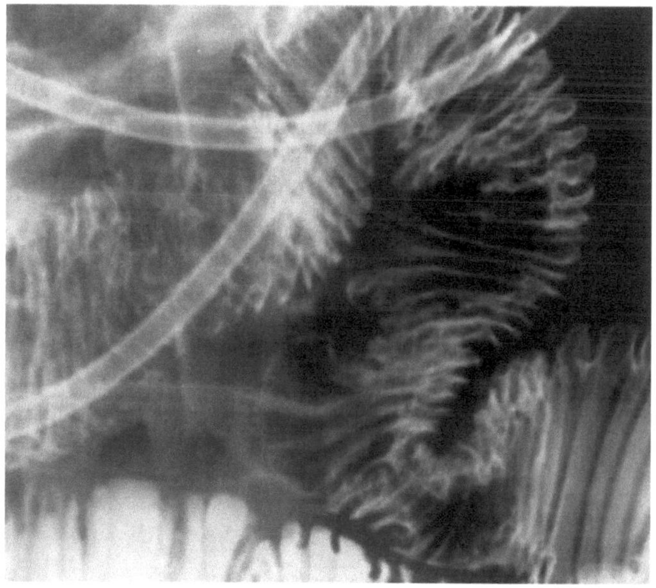

intraluminal pressure resulting in herniation of the intact mucosa through the hypertrophied bowel wall. These "false" diverticula are to be seen at the mesenteric border of the intestine (Fig. 4.3.-16). These may be differentiated from the "pseudodiverticula" in Crohn's disease found on the antimesenteric border. They are due to puckering of the antimesenteric wall vis-à-vis fibrotically healed ulcerations on the mesenteric border (Fig. 4.3.-17). Broad-based diverticular sacculations result from wall infiltrations in scleroderma (Fig. 4.3.-18).

4.4 Ileocecal Valve

The ileocecal valve resembles the lips into which the terminal ileum opens conically. This picture is presented in lateral view (Fig. 4.4.-1). En face viewing portrays a bulging ring (Fig. 4.4.-2). The thickness of the valve varies considerably. Alterations in form are caused by a lipomatosis (Fig. 4.4.-3) or inflammation (chapters 5.1 and 5.2). Destruction and deformation are mostly caused by Crohn's disease or tumors.

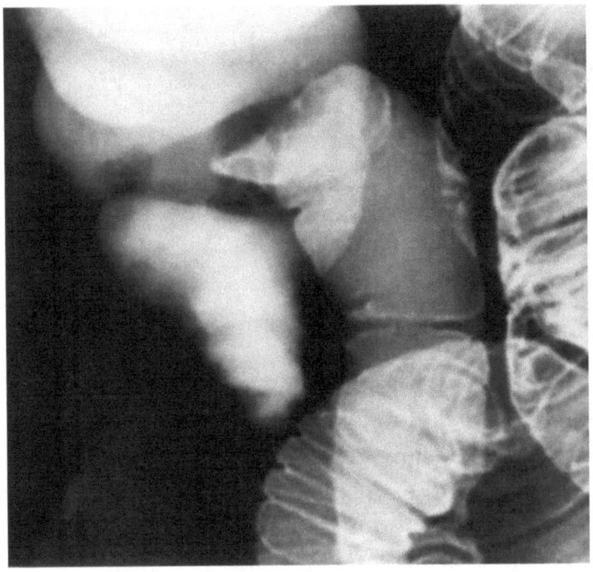

Fig. 4.4.-1. Normal ileocecal valve in lateral projection

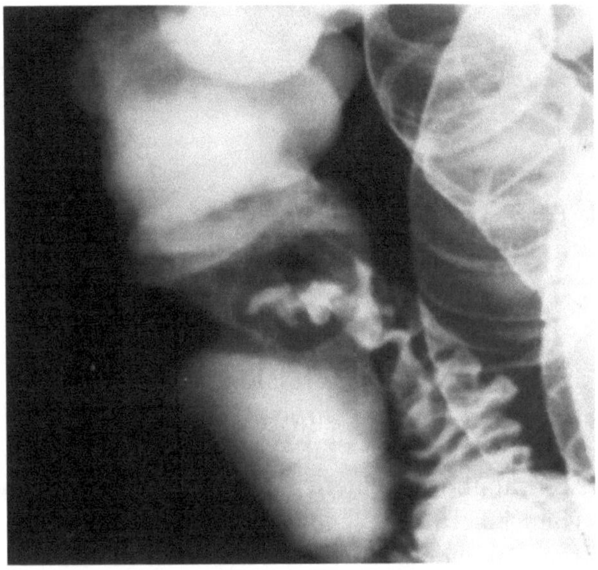

Fig. 4.4.-2. Normal ileocecal valve en face

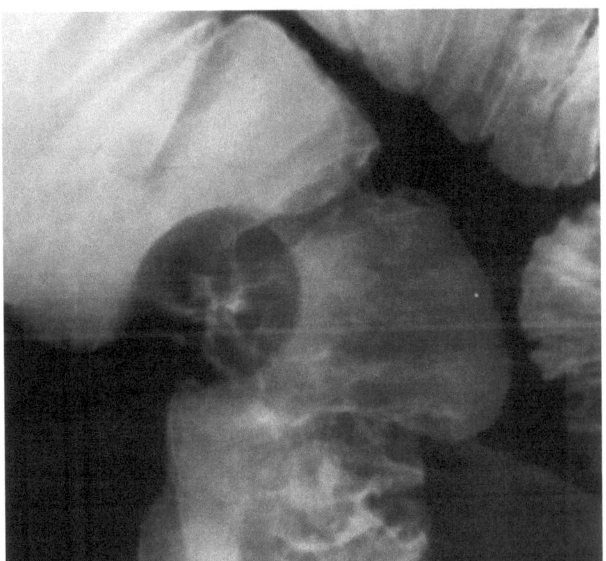

Fig. 4.4.-3. Lipomatosis of ileocecal valve

4.5 Motility Disorders

Motility disorders can be investigated by the enteroclysis technique. Contrast medium administered at a constant flow rate enables observation of the behavior of the small bowel. Although the investigational conditions are "nonphysiologic", they allow a conclusion concerning the intestinal motility, since this test for all patients is the same. Comparable examinations

Fig. 4.5.-1. Marked hyperperistalsis. In the barium phase, the contrast medium has almost reached the colon. Most of the bowel is in a state of contraction

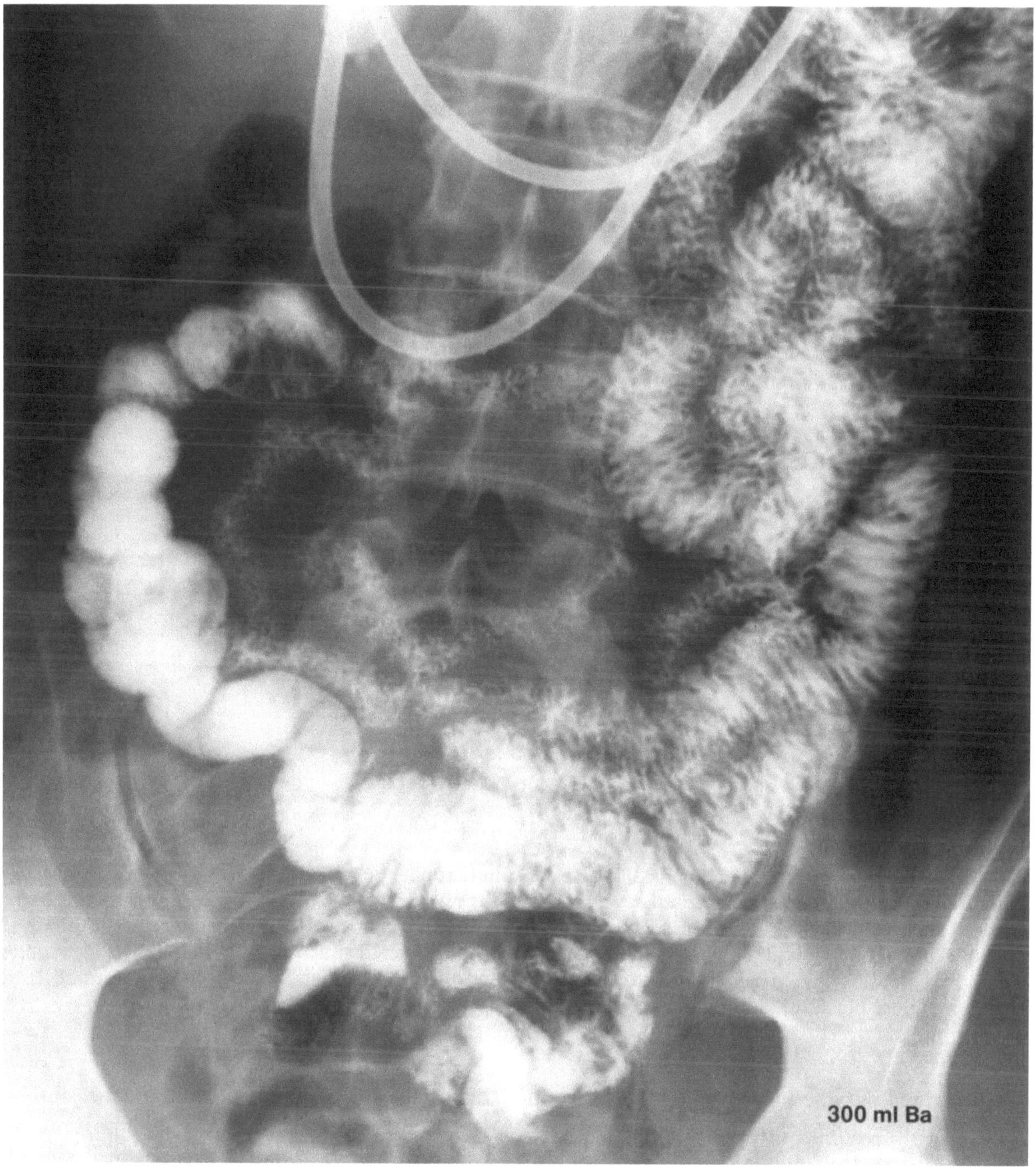

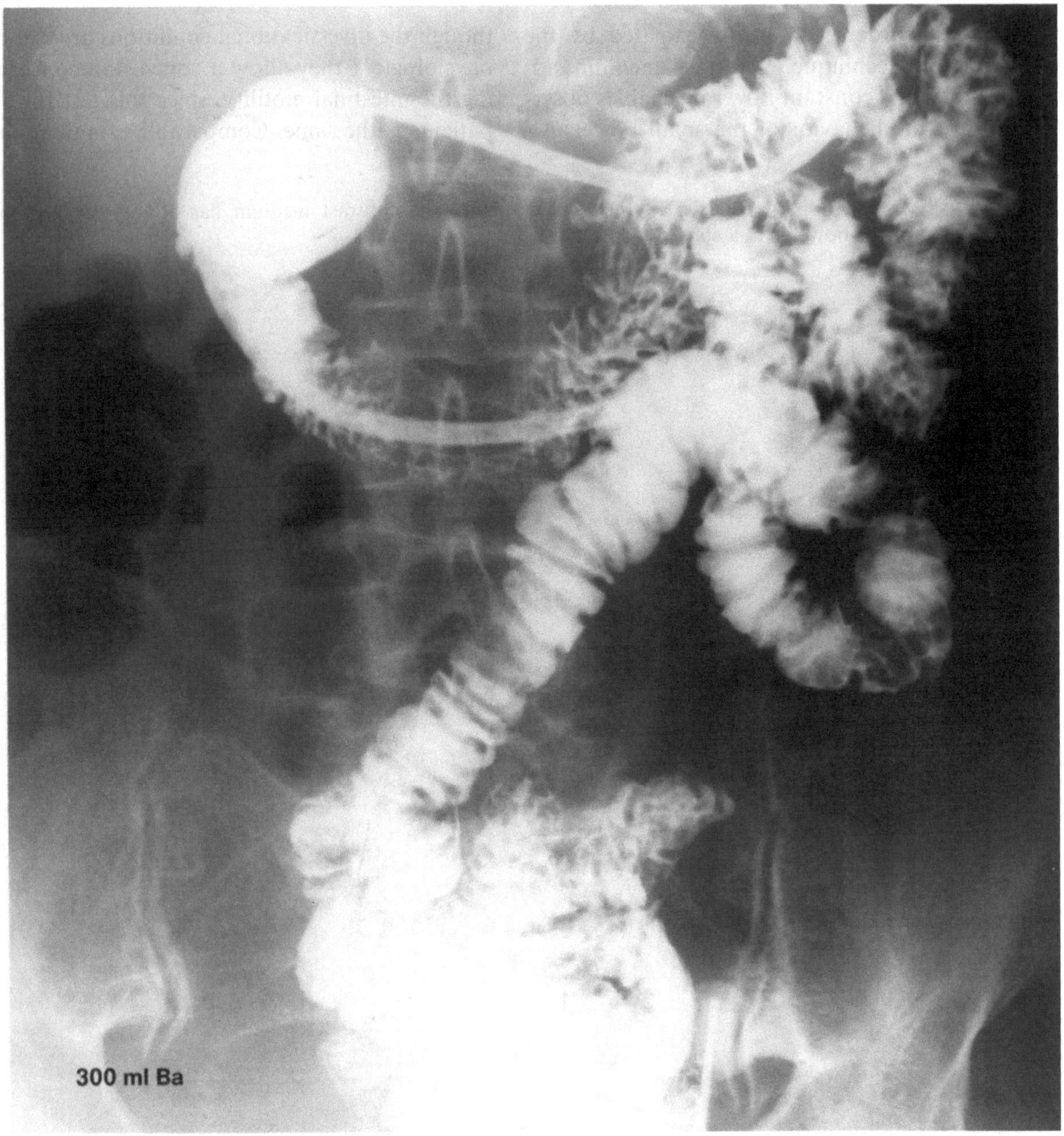

a

Fig. 4.5.-2 a to d. Example of hyperperistalsis as a concomitant phenomenon in enteritis in giardiasis. Investigation before and after treatment. *Pretreatment* (a and b) revealed moderate hyperperistalsis in the barium phase (**a**). The thickened folds are suggestive of inflammatory changes. In the methylcellulose phase (**b**), there is premature flocculation and inhomogeneous coating due to mucosal inflammation. *Posttreatment* (c and d) shows slight hyperperistalsis (**c**) in the barium phase. The folds are now nearly normal. In the methylcellulose phase (**d**), a normal mucosal coating may be observed

with varied flow rates have proved that the optimal investigational conditions were best obtained with a flow rate of 75 ml/min (Sellink and Rosenbusch 1981). Since general motility disorders are best recognizable in the jejunum, the barium phase is particularly important. The criteria for hypo- and hyperperistalsis were established according to the findings of Sellink

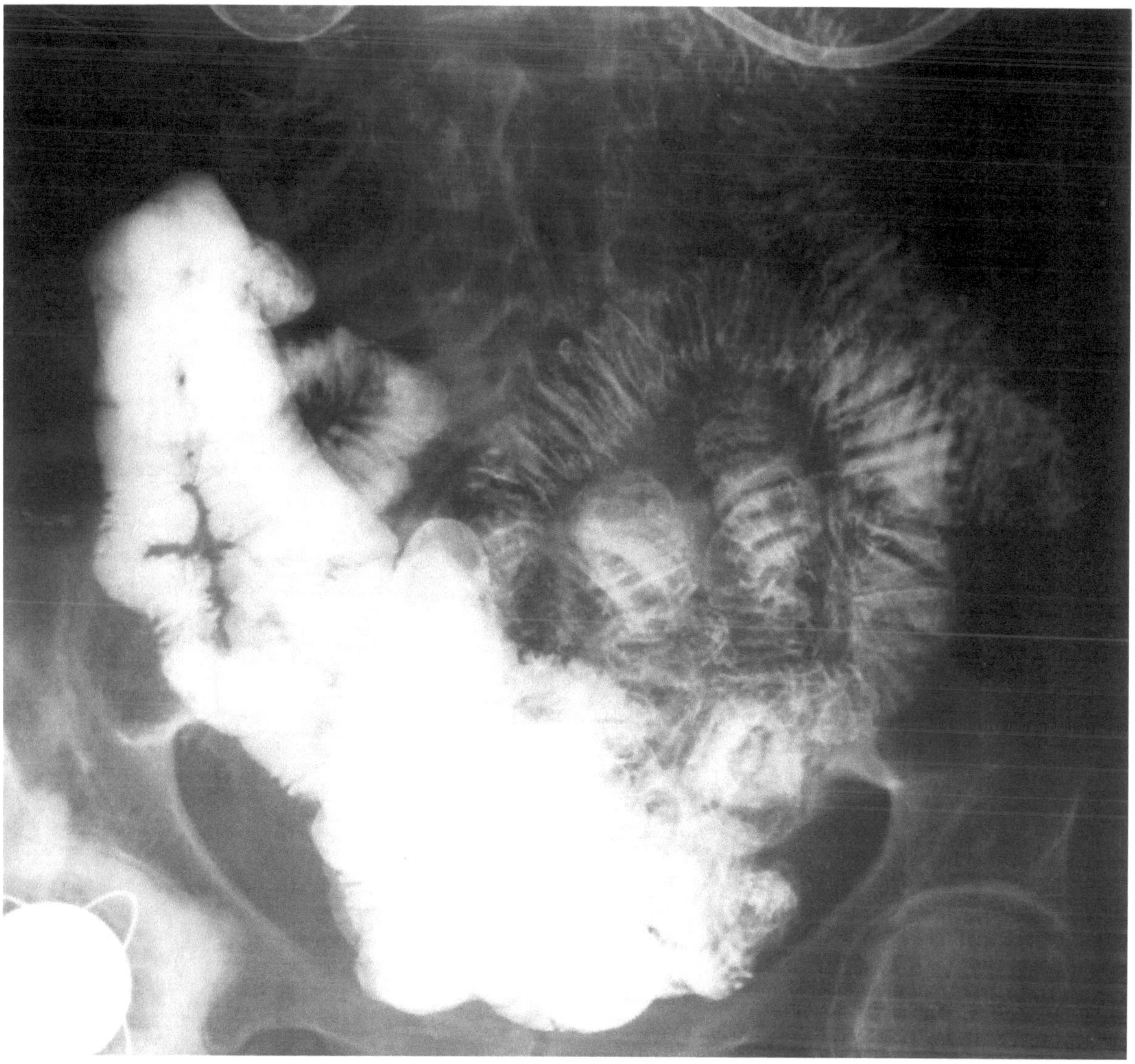

Fig. 4.5.-2b

(1976) and our own experiences. Examination fear and retching during intubation have no influence on the assessment of motility disorders.

In a normal small bowel peristalsis, roughly $^{1}/_{3}$ of the jejunal loops shown are contracted (see Fig. 2.7.-1). The methylcellulose phase often assists further interpretation. Survey radiographs are of particular importance here.

Motility disorders may be divided into two categories: general and local.

4.5.1 General Hyperperistalsis

In the barium phase, $^{2}/_{3}$ or more of the intestinal loops are in a state of contraction (Fig. 4.5.-1). The ileum is already almost filled and the cecum is sometimes reached (*intestinal hurry*). The hyperperistalsis is also maintained later in the methylcellulose phase (see Figs. 5.4.-1 and 2, pp. 132–135). The diameter of the intestinal loops is usually less than normal. In purely func-

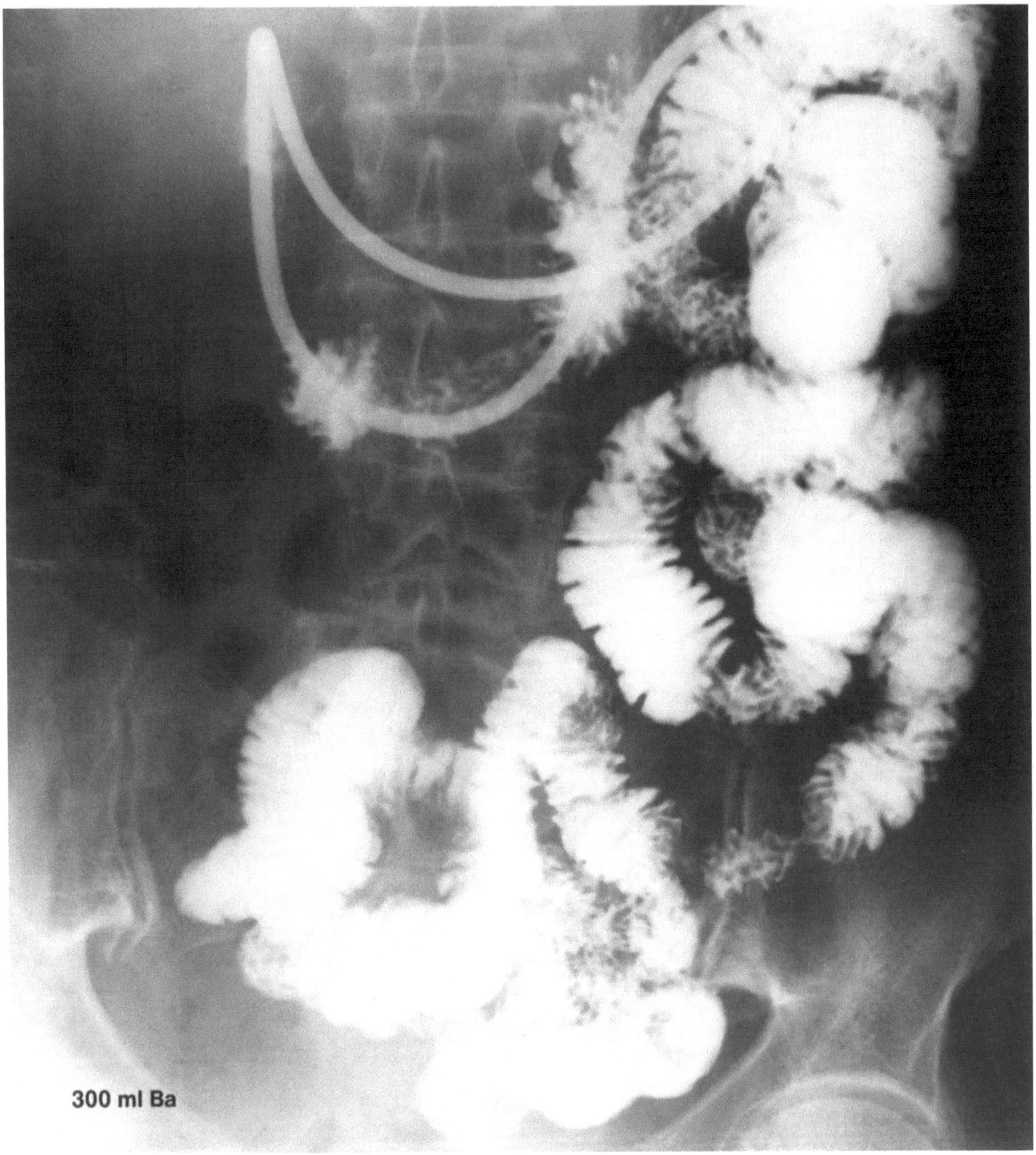

Fig. 4.5.-2c

tional hypermotility, the mucosal coating is normal or restored with renewed doses of barium and methylcellulose. On the whole, however, the coating is not maintained for as long as in normal peristalsis.

If the hyperperistalsis occurs as a consequence of or in concomitance with inflammation, impaired resorption or mucosal irritation, a reduced coating or premature flocculation in the methylcellulose phase is observed (Fig. 4.5.-2). In such cases, other intestinal alterations (fold thickening etc.) may be seen.

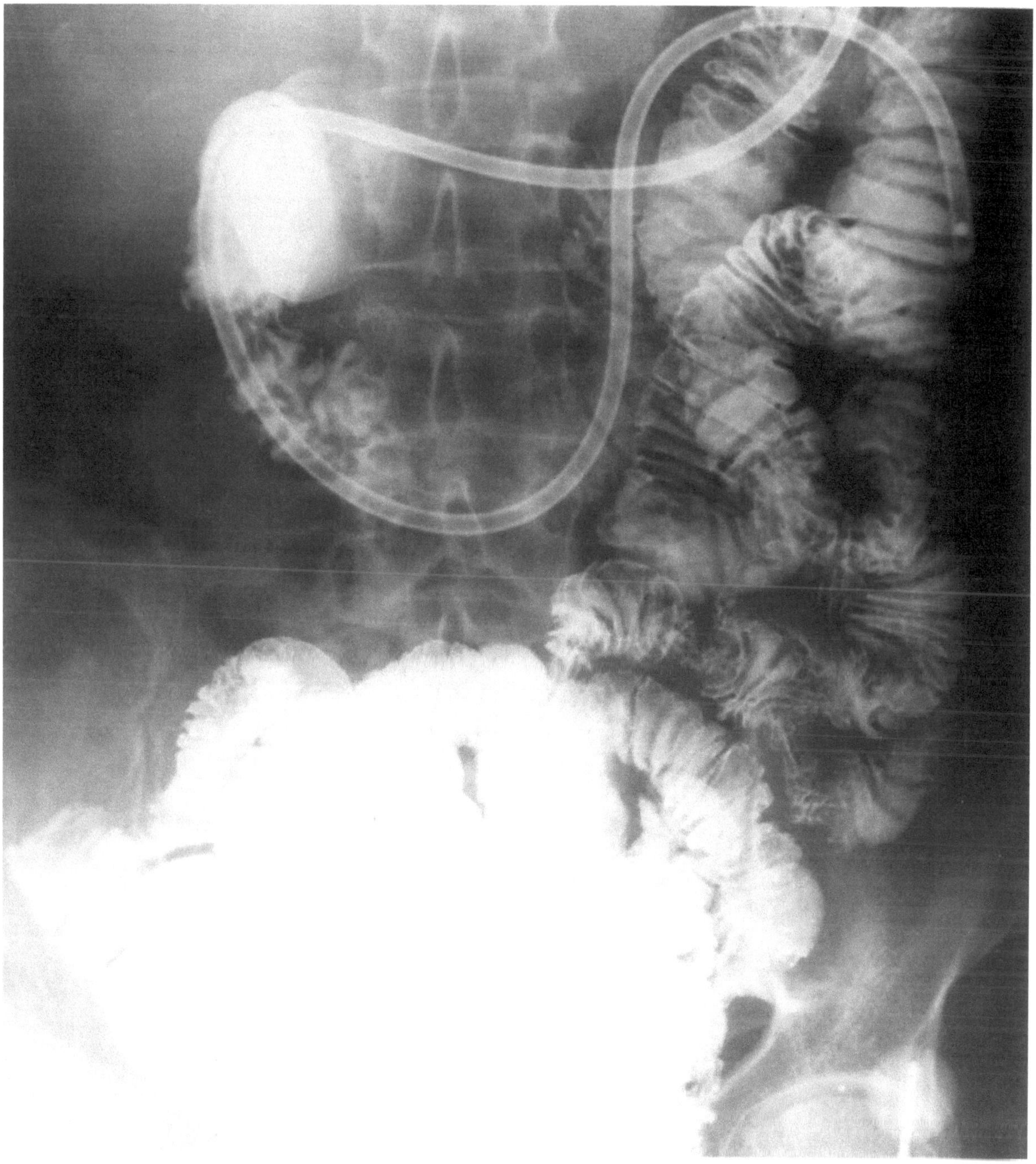

Fig. 4.5.-2d

4.5.2 General Hypoperistalsis

In the barium phase, only some of the proximal jejunal loops are filled and only a few bowel contractions are depicted. The bowel lumen is more or less grossly dilated and there may be gastric reflux. Occasionally, it is not possible to move the duodenal tube beyond the impression of superior mesenteric artery on the dilated duodenum (see Fig. 5.4.-4, p. 139). Hypoperistalsis may be assumed when the usual number of jejunal loops are filled but only a few contrac-

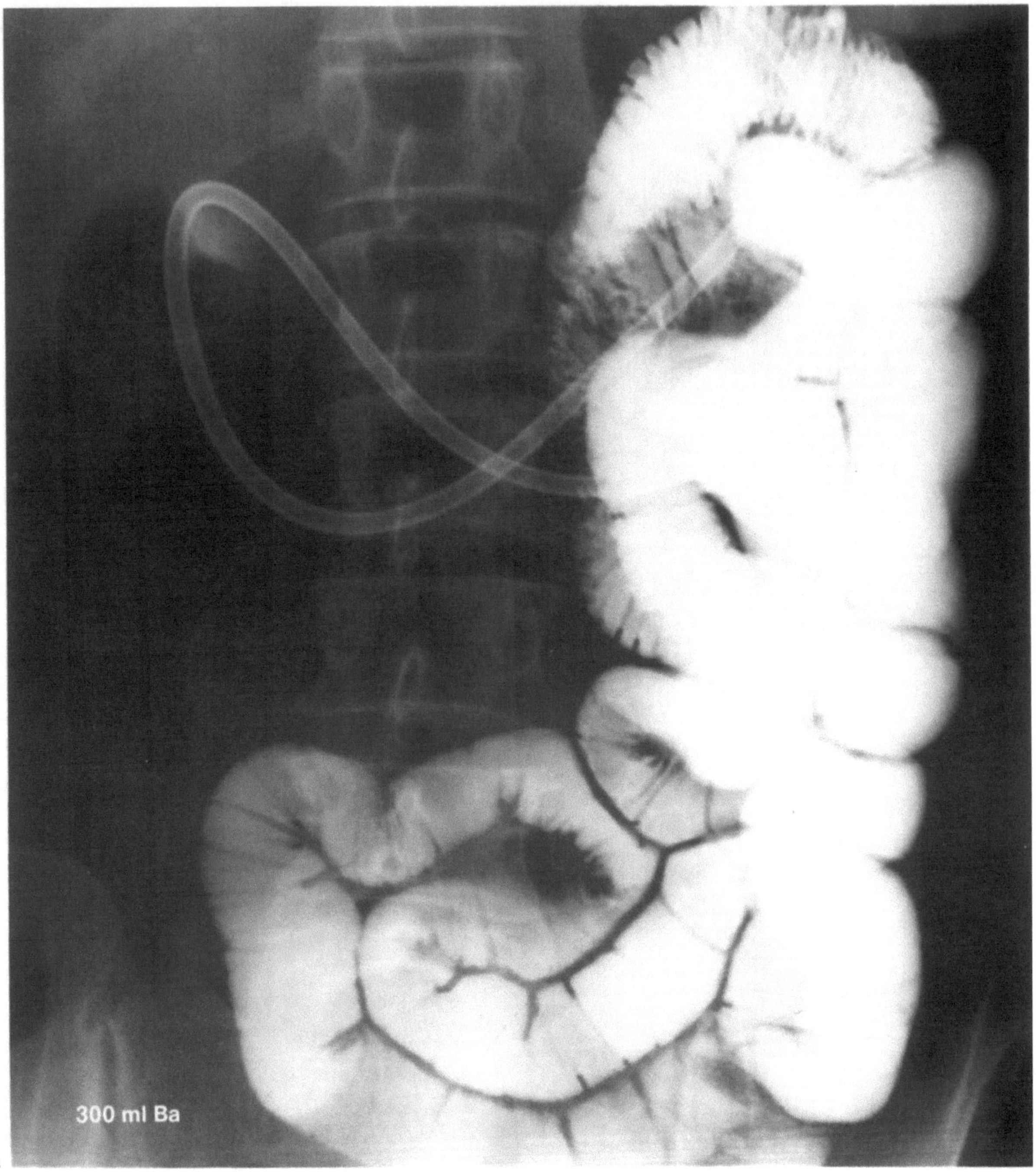

a

Fig. 4.5.-3 a and b. Hypoperistalsis. There are practically no contractions in the jejunum. The contrast medium has flowed through the bowel as through a rigid pipe. Significant rarification of the folds. Good mucosal coating in the methylcellulose phase (**b**)

tions are depicted. The number of folds is significantly reduced. In this case, the contrast medium is not actively transported by the small bowel. It travels as if flowing through a rigid pipe (Fig. 4.5.-3). A temporary hypoperistalsis in the jejunum can subside after a certain time. In such cases, the peristalsis in the ileum is normal or even increased (see Figs. 5.4.-5 and 6,

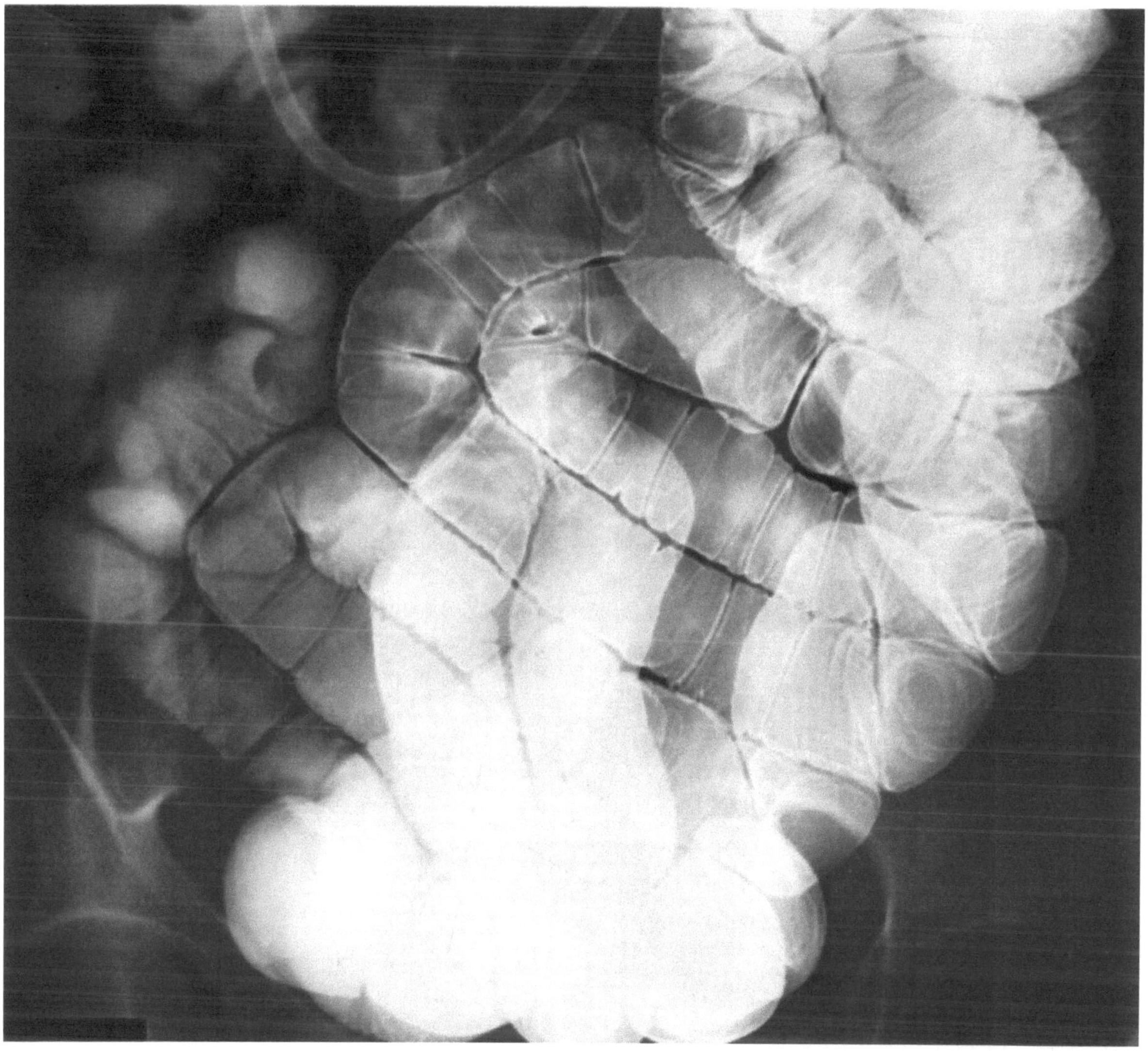

Fig. 4.5.-3b

pp. 140–141). Since general hypoperistalsis is mostly of functional origin, the coating is almost always optimal. Only in the case of increased amounts of intestinal fluid, e.g. in obstruction, there may be a hazy mucosal coating.

Hypoperistalsis can also develop in mechanical obstruction. In contrary to general hypoperistalsis (e.g. medication-induced) normal or even locally increased peristalsis in the proximal jejunum is present, depending on the severity, duration and localization of the ileus (Figs. 2.8.-3 to 5, pp. 19–25). The bowel loops may be normal or only somewhat dilated. In general hypoperistalsis the jejunum is dilated and dilatation decreases from proximal to distal (Fig. 5.4.-5, p. 140). In mechanical obstruction, on the other hand, there is increasing dilatation extending proximal to distal with loss of peristaltic movement. Only immediately close to the obstruction can a local hyperperistalsis be seen. In longstanding mechanical ileus after infusion of large amounts of fluid, distension of the jejunum with loss of peristalsis and interruption of prestenotic peristalsis are observed. This renders differentiation of paralytic ileus difficult or impossible.

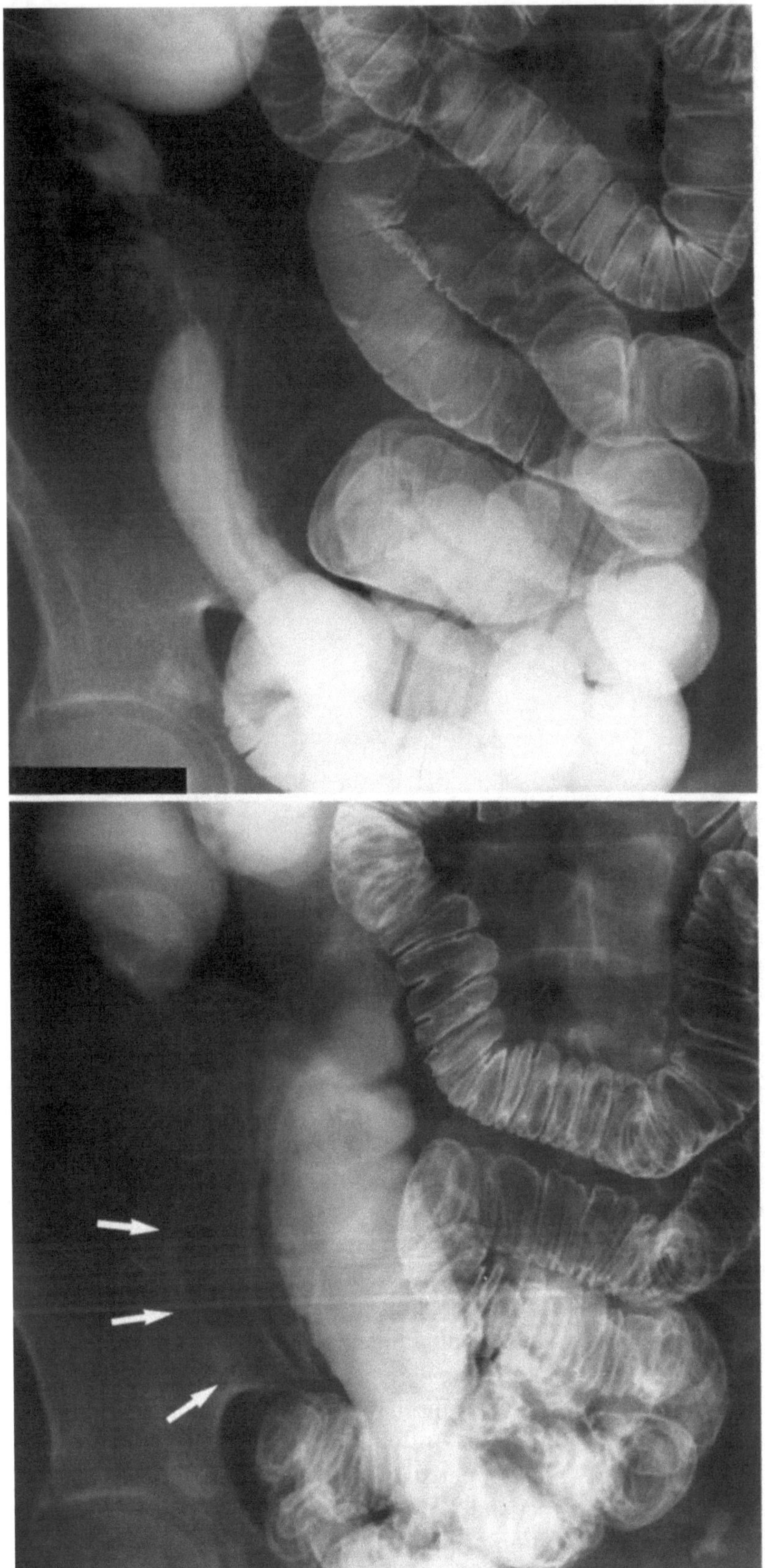

a
b

Fig. 4.5.-4a and b. String sign in Crohn's disease. Initially, the terminal ileum is not constricted (**a**). Several minutes later, it is highly contracted (→) (**b**). Due to the purely functional condition, there is no prestenotic dilatation. Contrast medium in the ptotic transverse colon

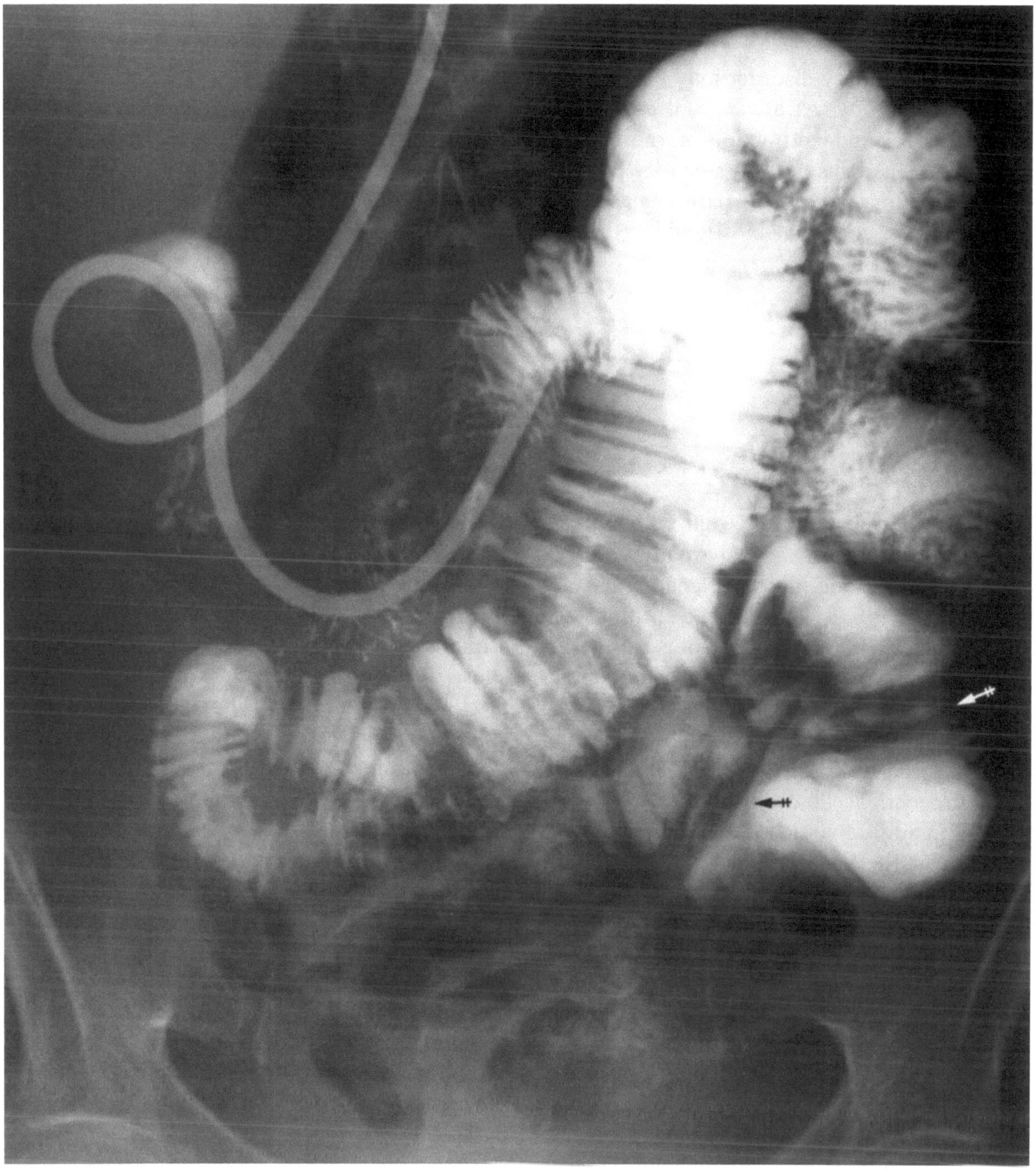

Fig. 4.5.-5. Local hyperperistalsis in an area of marked fibrous bands (⇸). Proximal dilatation and farther proximally hyperperistalsis in the jejunum

4.5.3 Nonpropulsive (Pendular) Peristalsis

This type of motility disorder may best be seen during fluoroscopy. At any rate, it can be observed as segmental contractions in radiographic pictures. Since this motility disorder presents in inflammatory or other pathological processes, mucosal coating is mostly reduced.

4.5.4 Local Motility Disorders

Local motility disorders are mainly recognizable during intermittent fluoroscopy and should be documented in several spot films for later interpretation. This group includes spastic contractions such as the string sign in Crohn's disease (Fig. 4.5.-4a, b), local hyperperistalsis in the presence of an obstruction (Fig. 4.5.-5) or in areas of previous surgery, hemorrhage, and in ischemic, tumorous or inflammatory processes in the abdomen (Fig. 5.4.-17, p. 159).

4.6 Mucosal Coating

Experience and results show that with our enteroclysis technique a normal small bowel always shows a good mucosal coating (Antes and Lissner 1983). This remains intact for 20–40 min. The initial barium bolus rinses surplus mucus and intestinal contents from the mucosa. The methylcellulose stabilizes the mucosal coating producing a translucent filling. Naturally, the barium mucosal coating is first washed off by the methylcellulose in the proximal jejunum. With additional doses of barium and continuation of the methylcellulose infusion, normal conditions are restored. If premature flocculation occurs or an initially poor mucosal coating persists, this can be regarded as *nonspecific enteritis or mucosal irritation* (Fig. 4.6.-1 and Fig. 4.5.-2). These flocculation and segmentation phenomena have been observed only in particular diseases of the small bowel or in diseases which have a secondary effect on the small intestine (Herlinger 1979). A diagnosis of malabsorption cannot be convincingly deduced from this entity.

Apart from these changes concerning the coating, one can observe other nonspecific signs of enteritis or mucosal irritation. These include thickening of the folds and intestinal wall, alterations of the surface, hyper- or pendular peristalsis – alterations which can only be recognized with certainty at short notice when the conditions for these examinations are optimal. Poor coating can result in misinterpretation or intensification of the thickening of folds and wall (Fig. 4.6.-2).

The impaired mucosal coating may only appear in sections of the small intestine. This is a sign of local mucosal irritation (Fig. 4.6.-3; see also Fig. 5.3.-15, p. 118).

We will refrain from listing diseases for which a reduced mucosal coating is observed as a nonspecific sign of enteritis or mucosal irritation since this phenomenon may present generally but also locally in concomitance with many diseases.

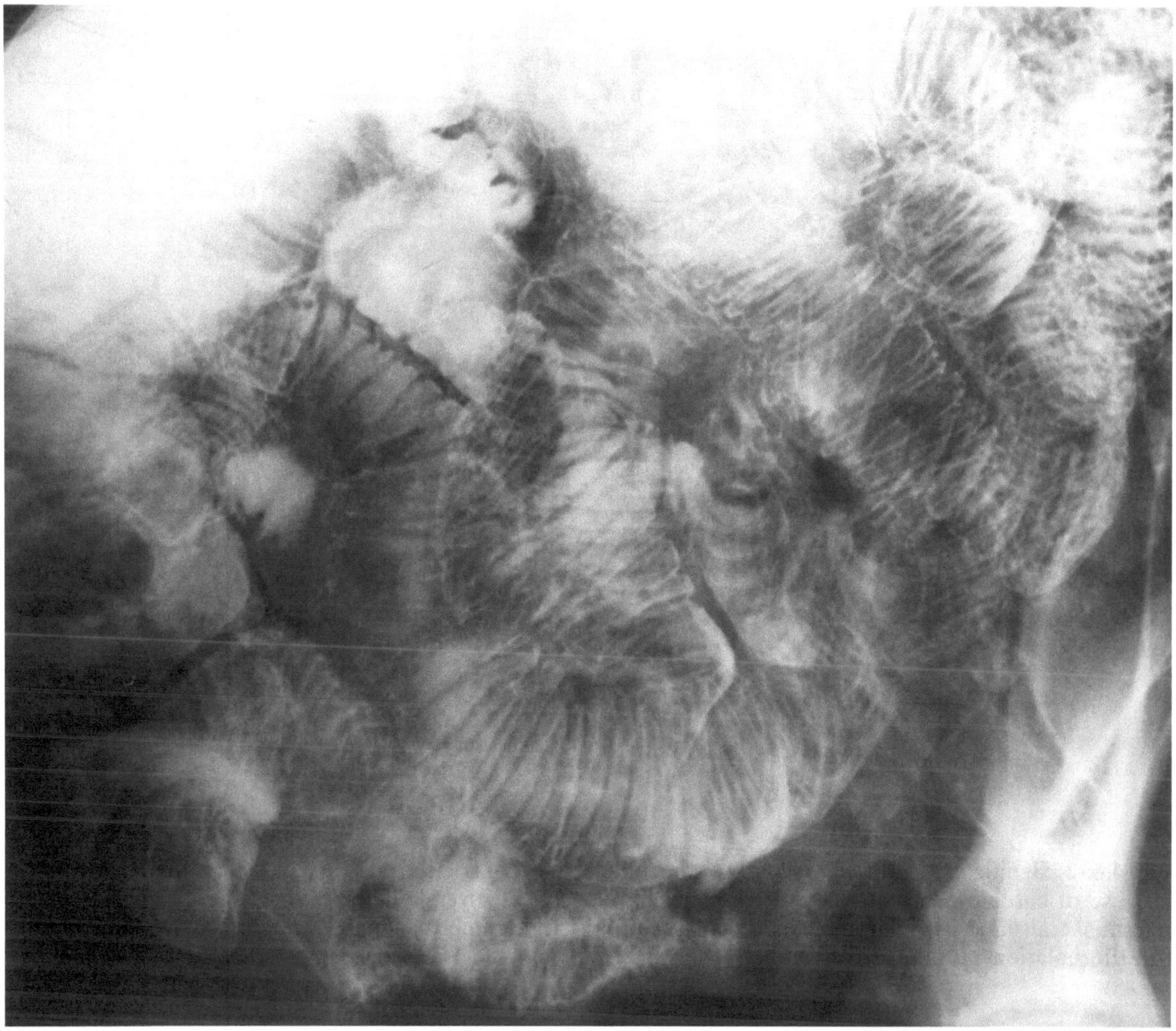

Fig. 4.6.-1. Reduced mucosal coating as a sign of nonspecific enteritis or mucosal irritation in a patient with exudative enteropathy. There is also a slight thickening of the folds and intestinal wall

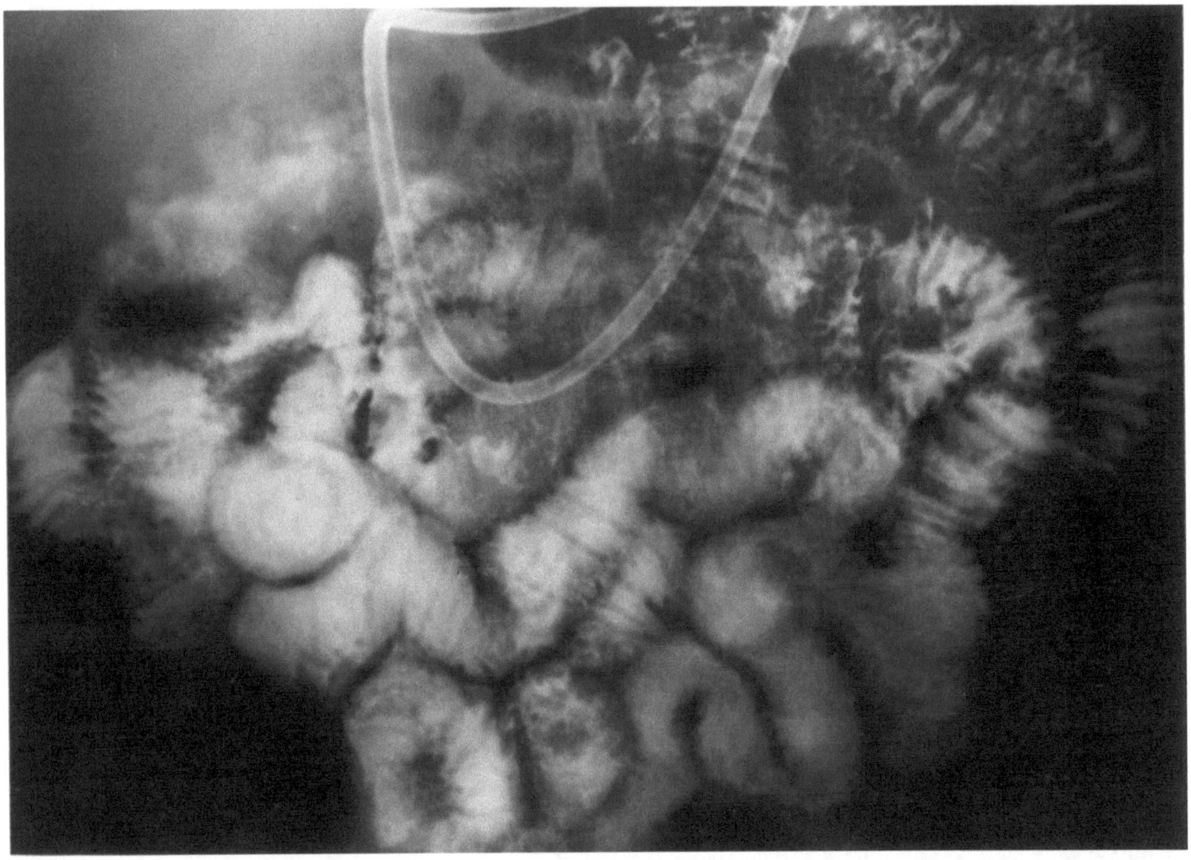

Fig. 4.6.-2. Significantly reduced mucosal coating and haziness of translucency in a patient with malabsorption because of chronic pancreatic insufficiency, insulin-dependent juvenile diabetes and alcoholism. Thickened intestinal walls and irregular and slightly enlarged folds. In the upper jejunum, where uncontrollable premature flocculation occurs, there is either intensified or simulated fold thickening (see also Figs. 5.4.-8 and 2.7.-5)

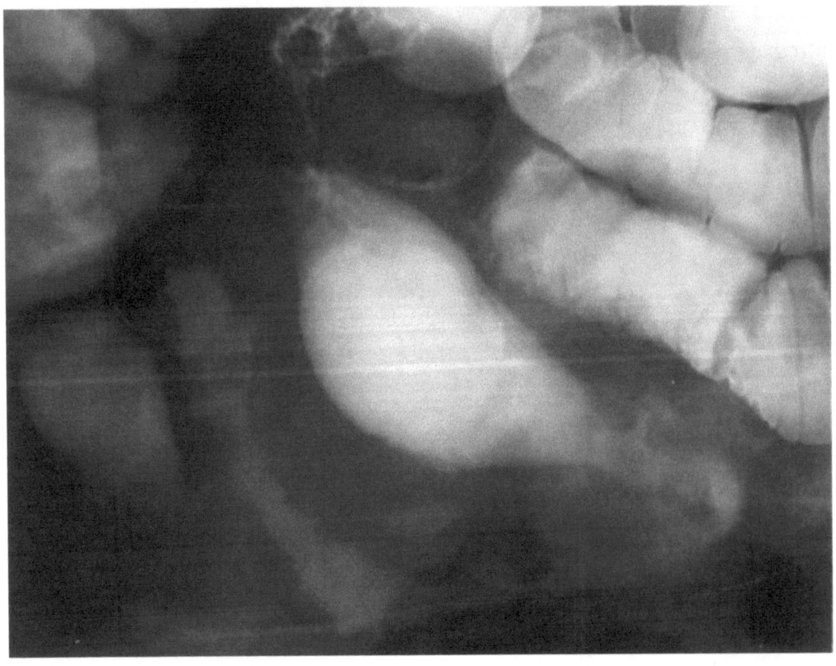

Fig. 4.6.-3. Locally reduced mucosal coating in the terminal ileum due to accompanying inflammatory changes in Crohn's disease (in addition: enterocutaneous fistula). Owing to the varied brightness between the normal loops and the bowel section with reduced mucosal coating, exposure problems often occur

5 Atlas of Small Bowel Diseases

5.1 Crohn's Disease

Crohn's disease is the best-known disease of the small bowel in western industrialized countries. Various double contrast methods have been established for roentgenological diagnosis of Crohn's disease (Ekberg 1977; Herlinger 1979; Nolan and Piris 1980; Kelvin and Gedgaudas 1981; Herlinger 1982).

Basically, Crohn's disease has to be regarded as a disease of the entire gastrointestinal tract with a tendency towards segmental distribution (Morson 1964). Extraintestinal pathology is common. The most frequently involved bowel segment is the terminal ileum, with or without involvement of the cecum whereas the jejunum and duodenum are only rarely involved.

The cause of Crohn's disease is unknown. Histologically, this disease begins in the lymph follicles of the intestinal mucosa and in larger Peyer's patches (Morson and Dawson 1979). Lymphedema and inflammatory infiltration of the submucosa and subsequently of all layers of the wall follow. This creates a granular or nodular mucosa. Small infiltrates with mucosal necroses form *aphthoid ulcers*. These early features (Figs. 5.1.-1 to 3 and 4.3.-12, p. 41) are already radiologically visible (Marshak 1975); see chapter 4.3.4. Lymphatic hyperplasia has to be differentiated (Fig. 5.2.-2, p. 86). The fine granulation and fissures can blur the mucosal contours.

These details along the contours are better visible in single contrast; superficial mucosal changes (e.g. aphthous ulcers, pseudopolyps) are better seen in double contrast and in a well-distended bowel (Fig. 5.1.-3).

The submucosal edema results in irregular thickening and/or smoothing of the folds (Fig. 5.1.-4). Similar alterations can be perceived in radiation enteritis, ischemia and yersiniosis. As the disease progresses, *linear ulcers* appear, spreading in a longitudinal and transversal direction (Fig. 5.1.-5). Even at an early stage, they may penetrate the deeper layers of the wall. These *ulcerous fissures* or spiculae may precede to collar button ulcers. In the case of penetrating wall defect sinus tracts, fistulae and abscesses may develop (Figs. 5.1.-6 and 7). Similarities may be observed in Behçet's disease.

Multiple longitudinal and transversal ulcers pervading an inflammatory, edematous mucosa form a *cobblestone pattern* (Figs. 5.1.-8 to 11). In an advanced stage of mucosal destruction the remaining mucosal islands are called *pseudopolyps* and in case of fibrotic transformation *fibrous plaques* (Figs. 5.1.-12 and 13).

Hypersecretion of the involved mucosa often causes a reduction of the mucosal coating or flocculation of the contrast medium. The diseased intestine tends towards hypermotility.

Segmental involvement is typical of Crohn's disease. Normal bowel (skip areas) may lie between diseased bowel segments (skip lesions) (Figs. 5.1.-14, 18 and 34). In most cases, distally located lesions are more severely involved than proximal lesions.

In a progression of Crohn's disease, all wall layers and the mesentery are thickened and the musculature becomes hypertrophic. The intestinal wall often retains its elasticity, as confirmed by the *string sign* (Figs. 5.1.-15 and 4.5.-4, p. 54). This is the momentary spasm of a diseased intestinal segment. For differentiation from other inflammatory processes, this phenomenon is typical for Crohn's disease. The other signs of transmural involvement (deep ulceration, fistulae, strictures and dilatations) are rarely seen in other diseases.

The spasm of the bowel referred to as string sign is a functional stenosis and causes no prestenotic dilatation. Increasing fibrosis of the intestinal wall, however, leads to *fixed stenosis* with obstruction (Figs. 5.1.-17 and 18; Fig. 2.8.-4c, p. 22). Shrinking of the ileocecal valve may also obstruct the transit.

Crohn's disease tends towards *asymmetrical involvement* (Fig. 5.1.-16). The preferred localization is the mesenteric border (Figs. 5.1.-6 and 7). Fibrosis leads to shrinking and straightening of the mesenteric attachment (Figs. 5.1.-13 and 22). As a result, the antimesenteric border becomes redundant and the intact intestinal wall puckers in a diverticula-like fashion. Peristaltic waves can proceed through these sacculations ("pseudodiverticula") (Fig. 5.1.-19). Advancement of fibrosis causes these eccentric sacculations to become fixed (Figs. 5.1.-20 to 22). One particular type is called *shell sign* (Sellink and Miller 1982) (Fig. 5.1.-20). On the other hand symmetrical ("aneurysmatic") dilatations (e.g. Fig. 5.1.-11) are caused by a disturbance of the neuromuscular function (Sartoris et al. 1984).

False diverticula form on the mesenteric border. They emerge as a result of herniation of the mucosa through the hypertrophied intestinal wall (Figs. 5.1.-23 and 4.3.-16, p. 44).

The inflammatory thickened mesenteric fatty and connective tissue and the adherent intestinal loops together form a conglomerate tumor which can be palpated as a mass. The "medial cecal defect" described by Berridge (1971), is caused by an impression of the cecum through this "conglomerate tumor" (e.g. Fig. 5.1.-20). The *omega sign* is a manifestation of a thickened intestinal loop gathered up in an arch or garland-like fashion by this fibrotic process (Fig. 5.1.-24).

Deep wall defects in Crohn's disease (Figs. 5.1.-6 and 7) often spread to adjacent structures. *Sinus tracts, fistulae* and *abscesses* appear, either ending blindly or penetrating into an adjacent intestinal loop or organ. A network of interconnecting sinus tracts/fistulae is called *fox-earth fistula* (Fig. 5.1.-25). Enteroenteral, enterocolic, and enterorectal fistulae are more frequent than those enterovaginal and enterovesical. Enterocutaneous fistulae mostly develop postoperatively (Figs. 5.1.-25 to 29). Fistula formation is an essential sign of activity in Crohn's disease.

A long-standing chronic Crohn's disease may destroy large parts of the bowel (Fig. 5.1.-30). The terminal stage reveals significantly distanced atonic intestinal loops with smooth, atrophic surfaces. The *bike-tire phenomenon* may be observed in a state of remission (Sellink and Miller 1982). This feature is due to the partial collapse of a smooth flaccid intestinal wall if the lumen is only moderately filled (Fig. 5.1.-31). Regeneration of the mucous membrane and intestinal wall is possible only where there is no marked fibrosis (Fig. 5.1.-33). Loss of larger portions of mucosa results in a malabsorption syndrome. The remaining small bowel mucosa is edematous due to protein deficiency (Fig. 5.1.-32). *Recurrencies* are frequent after surgery which mostly affect the anastomotic region (Figs. 5.1.-34 and 35). Carcinomatous degeneration in Crohn's disease is a rare complication (Feczko 1987).

In spite of typical radiological signs ir Crohn's disease, the differential diagnostic spectrum is wide. Inflammatory diseases of the smal bowel, e.g. nonspecific ileitis, Yersinia enteritis, radiation enteritis and tuberculosis, may show similar changes. Ischemic enteritis and tumors (particularly malignant lymphoma and metastatic peritoneal seeding) are mimicked by Crohn's disease (Fig. 5.1.-36).

The CT diagnosis (Figs. 5.1.-37 and 38) adds considerably more information about intestina wall thickening, mesenteric infiltration and extension of abscesses and fistulae (Frick et al. 1984). Wall thickening (targets) and conglomerate tumors can be diagnosed in early stages by ultrasound (Fig. 5.1.-39).

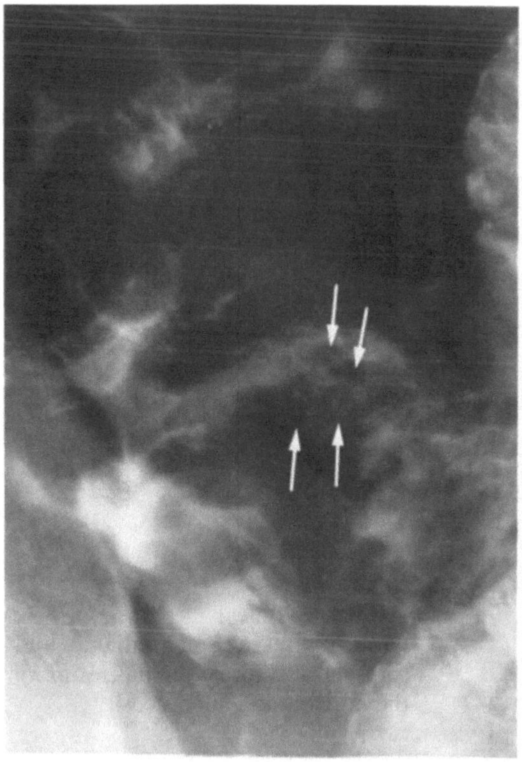

1

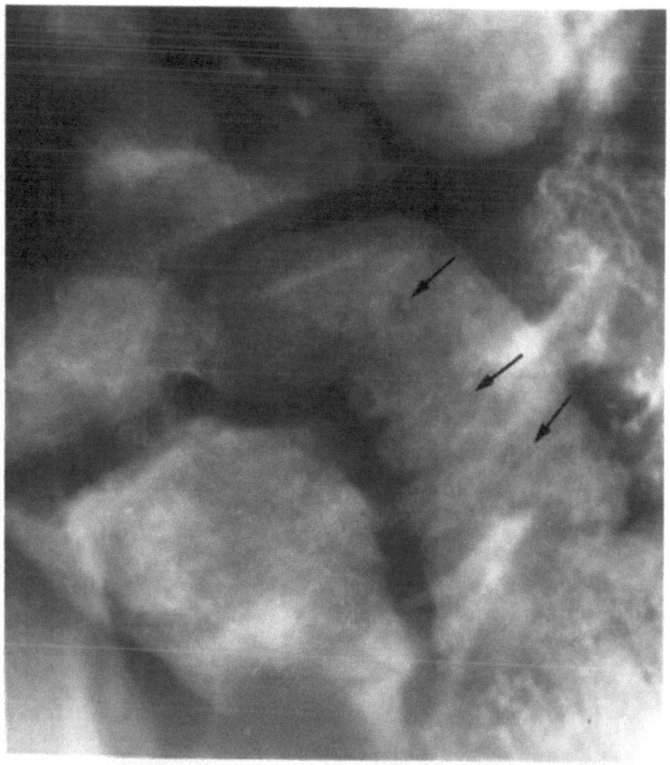

2

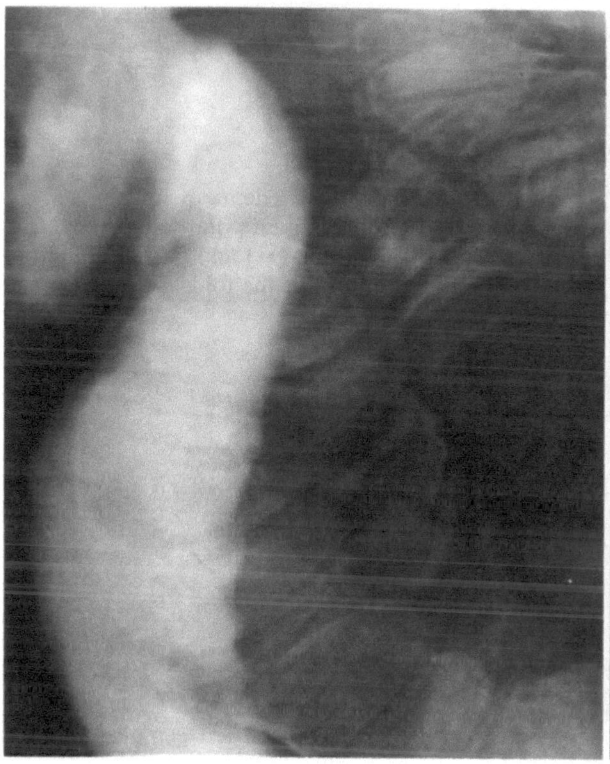

3a

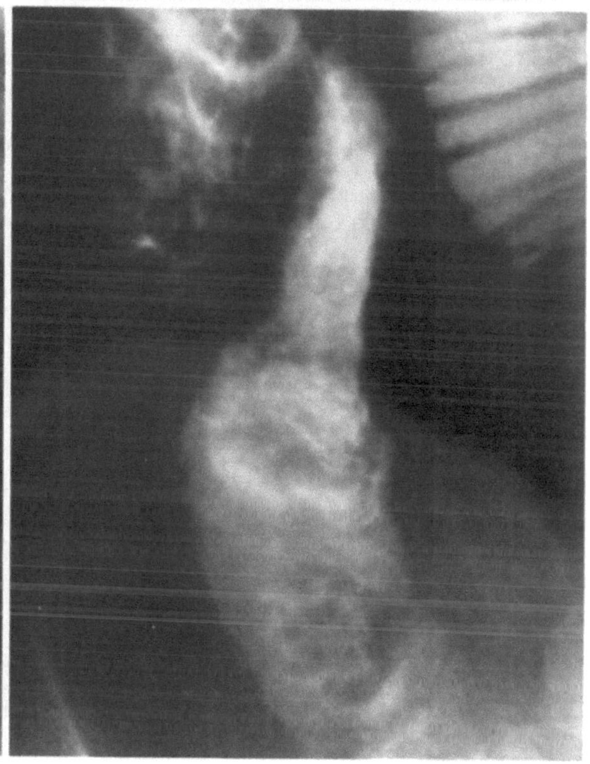

3b

Figs. 5.1.-1 to 3. Early manifestation of Crohn's disease. Three different patients present a nodular mucosa and aphthoid ulcers (→). In double contrast (Fig. 5.1.-3b), details of the mucosa are more visible than in single contrast (Fig. 5.1.-3a)

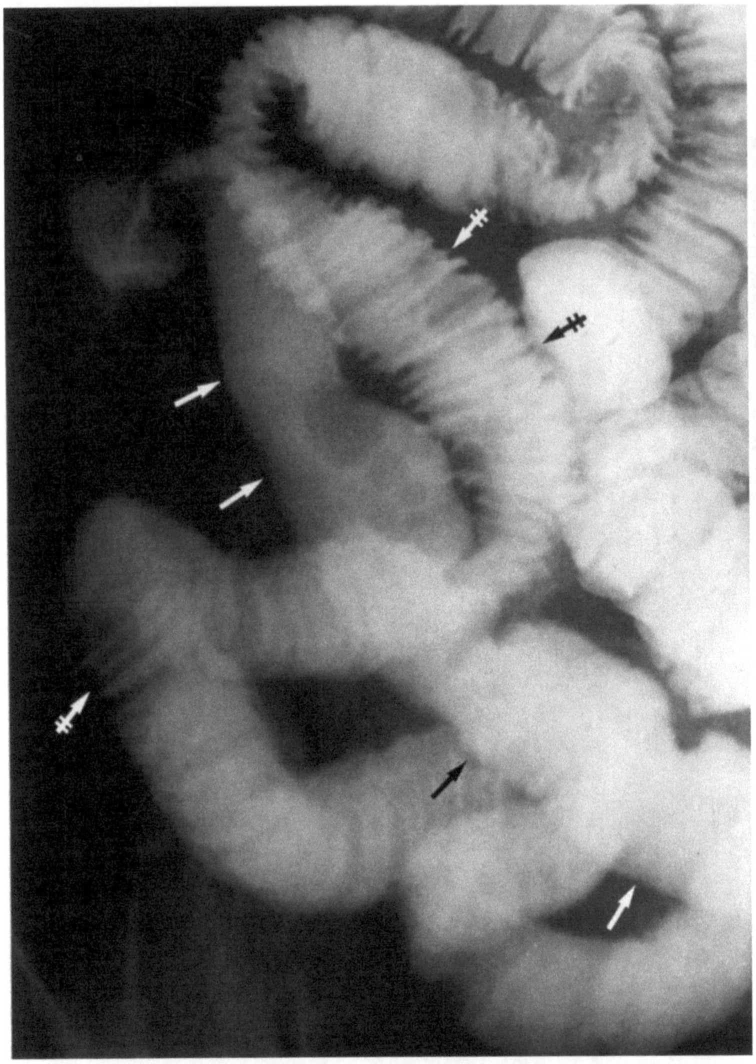

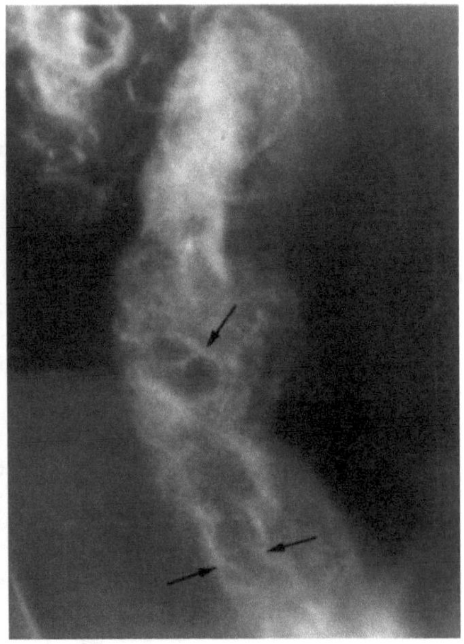

Fig. 5.1.-5. Linear ulceration in Crohn's disease. Longitudinally and transversally spreading ulceration of the mucosa and submucosa

Fig. 5.1.-4. Edema of folds in Crohn's disease. Partially irregular thickening (⇸) and partial obliteration (→) of the folds

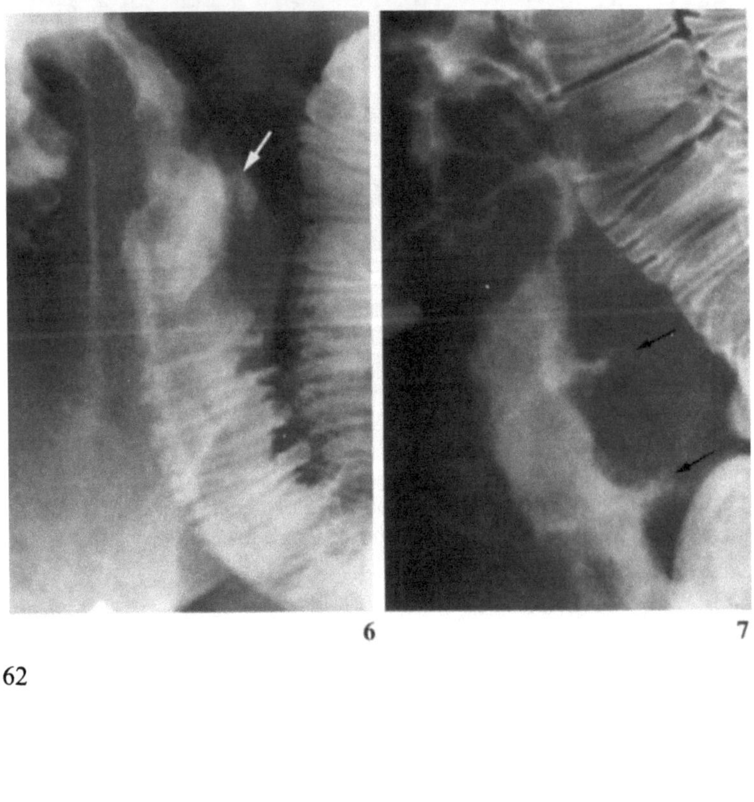

6 7

Figs. 5.1.-6 and 7. Deep ulcerations and collar button ulcer (→ in Fig. 6) in Crohn's disease. Ulceration on the mesenteric border in two different patients. Penetration of the entire intestinal wall is regarded as a prestate for fistulae

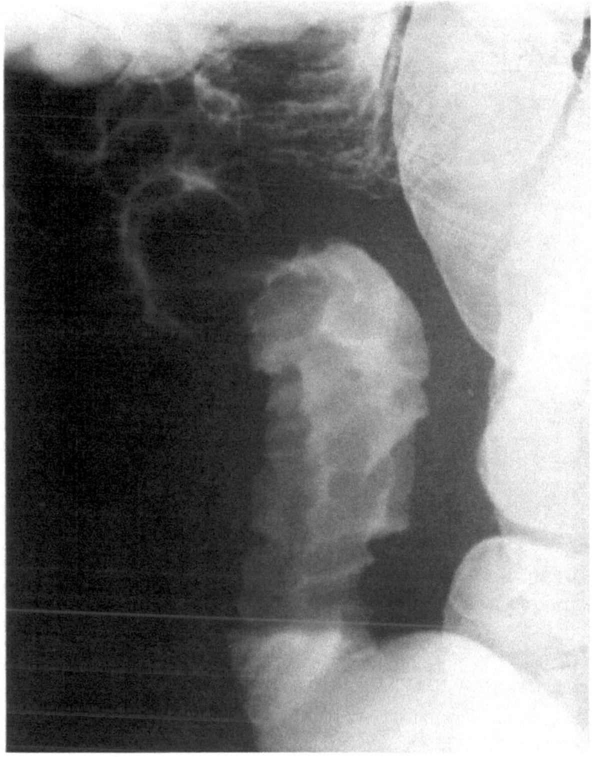

8

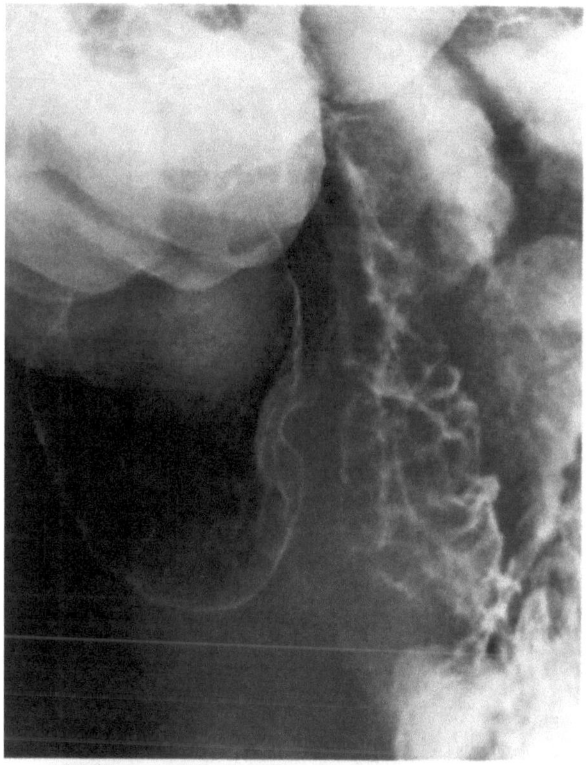

9

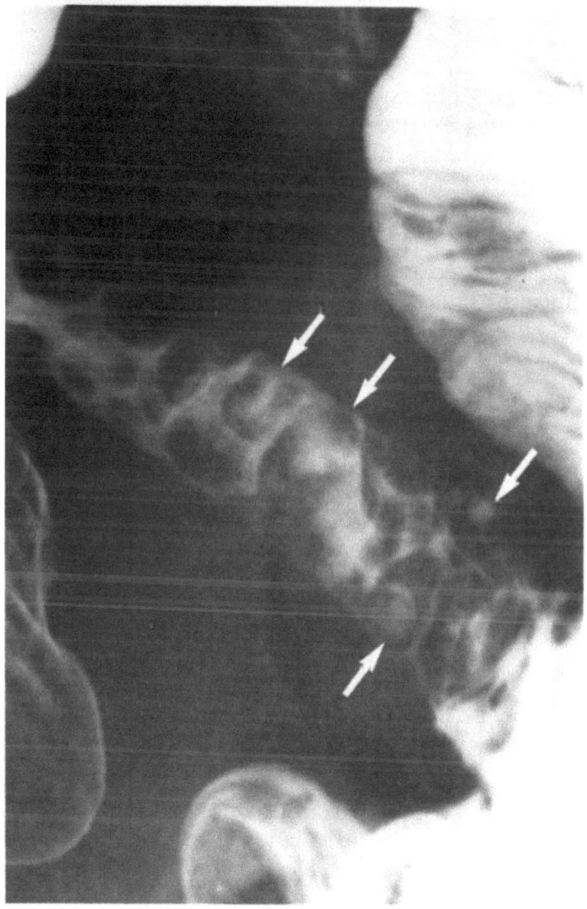

10

Figs. 5.1.-8 to 10. Cobblestoning of the terminal ileum in Crohn's disease (three different patients). The pattern is formed by longitudinal and transversal ulceration in an edematous mucosa. Central ulcerations (→) in Fig. 5.1.-10

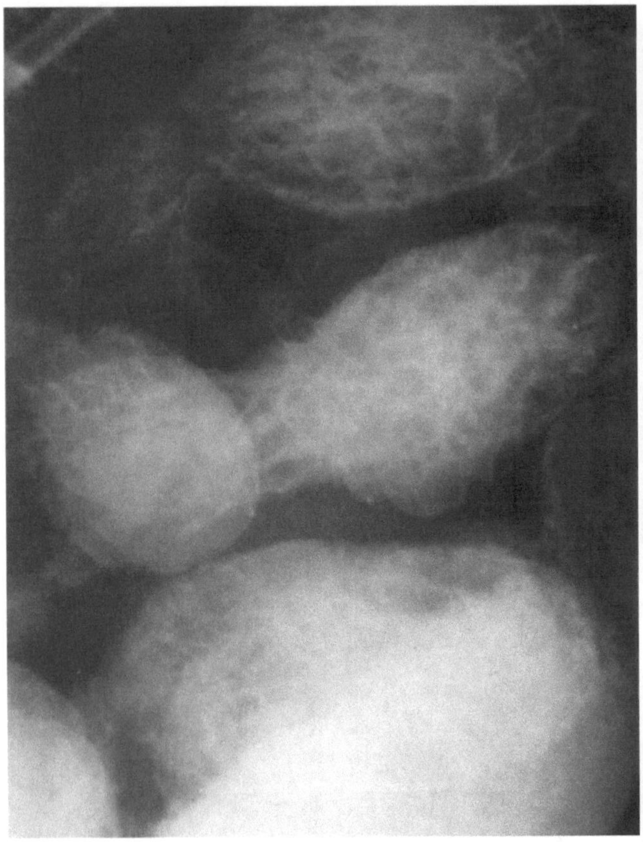

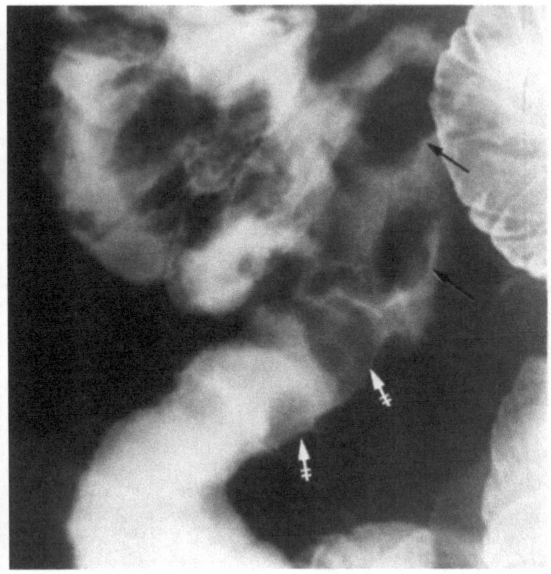

Fig. 5.1.-12

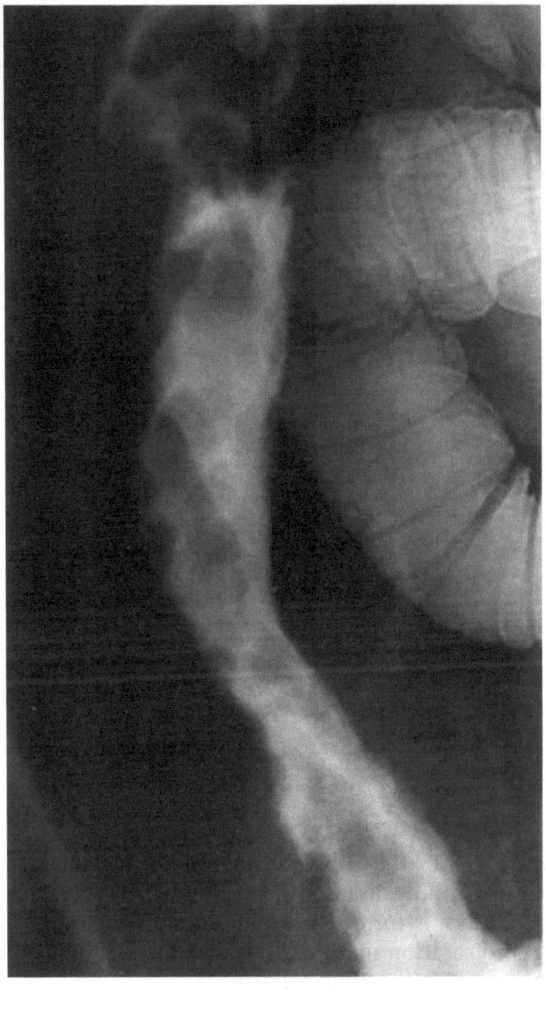

Fig. 5.1.-11. Cobblestoning in advanced stage of Crohn's disease. Ulceration between the mucosal islands. Alternating dilated and narrowed bowel sections

Fig. 5.1.-12. Fibrous plaques in Crohn's disease. Granulated mucosa with pseudopolyps (⇸) as well as fibrous plaques (→). (Only to be differentiated histologically)

Fig. 5.1.-13. Pseudopolyps in advanced Crohn's disease. Irregularly dispersed islands of residual mucosa between atrophic mucosa. Destruction of the ileocecal valve. Straightening of the mesenteric border

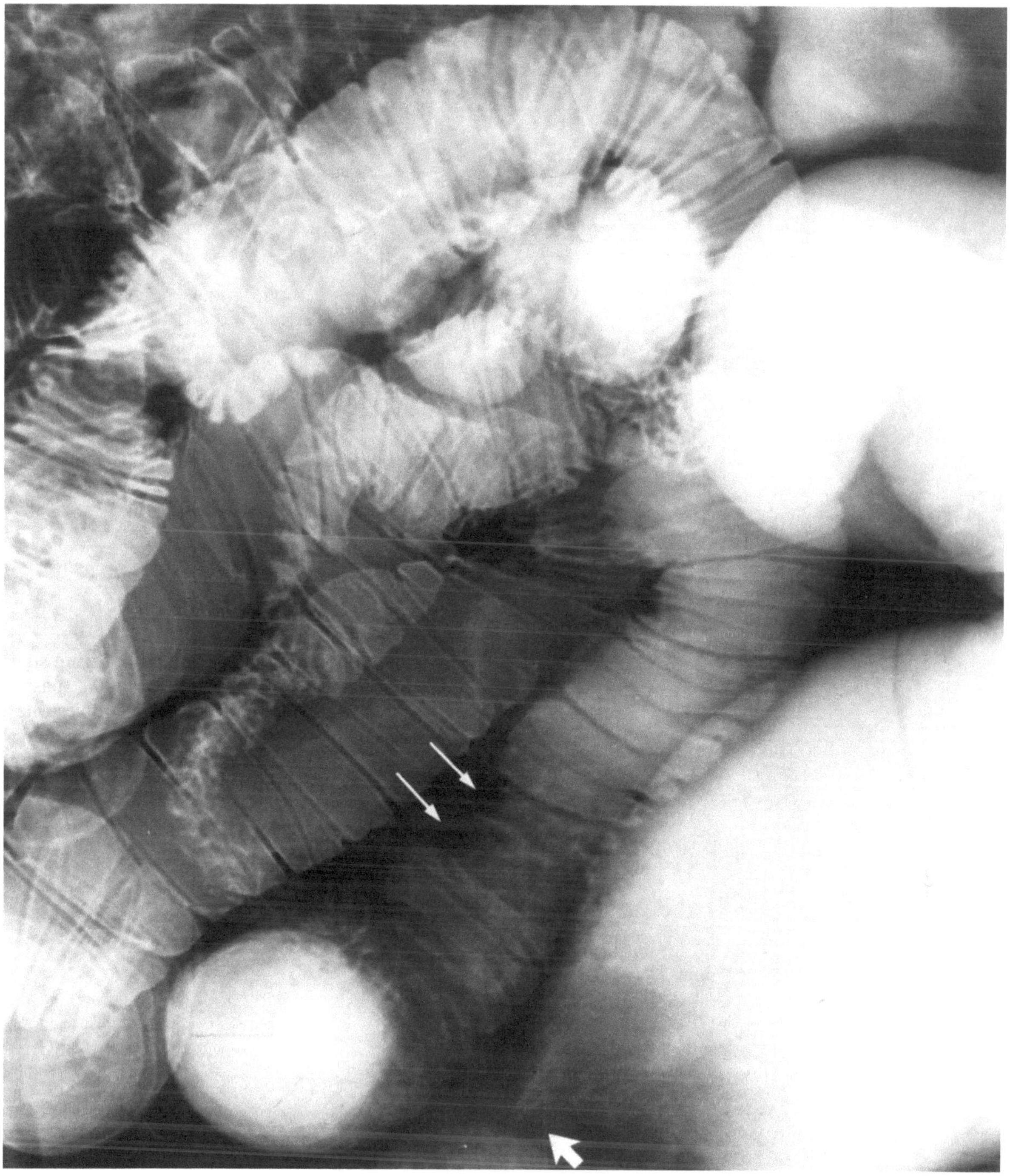

Fig. 5.1.-14. Segmental involvement in Crohn's disease. Between the normal loops there is a short, affected segment (→) with thickening of the wall and destruction of the mucosa. Advanced stenosis of a further skip lesion with prestenotic dilatation (➡)

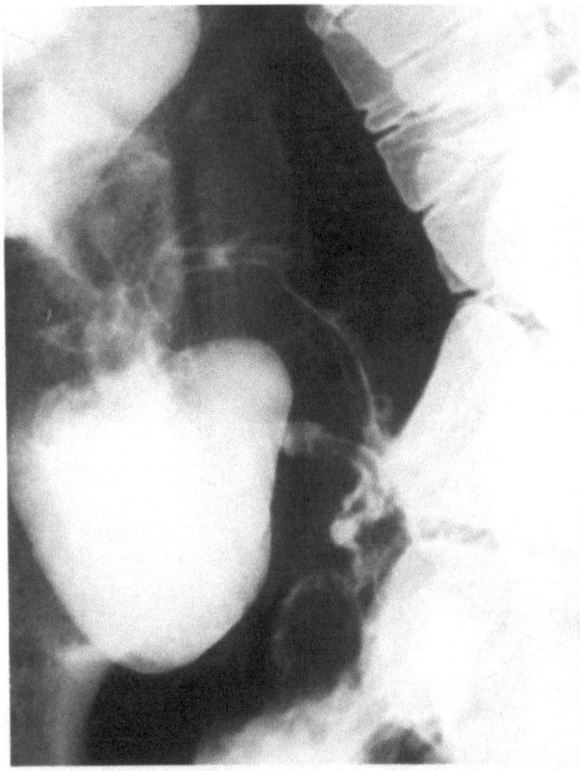

a

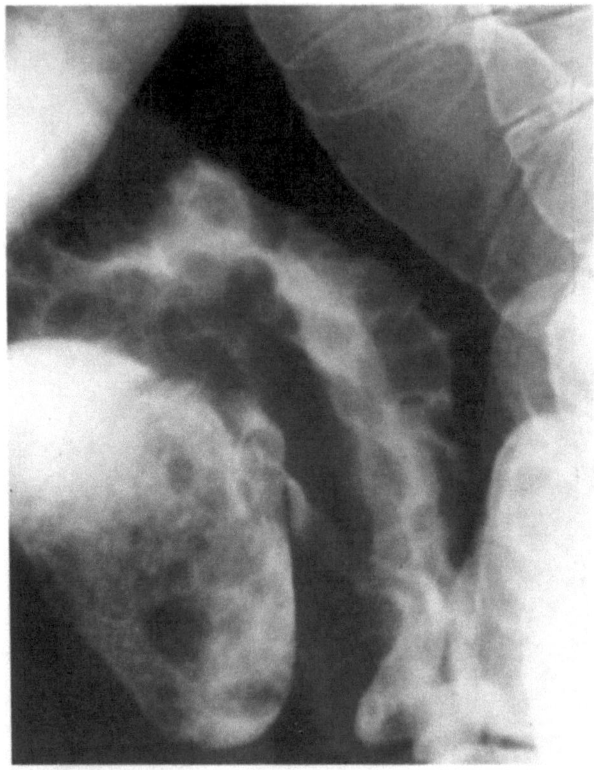

b

Fig. 5.1.-15a and b. String sign in Crohn's disease. The spasm (**a**) obliterates the cobblestone pattern of the terminal ileum, which is best visible in double contrast (**b**)

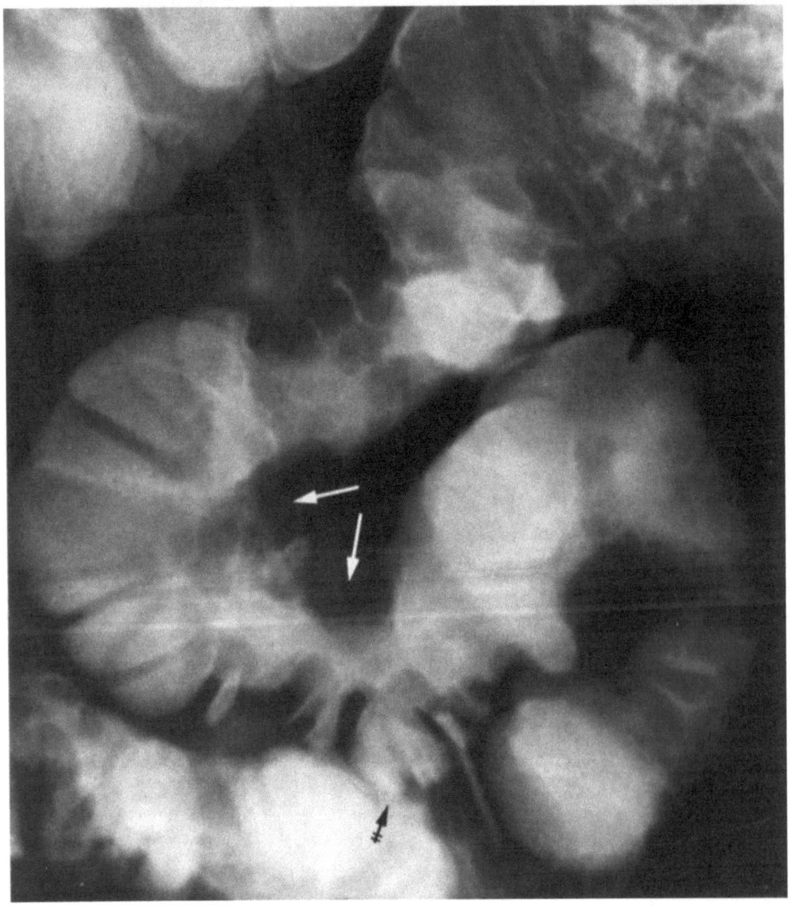

Fig. 5.1.-16. Asymmetrical involvement in Crohn's disease. Because of involvement of the mesenteric border with ulceration and fibrosis (→), diverticula-like sacculations develop on the opposite side (↠)

Fig. 5.1.-17. Fixed stenosis in Crohn's disease. Fibrosis of the intestinal wall causes narrowing of the terminal ileum with prestenotic dilatation. Involvement of the colon and ileocecal valve

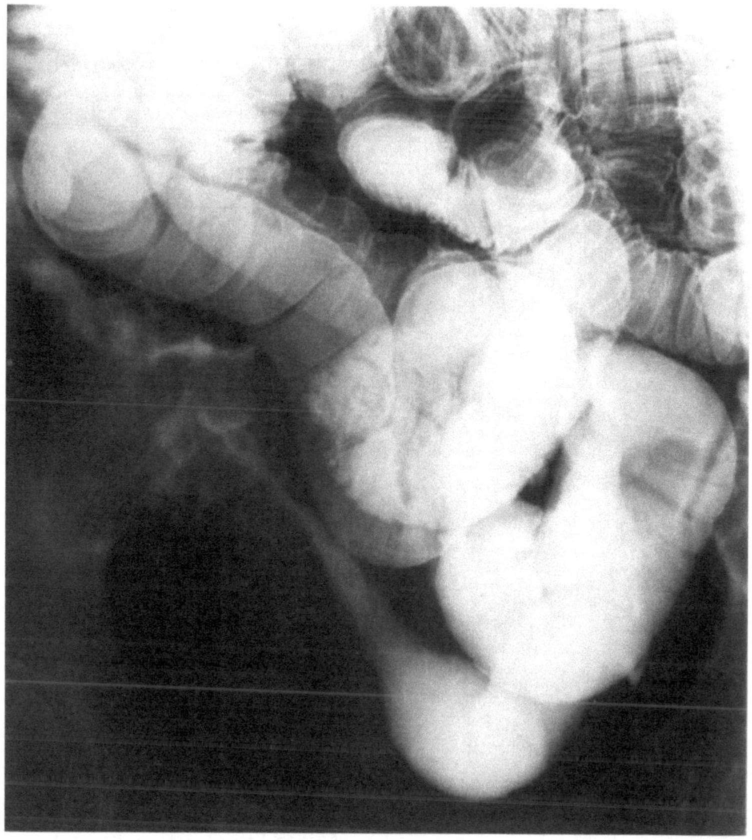

Fig. 5.1.-18. Solitary stricture in Crohn's disease. The fixed stenosis causes obstruction (→). The stricture is probably due to a healed up fibrotic ulcer. String sign in the terminal ileum (⇒)

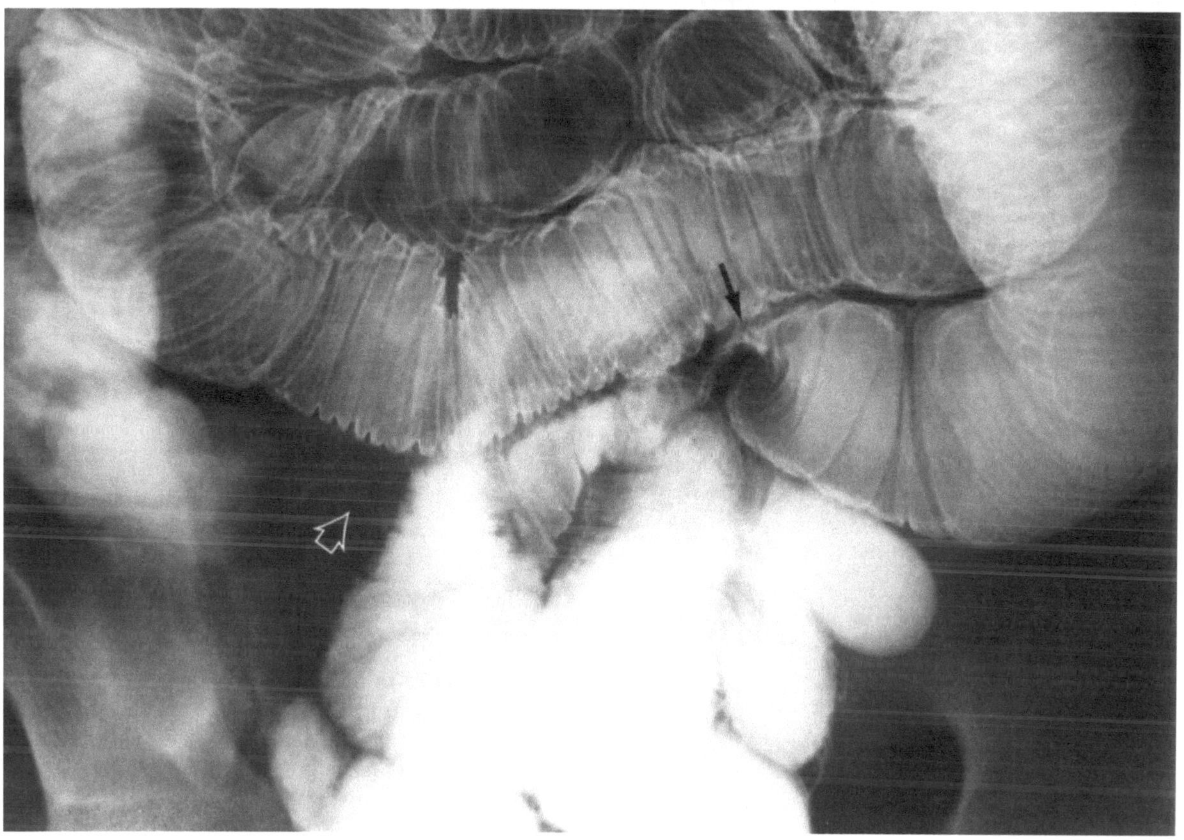

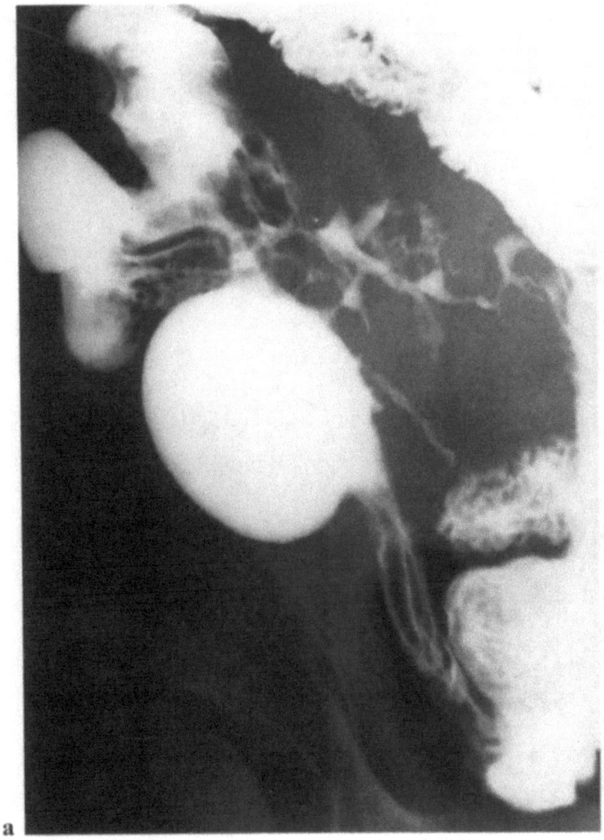

a

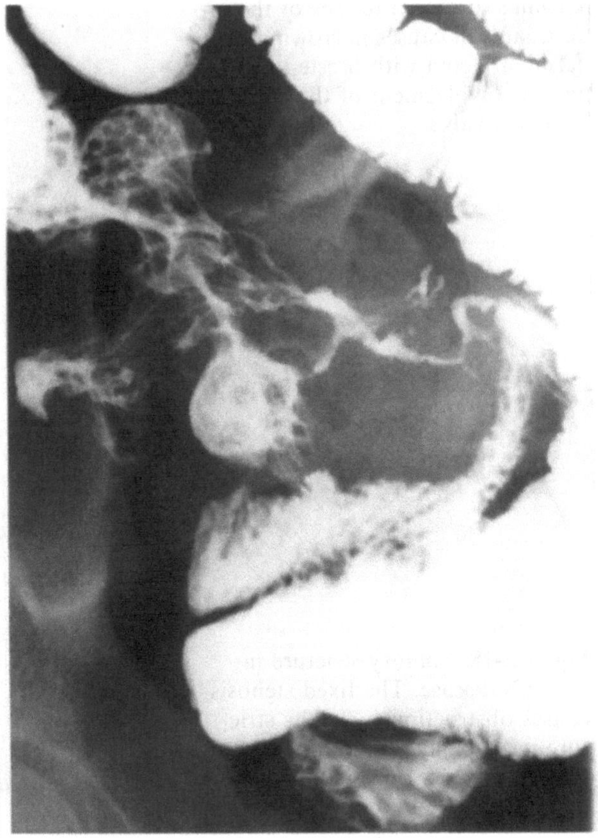

b

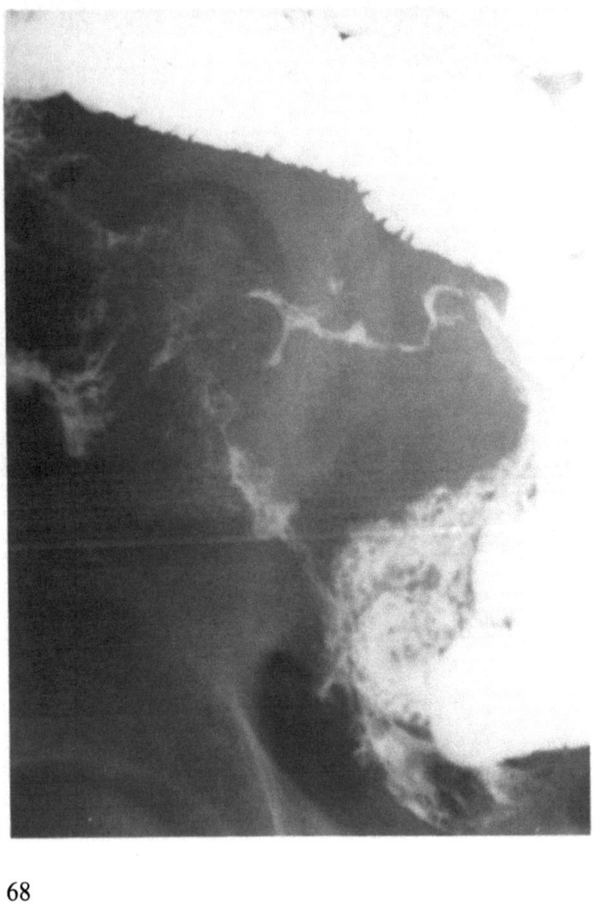

c

Fig. 5.1.-19 a to c. Sacculation of bowel wall in Crohn's disease. Example of diverticula-like sacculation of intact intestinal wall on the antimesenteric border ("pseudodiverticulum"). The spot films during fluoroscopy show the different phases of dilatation. Additional string sign and fistulous tract

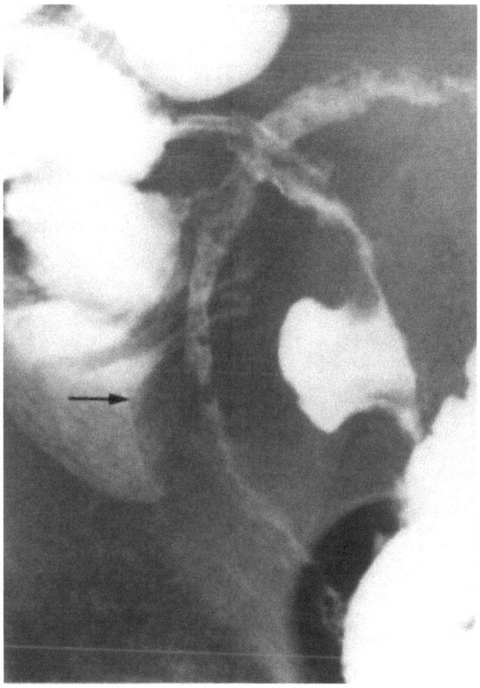

Fig. 5.1.-20. Shell sign in Crohn's disease. Fixed asymmetrical sacculation of the intestinal wall on the antimesenteric border. String sign. "Medial cecal defect" (→)

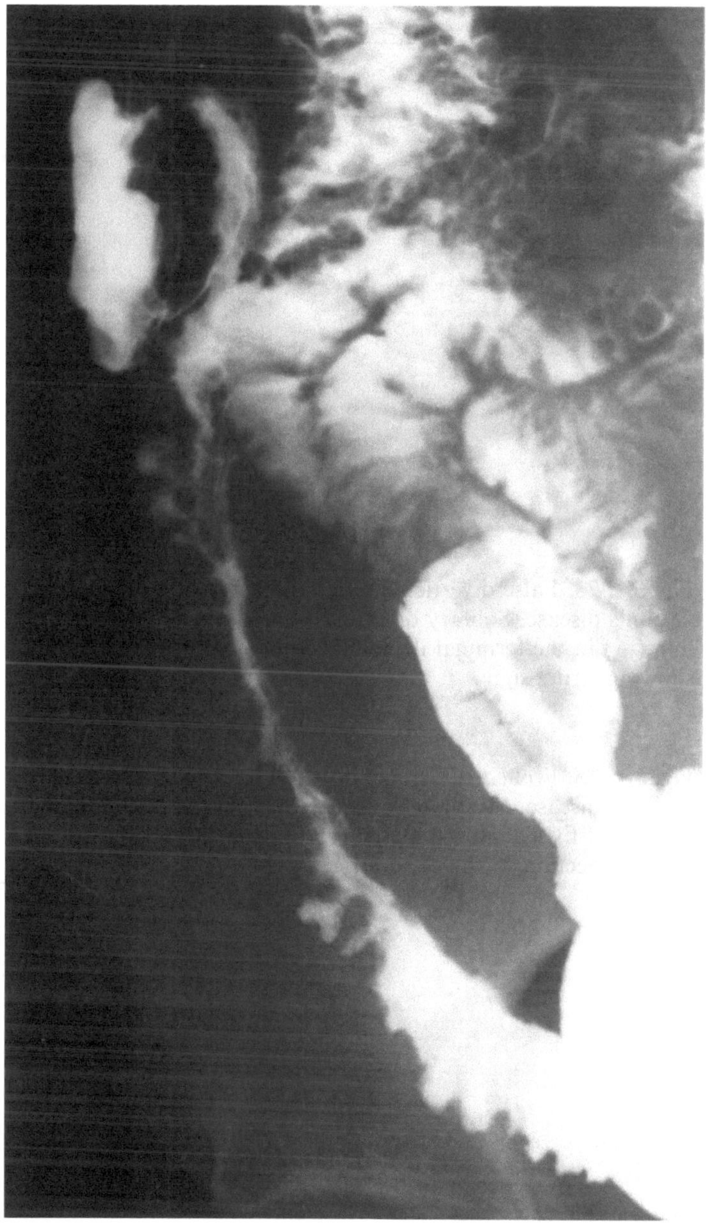

Fig. 5.1.-22. Sacculation on the antimesenteric border in Crohn's disease. Diverticula-like alterations due to asymmetric fibrosis

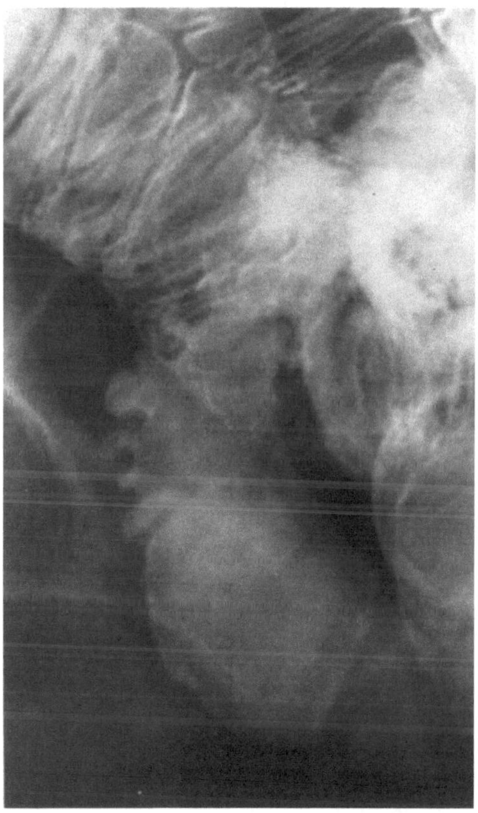

Fig. 5.1.-21. Sacculation of the intestinal wall on the antimesenteric border in Crohn's disease. Diverticula-like alterations due to asymmetric fibrosis

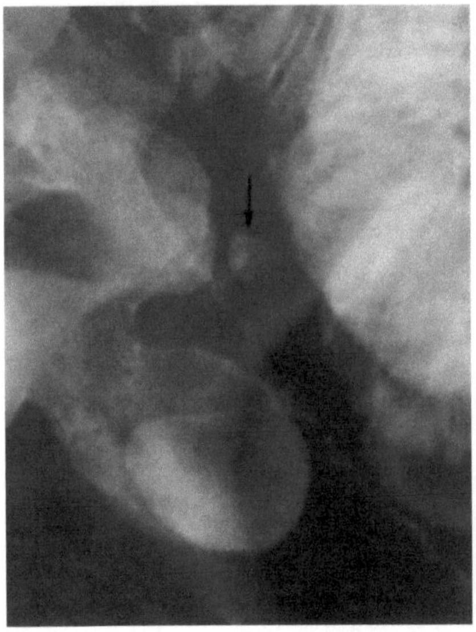

Fig. 5.1.-23. False diverticulum in Crohn's disease. Solitary diverticulum (→) in the terminal ileum showing string sign

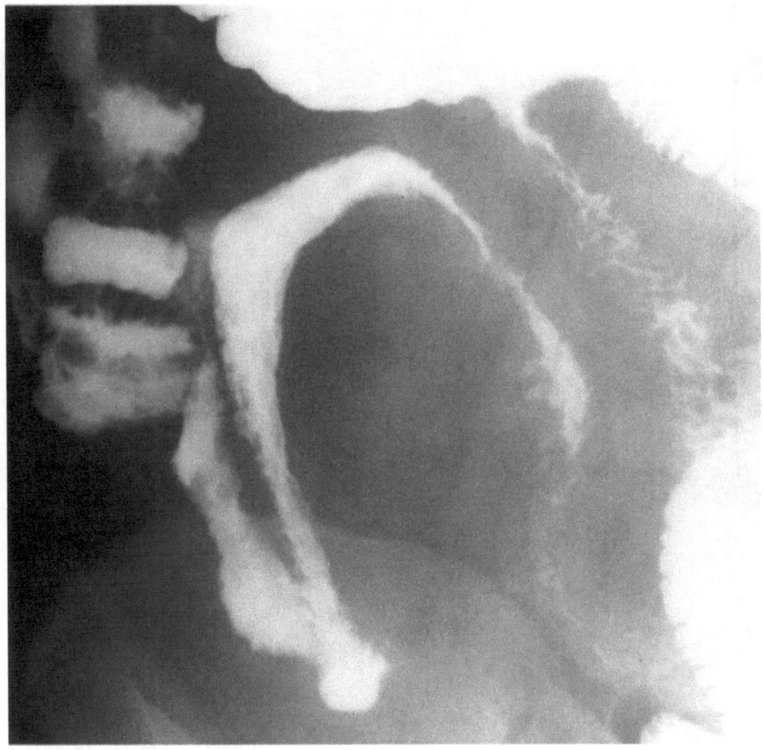

Fig. 5.1.-24. Omega sign in Crohn's disease. Due to induration and shrinking of the mesentery, the narrowed terminal plus preterminal ileum is gathered up in an arch or garland-like fashion

Fig. 5.1.-25. Fox-earth fistulae in Crohn's disease. Multiple sinus tracts and fistulae in the mesentery with connection to the cecum

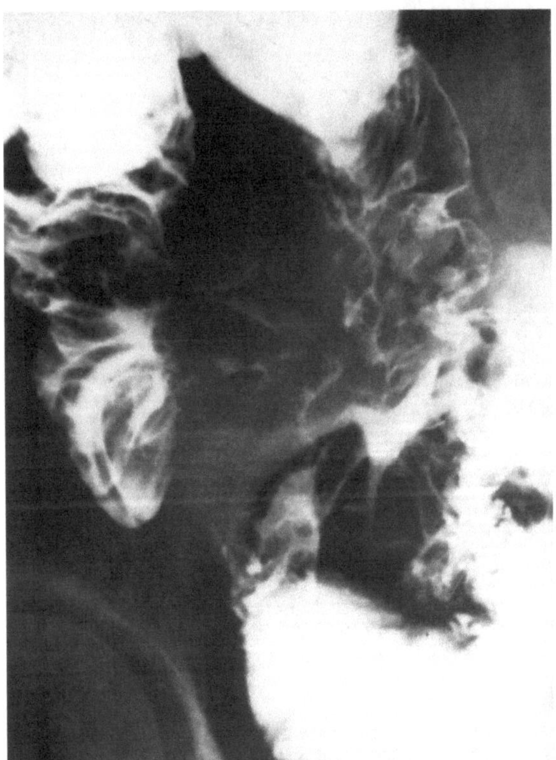

Fig. 5.1.-26. Enterocolic fistula in Crohn's disease. Fistula from the ileum to the cecum (→). String sign of the terminal ileum (⇒). Destruction of the ileocecal valve (>)

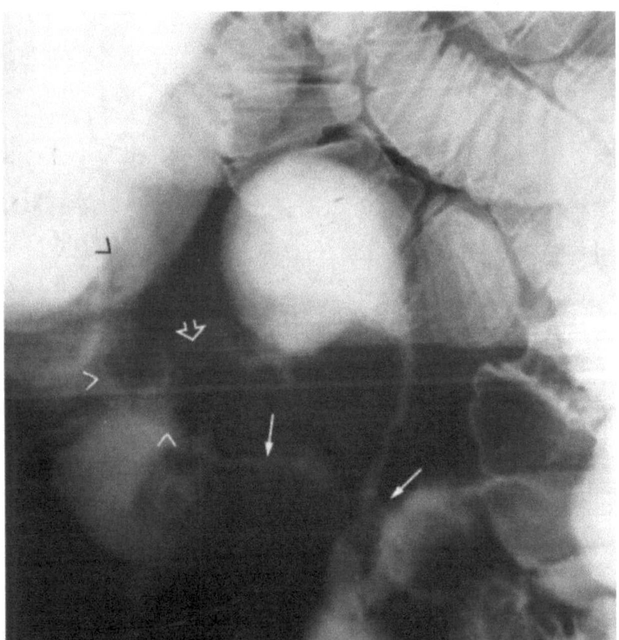

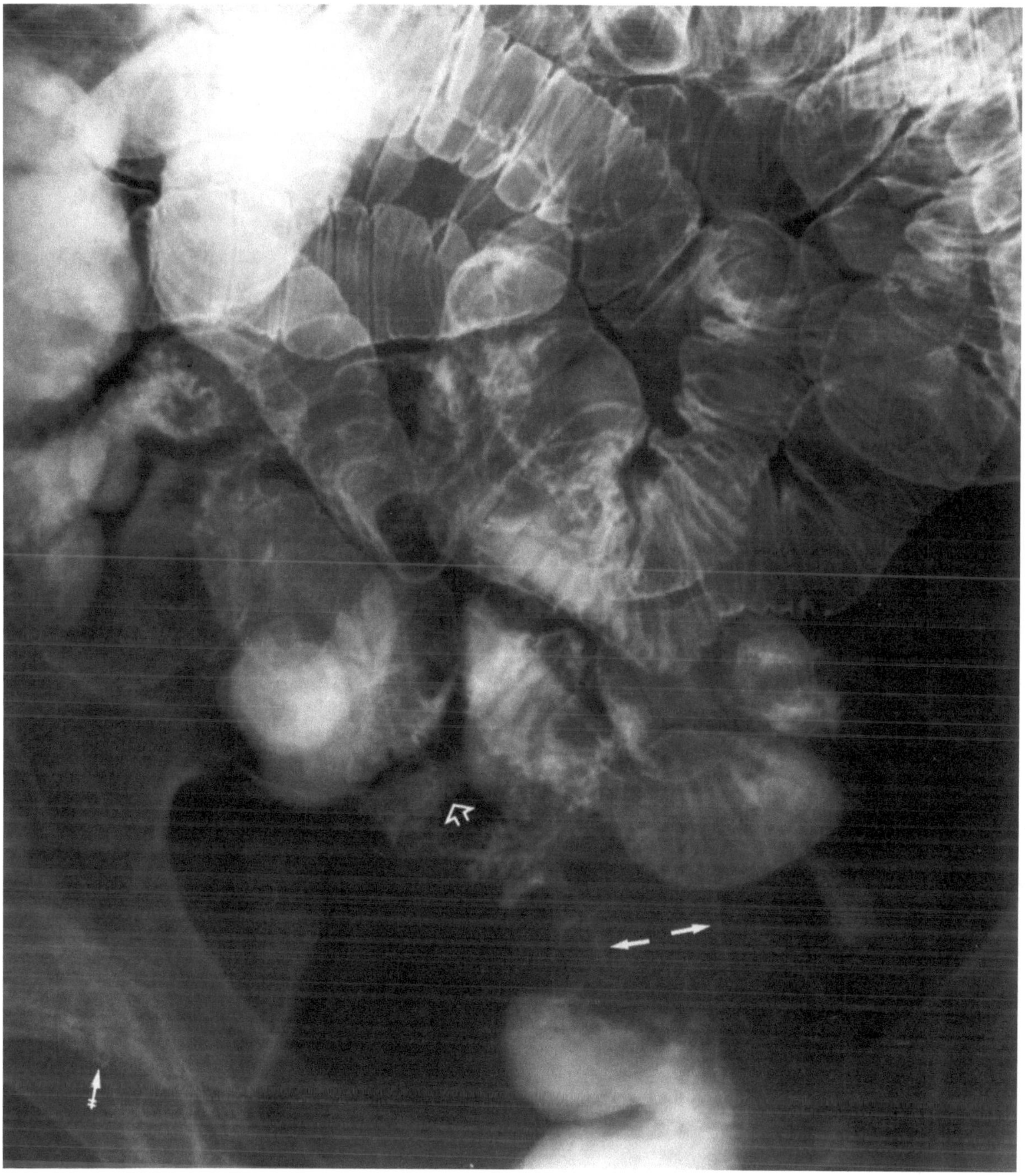

Fig. 5.1.-27. Enterorectal and enterocutaneous fistulae in Crohn's disease. Early appearance of contrast medium in the rectum through fistulae (→) from the preterminal ileum. Broader fistula from the ileum to the skin (⇒). Contrast medium in surgical dressing (⇸)

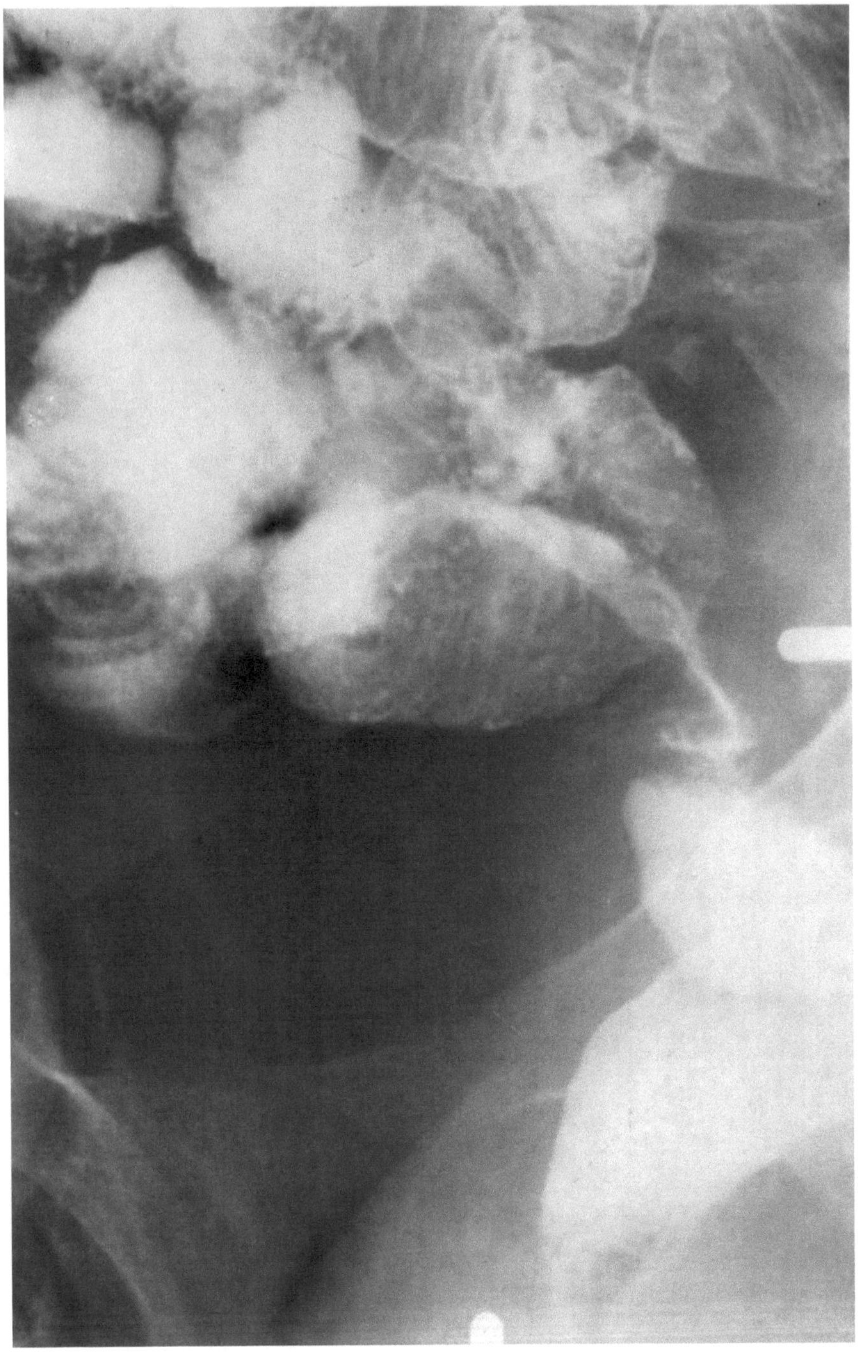

Fig. 5.1.-28. Ileorectal fistula

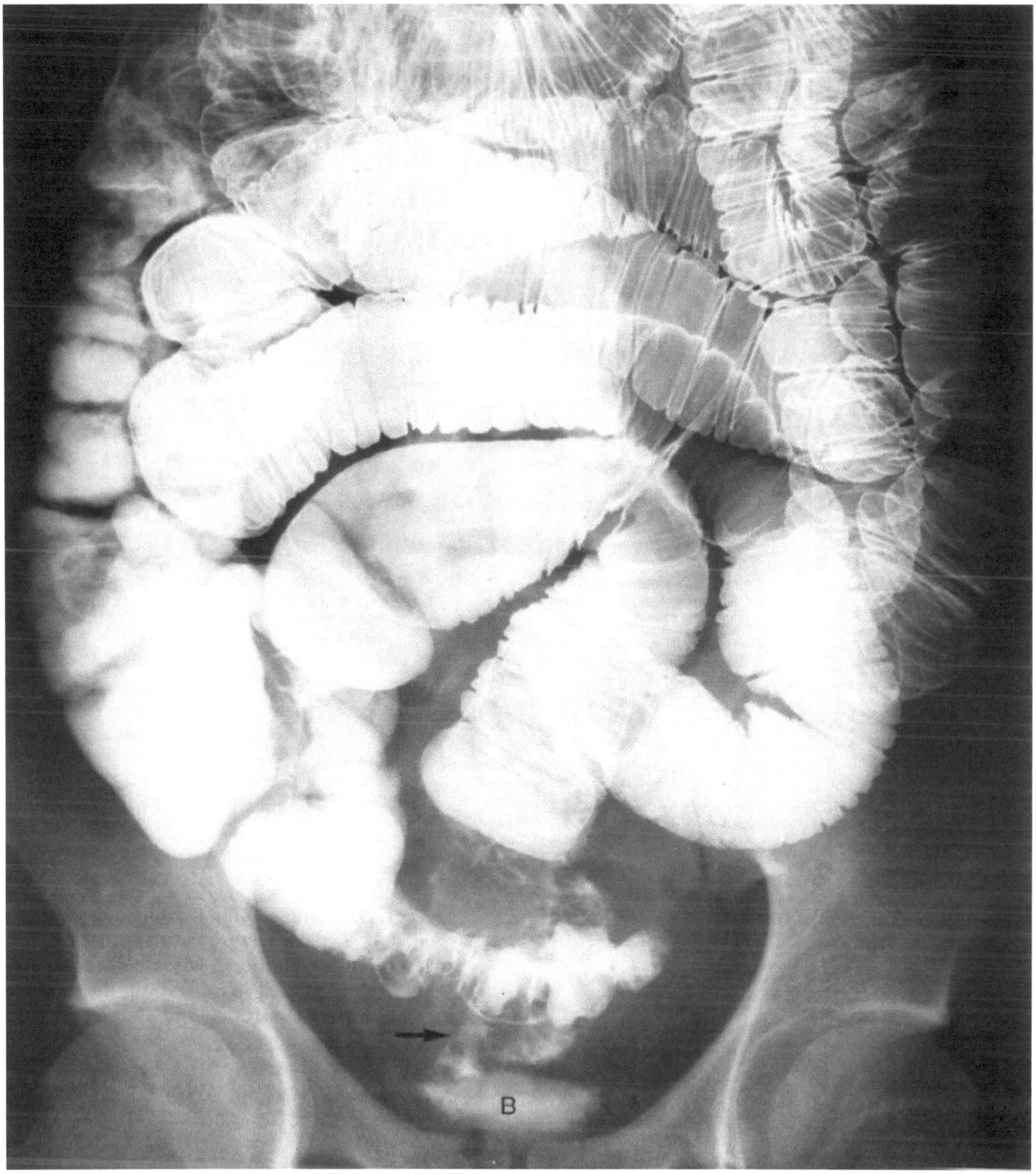

Fig. 5.1.-29. Enterovesical fistula in Crohn's disease. Broad fistula (→) from the ileum to the bladder (B)

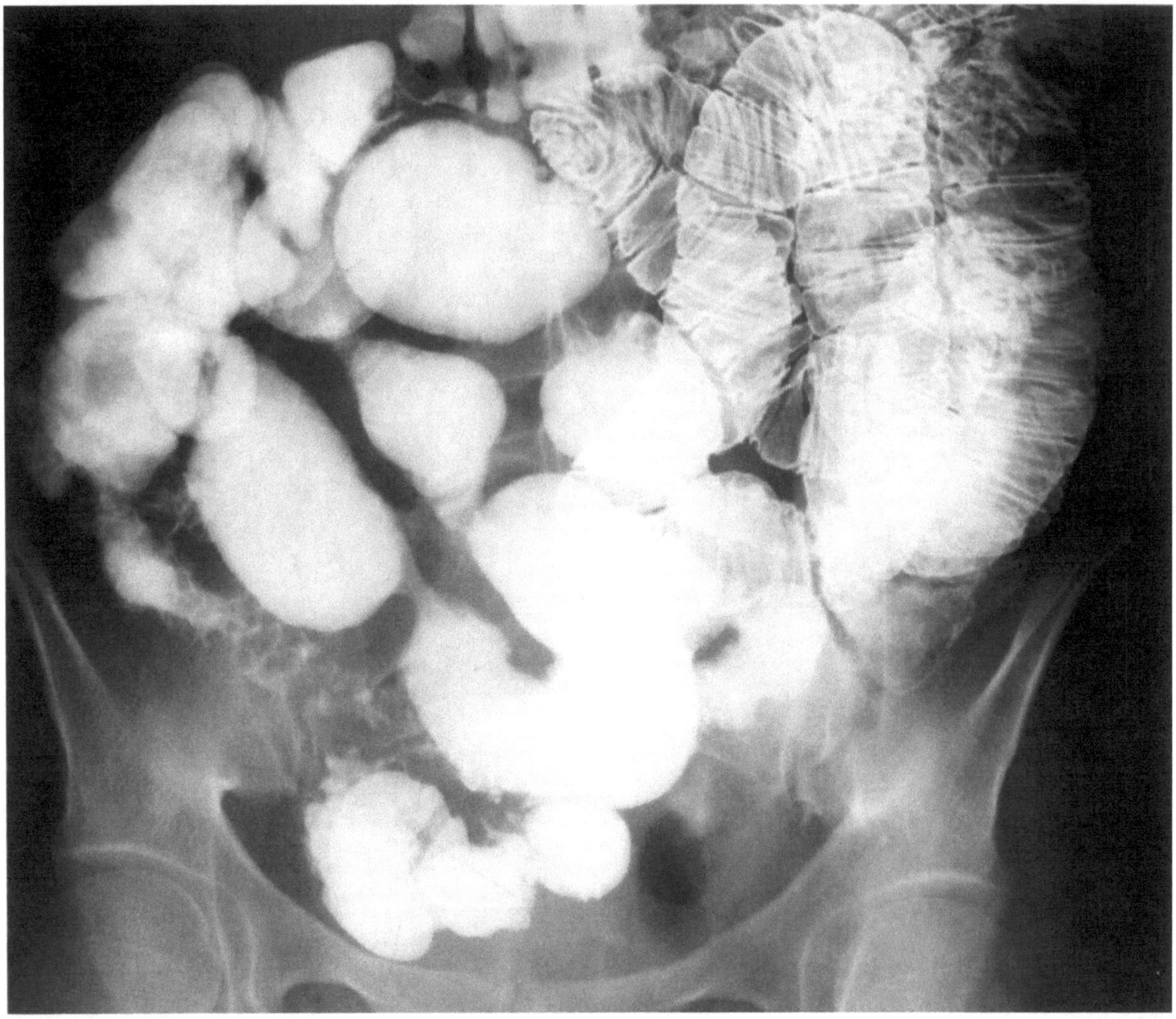

Fig. 5.1.-30. Long-standing Crohn's disease of the ileum. Typical picture with alternating strictures and dilatations. Disease duration 5 years. At the time of investigation, the patient had 3–6 watery stools/day and abdominal pain

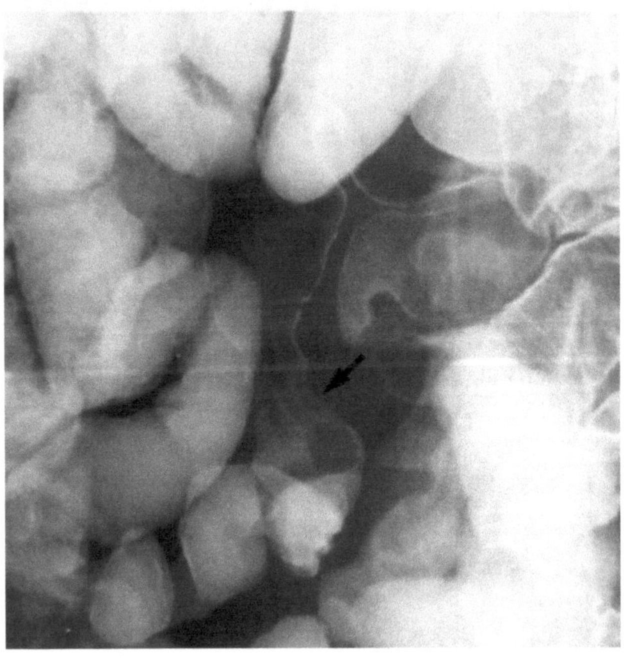

Fig. 5.1.-31. Bike-tire phenomenon in Crohn's disease in remission. Atrophic, smooth mucosa with parallelling folds of a flaccid, partially collapsed intestinal wall

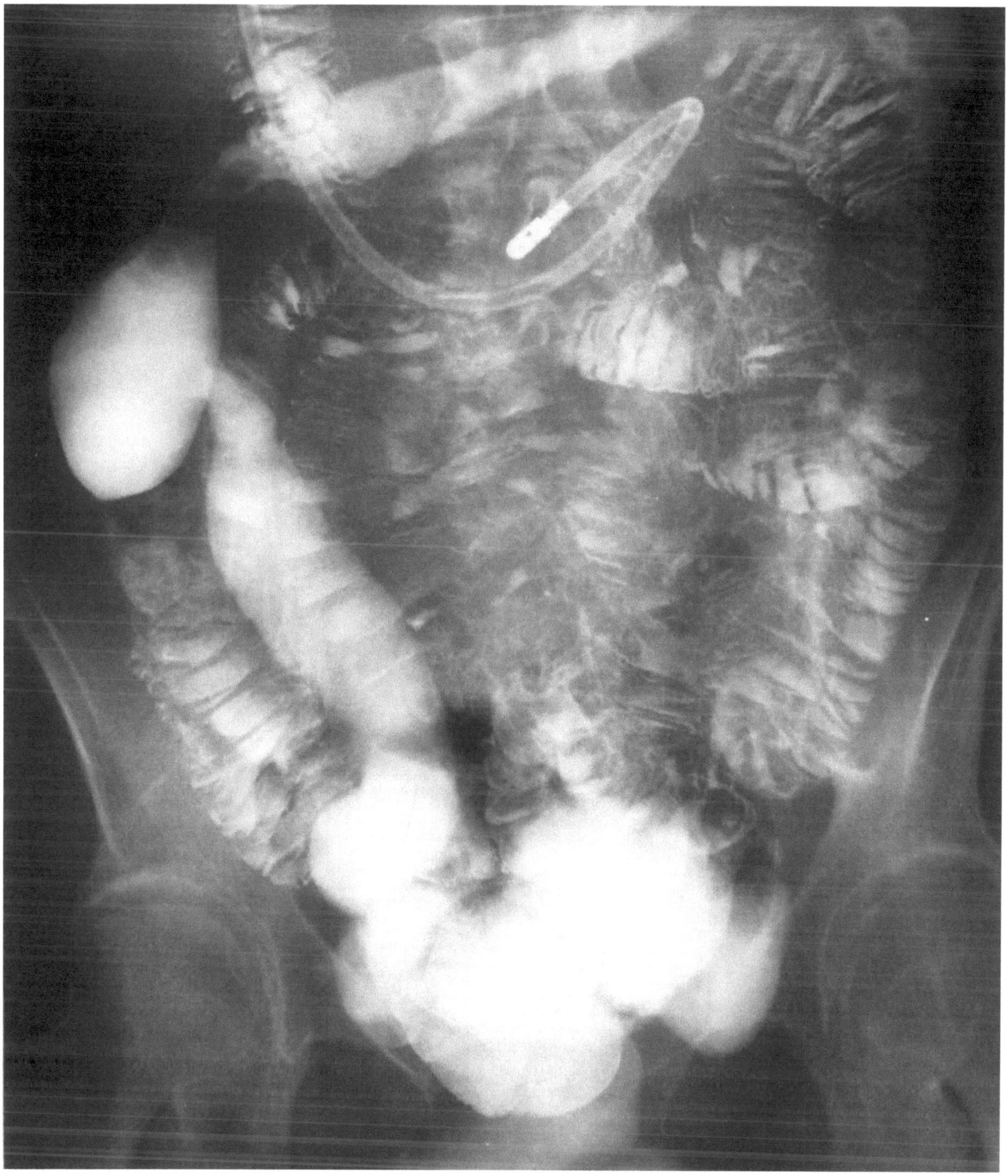

Fig. 5.1.-32. Crohn's disease with malabsorption syndrome. Extensive disease with dilatation of the distal ileum. Greatly reduced mucosal coating which is usual in the malabsorption syndrome

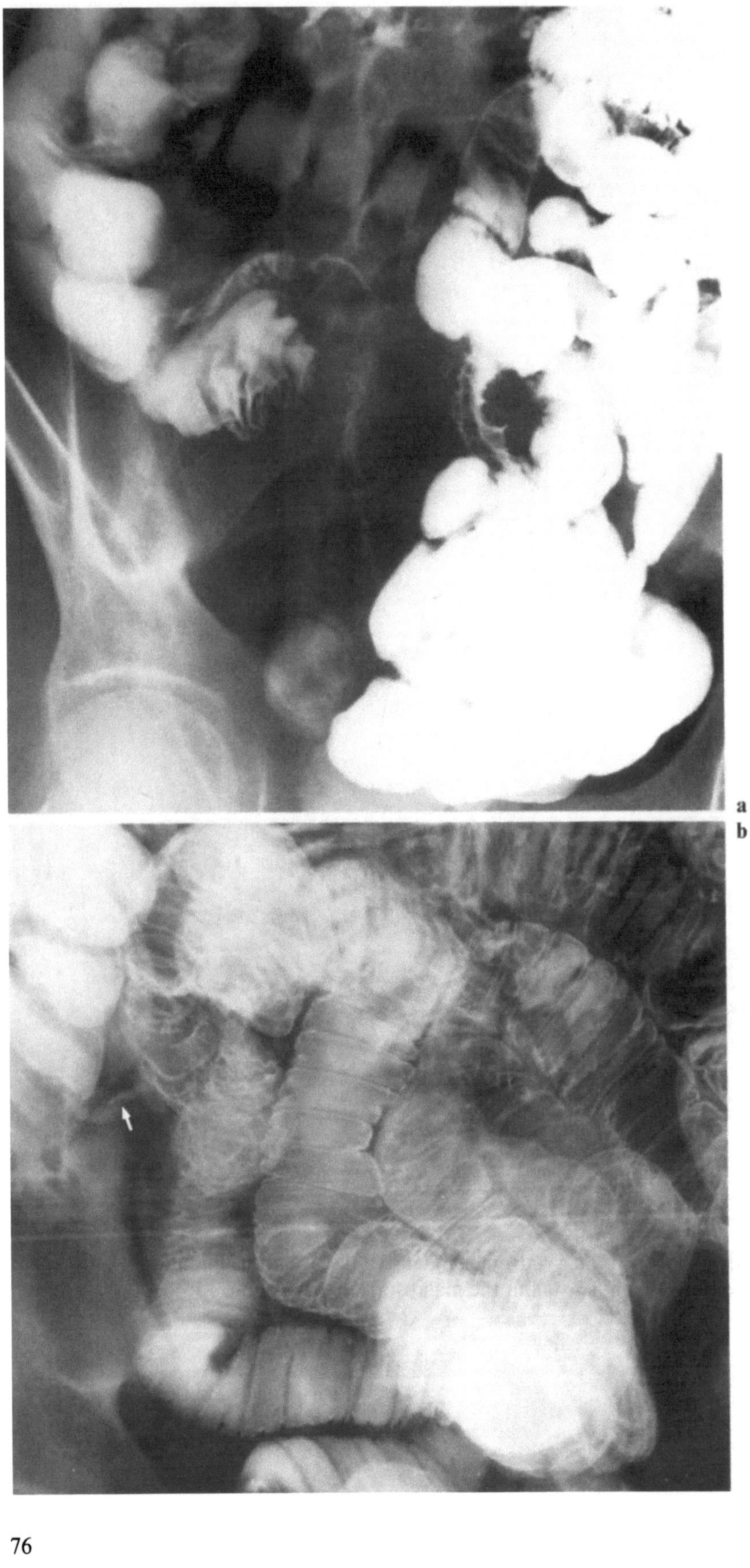

Fig. 5.1.-33 a and b. Crohn's disease in remission. **a** String sign of the distal ileum. Thick ening of the intestinal wall and mesentery. Skip lesion in the proximal ileum. **b** After a year's therapy, no detectable accompanying tumor. String sign (→) as evidence of residual disease in the presently asymptomatic patient

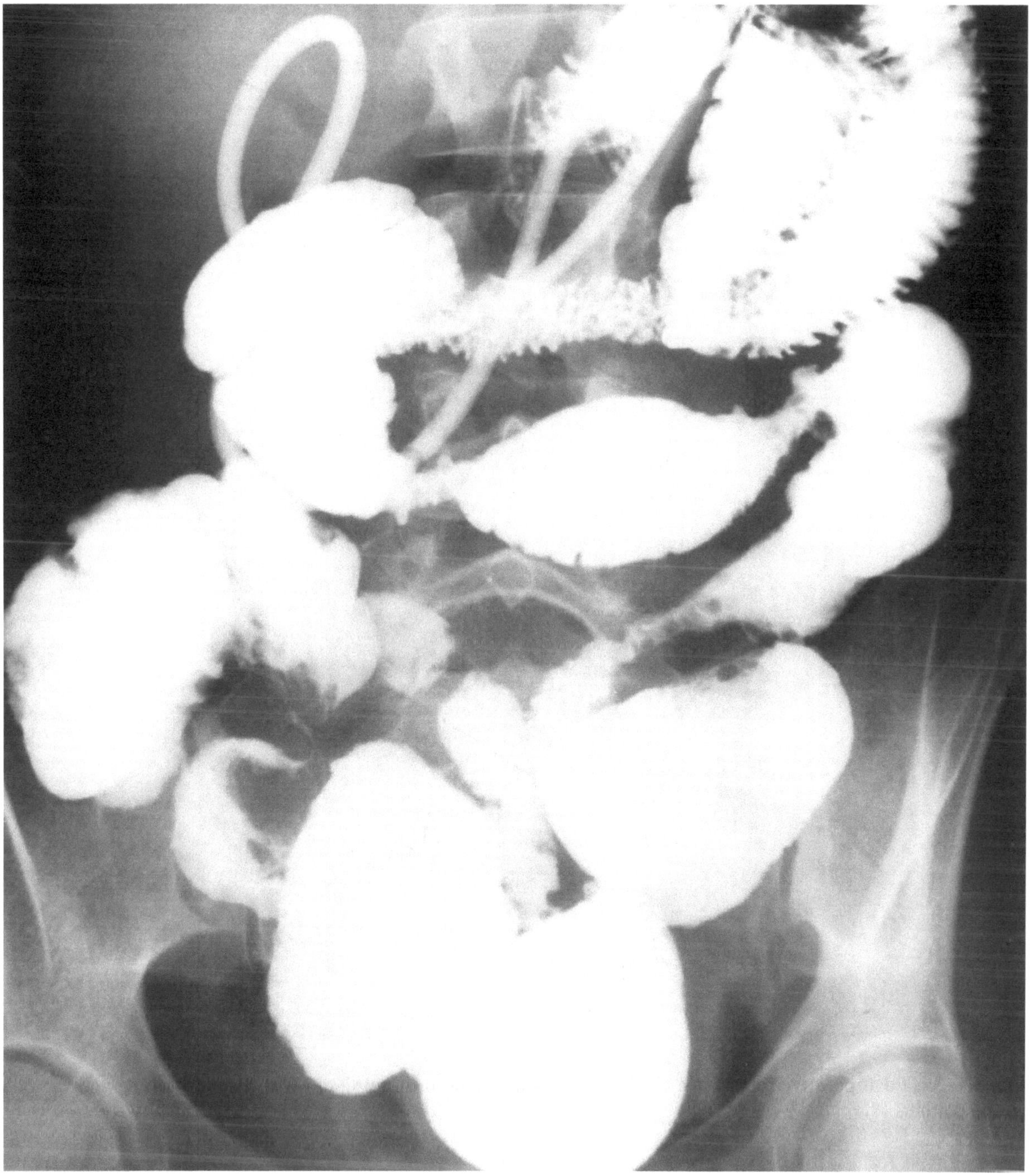

Fig. 5.1.-34. Short bowel in Crohn's disease. After repeated small bowel resections and ileoascendostomy, only a few diseased bowel loops remain

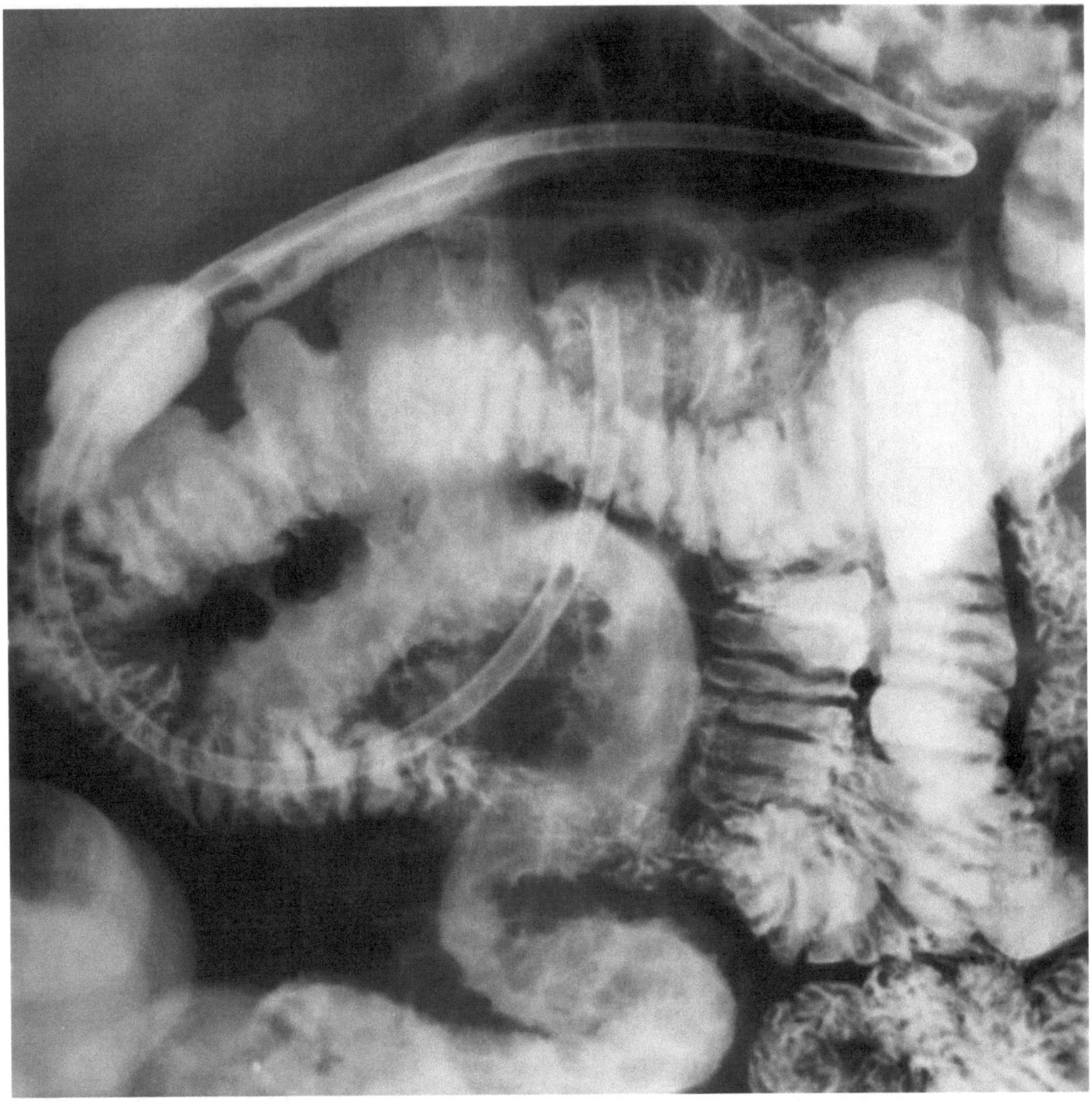

Fig. 5.1.-35. Postoperative recurrence of Crohn's disease. Neoterminal ileum with pseudopolyps and fistulae to the colon

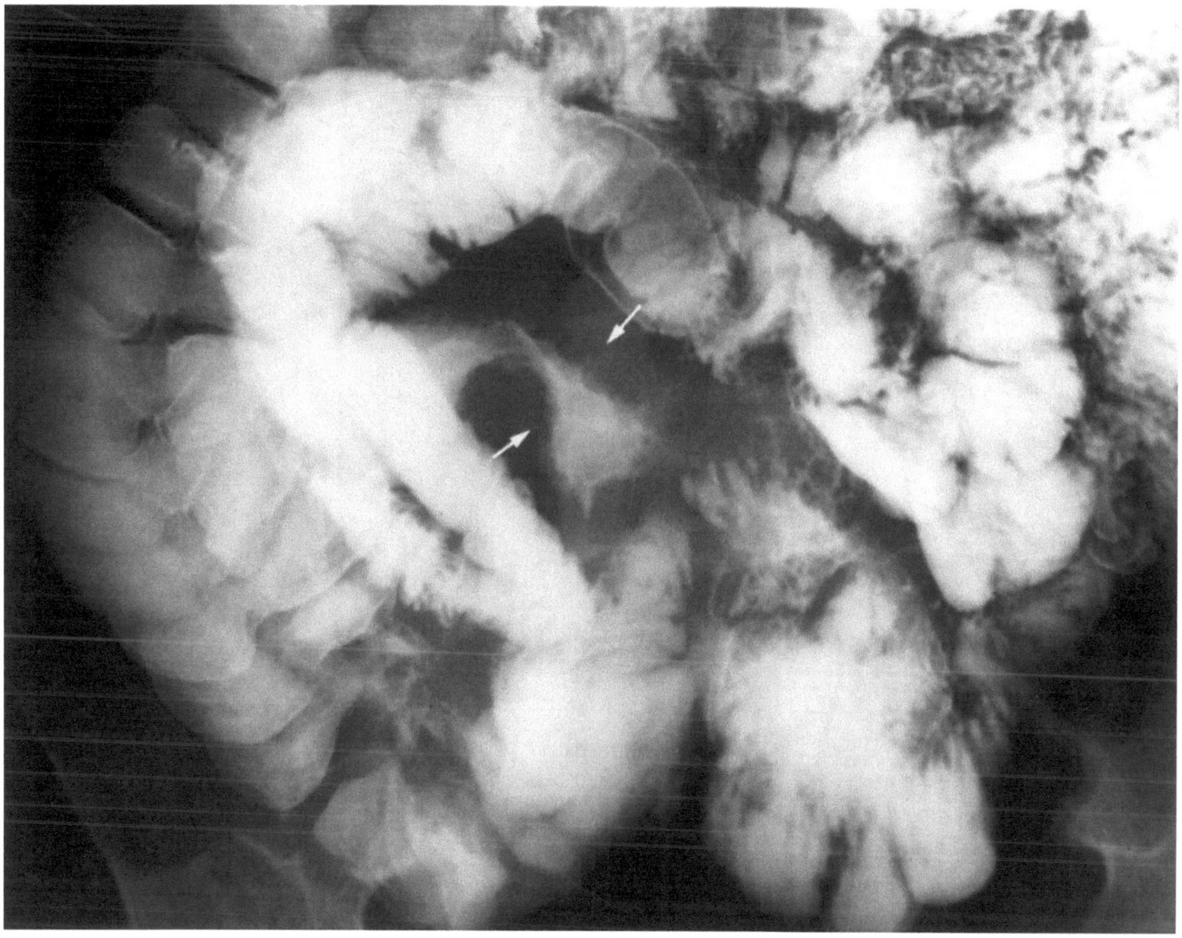

Fig. 5.1.-36. Crohn's disease of the ileum. Destruction of the mucosa with cobblestoning and stenosis. Thickened wall due to the inflammatory tumor (→). The picture simulates a malignant lymphoma

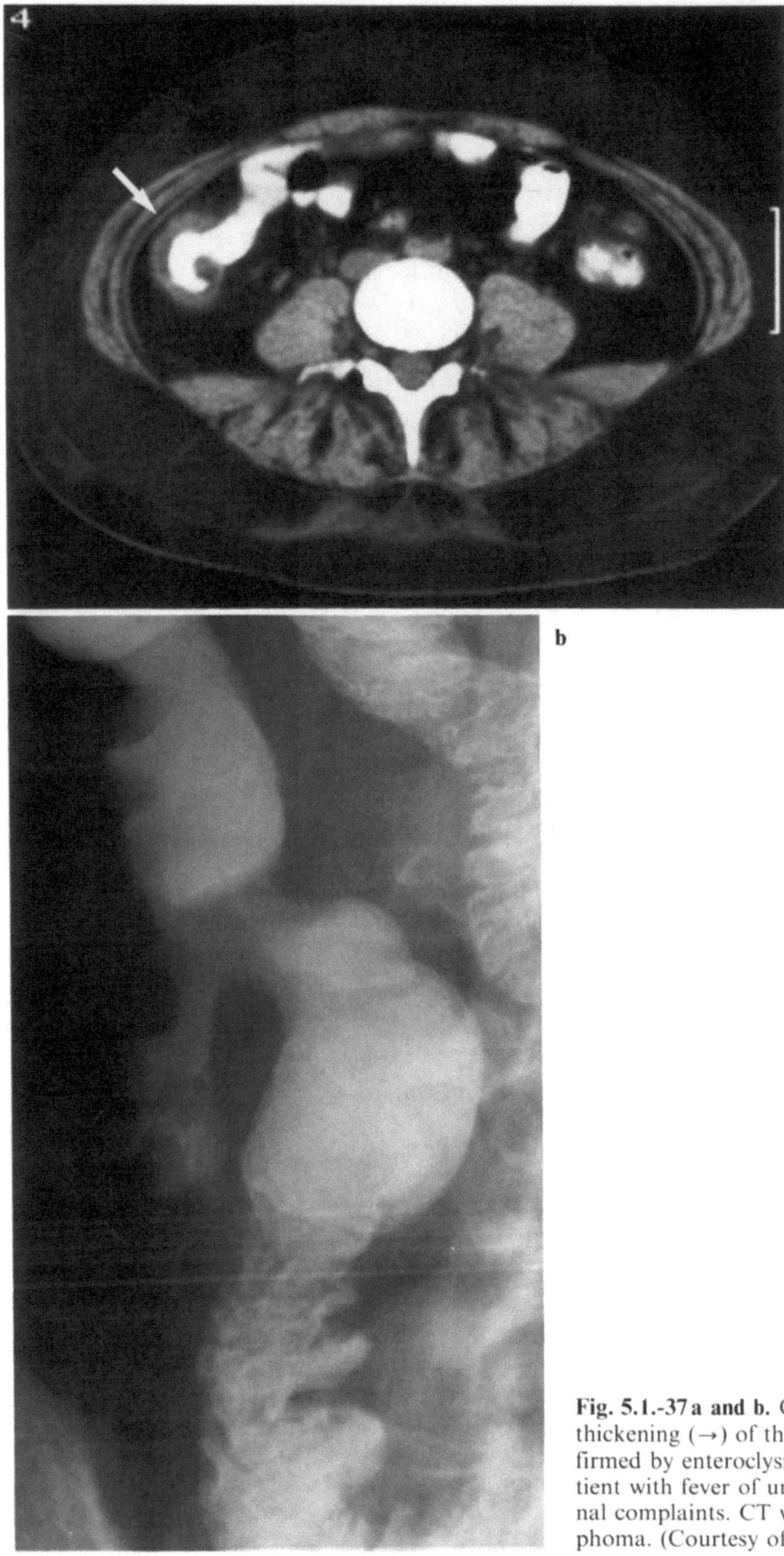

a

b

Fig. 5.1.-37 a and b. CT in Crohn's disease. Wall thickening (→) of the ileocecal region (**a**), confirmed by enteroclysis (**b**). 21-year-old adipose patient with fever of unknown origin without abdominal complaints. CT was performed to rule out lymphoma. (Courtesy of Dr. Randolf, Isny, Germany)

38 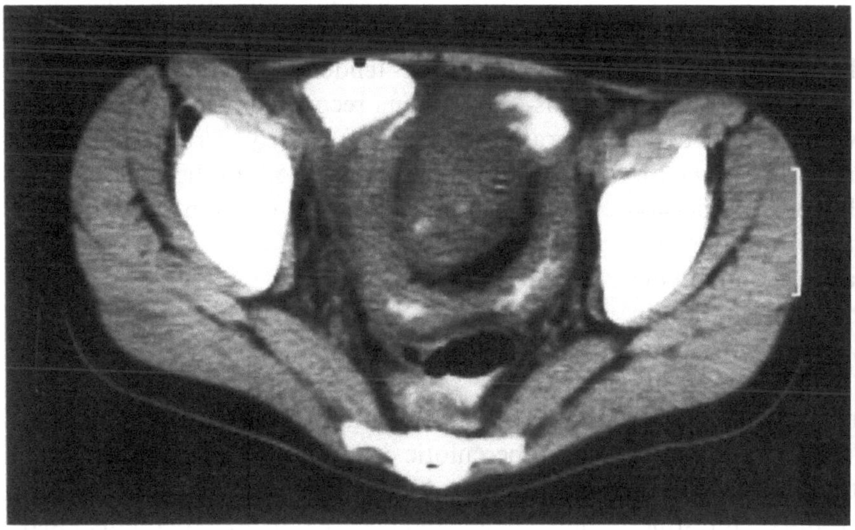

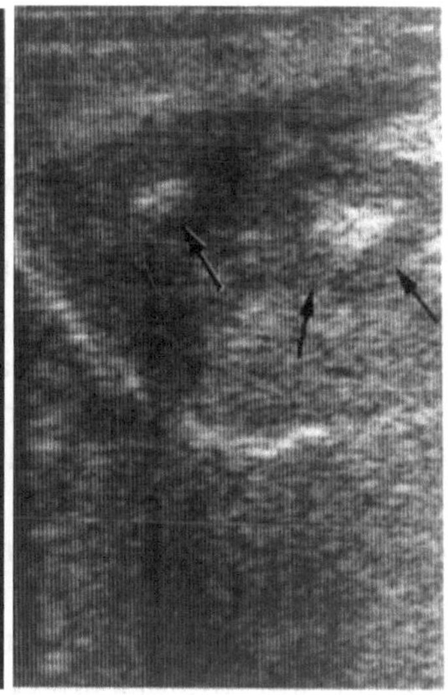 39

Fig. 5.1.-38. CT in Crohn's disease. CT shows impressively the inflamed, thickened intestinal wall in relation to the lumen

Fig. 5.1.-39. Ultrasound in Crohn's disease. Large conglomerate tumor with target lesion due to thickened, inflamed intestinal loops (→)

5.2 Inflammatory Diseases apart from Crohn's Disease

In radiological literature Crohn's disease is the most frequently reported chronic inflammatory condition of the small bowel. Less attention has been devoted to other inflammatory processes or inflammatory-like diseases of the small bowel.

Radiologic changes are often nonspecific, making differential diagnosis difficult. With careful examination technique and sound clinical knowledge, however, differential diagnosis may be approximated. Some inflammations, e.g. chronic radiation enteritis, do portray characteristic changes.

Interpretation of films should mainly include fold and surface changes, mucosal coating and disturbance of intestinal motility. Poor mucosal coating often combined with disturbed motility, indicates actively inflamed mucosa or intestinal wall changes. The same radiological picture may be perceived in motility disorders, which correspond with maldigestion. Clinically, both often present the same symptom: diarrhea. Some of the inflammatory bowel diseases presented in this chapter could also be demonstrated in chapter 5.4.2.

5.2.1 Lymphofollicular Hyperplasia

Multiple, 1–2 mm sized, evenly dispersed elevations, especially in the terminal ileum, correspond to enlarged lymph follicles in the mucosa. In asymptomatic children and adolescents, they present as coincidental findings and bear no pathological significance (Wells 1948; Lasserich 1953). In the double contrast examination, these hyperplastic lymph follicles can often be observed in older people as well (Figs. 5.2.-1, 4.3.-6 and 4.3.-7, p. 39).

They are only of pathological significance, if other signs of disease, e.g. diarrhea, pain, fever or general symptoms are present. Additional signs of nonspecific enteritis or mucosal irritation and/or pathologically enlarged lymph follicles are usually observed in these cases (Fig. 5.2.-2).

The term "nonsclerosing ileitis" has been introduced for this condition (Golden 1945; Prévôt 1950). This entity is now considered to be caused by infection with Yersinia or other organisms (Brombart 1980). Other possibilities for lymphofollicular enlargement are intestinal tuberculosis, early Crohn's disease, accompanying reaction in parasitic disease or inflammation in the pelvis and abdomen, malignant lymphoma, intestinal nodular lymphatic hyperplasia in hypogammaglobulinemia (Marshak et al. 1974; Hermans et al. 1966) (Fig. 5.2.-2), Whipple's disease, mastocytosis and last but not least artifacts in an insufficiently cleansed intestine. Lymph follicles may also be simulated by orthograde viewing of contracting folds.

5.2.2 Nonspecific Ileitis

This term denotes alterations at the terminal and preterminal ileum which correspond with thickening of folds and superficial changes, uncharacteristic of Crohn's disease. The bowel wall is not considerably thickened. The adjacent small bowel loops may be more or less pushed aside from the terminal ileum by the reactive, enlarged mesenteric lymph nodes. A local hyperperistalsis is usually observed, but there is no typical string sign (Figs. 5.2.-3 and 4). The mucosal coating may be impaired.

Yersinia organisms are often found as cause of this nonspecific inflammation (Figs. 5.2.-3 to 5). Evidence is supplied by determination of the antibody titers, or by bacteriology, in the early phase. Other possible agents are Campylobacter (Fig. 5.2.-6), Chlamydia and Aeromonas. Patients mostly complain of abdominal cramps, diarrhea, fever and general symptoms. Appendectomy is often performed as a result.

The radiological changes are nonspecific but nevertheless rather uniform. This also correlates with the nonspecific macroscopic and histologic picture. The radiologist must mention the differential diagnosis of these agents, so that specific bacteriological and serological examinations may ensue. In several of our cases of "nonspecific ileitis" this was not done and so there was no evidence of an organism. On account of the self-healing tendency of these inflammations, the patients recovered after symptomatic therapy (Fig. 5.2.-7). Early Crohn's disease, especially in the presence of aphthoid ulcers, has to be mentioned in the differential diagnosis (Fig. 4.3.-13, p. 41).

5.2.3 Tuberculosis

Since the introduction of pasteurized milk and antituberculotic drugs, bowel tuberculosis is seldom found in industrialized countries. The terminal ileum and ileocecal region are predisposed for this disease. Initially, the infected and enlarged Peyer's patches resemble nonspecific ileitis (Fig. 5.2.-8) or lymphofollicular hyperplasia. Tuberculous mucosal infiltrations may ulcerate. The picture then simulates aphthous ulcerations in Crohn's disease (Fig. 5.2.-9a). The differentiation between these two clinical entities may be impossible. Thus, before Crohn et al. (1932) reported their findings, many cases of inflammation of the terminal ileum were diagnosed as tuberculosis when in fact Crohn's terminal ileitis was the case. Typhoid and sarcoidosis may produce similar pictures. With appropriate therapy, primary intestinal tuberculosis may recede completely (Fig. 5.2.-9b). In case of marked ulceration, it is almost impossible to differentiate between tuberculosis, Crohn's disease and carcinoma (Fig. 5.2.-10).

5.2.4 Radiation Enteritis

The small bowel is relatively radiosensitive. Acute reactions to irradiation are generally no indication for a contrast medium investigation. An exposure of 45 Gy or more causes chronic radiation damage (Rubin and Casarett 1968; Strockbine et al. 1970; Graham and Villalba 1963). It mostly takes one to two years for the symptoms to show up (Graundins 1969; De Cosse et al. 1969). Sometimes, the first symptoms appear after 10 years or later (Chau et al. 1962). The frequency of radiation damage accounts for 0.6–17% in tumor irritation of the pelvis and/or the abdomen (Rogers and Goldstein 1977; Bruneton et al. 1982). Previous surgery, inflammations in the pelvis, atherosclerosis and diabetes increase the risk of severe radiation reaction (Neumeister and Pfeiffer 1966; Mason et al. 1970). The mobility of the intestinal loops in the small pelvis is reduced by adhesions. The ileum is therefore more often affected since irradiation is performed more often in the pelvis (gynecological tumors) than in the upper abdomen region.

The bowel responds to the irradiation with alterations in the mucosa, the vessels and tissues of the deeper wall layers. The mucosal damage may recede whereas the radiation effect on the intestinal wall progresses, resulting in obliterative endarteritis and fibrosis (Joelsson et al. 1971; Mason et al. 1970). Macroscopically, dense peritoneal adhesions, thickened, shrunken mesentery with taut, gathered up intestinal loops and thickened, swollen bowel wall are to be seen. The lumen may be narrowed to an advanced stricture. The mucosa is edematous or smooth and atrophic. Ulceration may be present. Which of these changes predominates will depend on the stage of inflammatory activity, i.e. whether this is a case of chronically active radiation enteritis or fibrosis.

This correlates to the radiological picture. In a less severe involvement, there are spastic contractions and restricted distension of the intestinal lumen, sometimes accompanied by local hyperperistalsis and slightly thickened folds (Fig. 5.2.-11). In a further advanced stage, the folds are thickened and irregular with compressed interfold spaces, thus appearing like deep spiculae (Fig. 5.2.-12). The distance between the adjacent loops is widened on account of the thickened intestinal wall. The bowel loops are fixed and gathered up due to the shrivelled, thickened mesentery and the adhesions of the serosa. The folds may be distorted ("tacked down"; Herlinger 1969). The mobility is therefore diminished or abolished. The passage of the contrast medium through these adherent, rigid loops is considerably delayed, especially when there are additional strictures. The proximal intestinal loops are then dilated. An edematous mucosa may simulate a cobblestone pattern. In atrophy of the mucosa, there is more or less loss of folds and the surface is smooth (Figs. 5.2.-12 to 14). The mucosal coating may be reduced because of bowel fluid retention, edema and inflammation (Fig. 5.2.-14). In advanced cases of radiation damage, ulcers form which can result in hemorrhage, perforation, fistula formation of adjacent organs or high grade strictures (Fig. 5.2.-15).

The radiologic changes in radiation enteritis mostly allow a specific diagnosis (Antes and Lissner 1983). Difficulties may arise in the differential diagnosis concerning peritoneal carcinomatosis, especially when irradiation has been carried out previously. Crohn's disease may produce similar pictures.

5.2.5 Other Inflammatory Conditions

Here, changes in the small bowel are described, which are brought about by various agents or inflammations of as yet unknown etiology.

The clinical symptoms are mostly chronic diarrhea, nonspecific abdominal complaints and occasional malabsorption.

Radiological pictures mostly show a *nonspecific enteritis or mucosal irritation* of the entire small bowel or of individual sections. This is often accompanied by a disturbed motility. These alterations usually recede with treatment (Figs. 5.2.-21 and 22, and 4.5.-2a to d, pp. 48–51).

These diseases bear similarities regarding the clinical symptoms and radiological changes, which are described in chapter 5.4 (motility disorders). This fact is particularly significant for the differential diagnosis.

5.2.5.1 Bacterial and Viral Enteritis

Bacterial organisms such as Salmonella, Shigella and E. coli are the most frequent. In viruses, the Rota virus is the most important (Ruppin 1980). Most agents have an enterotoxic effect and do not cause morphologically confirmable mucosal damage. Accordingly, radiological pictures mostly portray a *nonspecific en-*

teritis or mucosal irritation with more or less marked disturbed motility (general or local hyperperistalsis or nonpropulsive peristalsis; Figs. 5.2.-16 and 17). Anatomic causes (e.g. small bowel diverticula, loss of ileocecal valve, fistulae, afferent loop syndrome) or functional disorders (e.g. intestinal pseudoobstruction, scleroderma, immune defect) can cause bacterial overgrowth of the small bowel, resulting in chronic diarrhea and malabsorption (Fig. 5.2.-18).

5.2.5.2 Eosinophilic Enteritis

Histologically, this disease is characterized by marked eosinophil cell infiltration in all layers of the intestinal wall. The jejunum and gastric antrum are the most frequent localizations. In most cases, blood eosinophilia is present. The origin of the disease is unknown; food allergy is considered to be the prime cause. The clinical symptoms are abdominal pain, malabsorption and diarrhea. Radiological findings portray irregularly thickened and deformed folds, which may also result in narrowing of the lumen. Infiltrations and damage of the muscular layers result in local dilatation and thickening of the wall. Ulcerations, strictures and fistulae are rare. Malignant lymphoma, Crohn's disease or a nonspecific inflammation (e.g. yersiniosis) (Figs. 5.2.-19 and 20) have to be considered in the differential diagnosis.

5.2.5.3 Whipple's Disease

The origin of this rare disease is still unknown; a bacterial infection is considered to be the cause. This disease, also known as *intestinal lipodystrophy*, mainly occurs in middle-aged men. The clinical symptoms are chronic diarrhea, abdominal discomfort, malabsorption, joint pain, weight loss and malaise. Pathologic-anatomically, there is lymphadenopathy, hyperpigmentation, hepatosplenomegaly and joint effusion. The small bowel biopsy reveals swollen villi and in the broadened lamina propria, groups of foamy macrophages containing PAS-positive material, the so-called *lipogranulomata*. These and bacterial structures may also be found in other organs and in lymph nodes. With appropriate antibiotic therapy, remission can be achieved.

In enteroclysis, morphological and functional alterations may be found (Antes and Kruis 1982). The inflamed mucosa and mural infiltration result in a fine granular surface, thickened folds and nodular wall infiltrations. Enlarged mesenteric lymph nodes may displace or compress the bowel. In a florid stage of the disease, there is an additional sign of *nonspecific enteritis or mucosal irritation* with hyperperistalsis (Fig. 5.2.-21). After therapy and in remission, the alterations recede largely (Fig. 5.2.-22).

5.2.5.4 Small Bowel Ulcer

The primary nonspecific small bowel ulcer is rare. The favorite localizations are the upper jejunum and lower ileum. These nonspecific ulcers – mostly solitary (Evert et al. 1948) but occasionally multiple – originate from local ischemia in arteriosclerosis, vasculitis or vascular spasm, bacterial lesions, foreign bodies, ectopic gastric mucosa or Zollinger-Ellison syndrome. In the sixties, KCl tablets, dissolving in the small bowel, were also one of the causes. Other medicaments too, e.g. chlorpromazine, digitalis, indomethacin and steroids, are said to cause ulcers (Sturges and Krone 1973). The real cause, however, may often remain unknown. There is histological correlation with the gastric ulcer or duodenal ulcer. Inflammation and reactive connective tissue growth can cause strictures.

Clinically, there is often uncharacteristic abdominal complaints and signs of obstruction only. Complications include bleeding, penetration and perforation.

Radiographs show one or more short strictures with prestenotic dilatation (Fig. 5.2.-23). The ulcer does not always have to be depicted, as it is often scarred causing constriction (see Fig. 2.8.-3, p. 19)

5.2.5.5 Parasites/Worms

Giardia lamblia and worms are the most frequent pathogenic parasites in the small bowel.

Giardiasis (Lambliasis): The pathogen is the flagellated single-cell Giardia lamblia, which mostly invades the duodenum and jejunum and may result in endemic or epidemic diarrhea. There are also asymptomatic carriers, however. Increased infection susceptibility has been reported in hypo- or dysgammaglobulinemia (Ament and Rubin 1972). Therefore it cannot be clearly differentiated whether a nodular lymphatic hyperplasia in giardiasis in the jejunum is a consequence of an infection or the manifestation of an immunoglobulin disease.

In a condition of nonspecific enteritis or mucosal irritation of the upper small bowel with hyperperistalsis, with or without recognizable lymphofollicular hyperplasia, differential diagnosis must include the possibility of lambliasis (Figs. 5.2.-24 and 4.5.-2, pp. 48–51).

Worms: Ascaris and tape worms are the most frequently found worms in the small intestine. Enteroclysis can detect these intestinal parasites without difficulties (Fig. 5.2.-25).

5.2.5.6 Miscellaneous

Due to the close contact with other abdominal organs, inflammatory processes may also involve the small bowel (Fig. 5.2.-26).

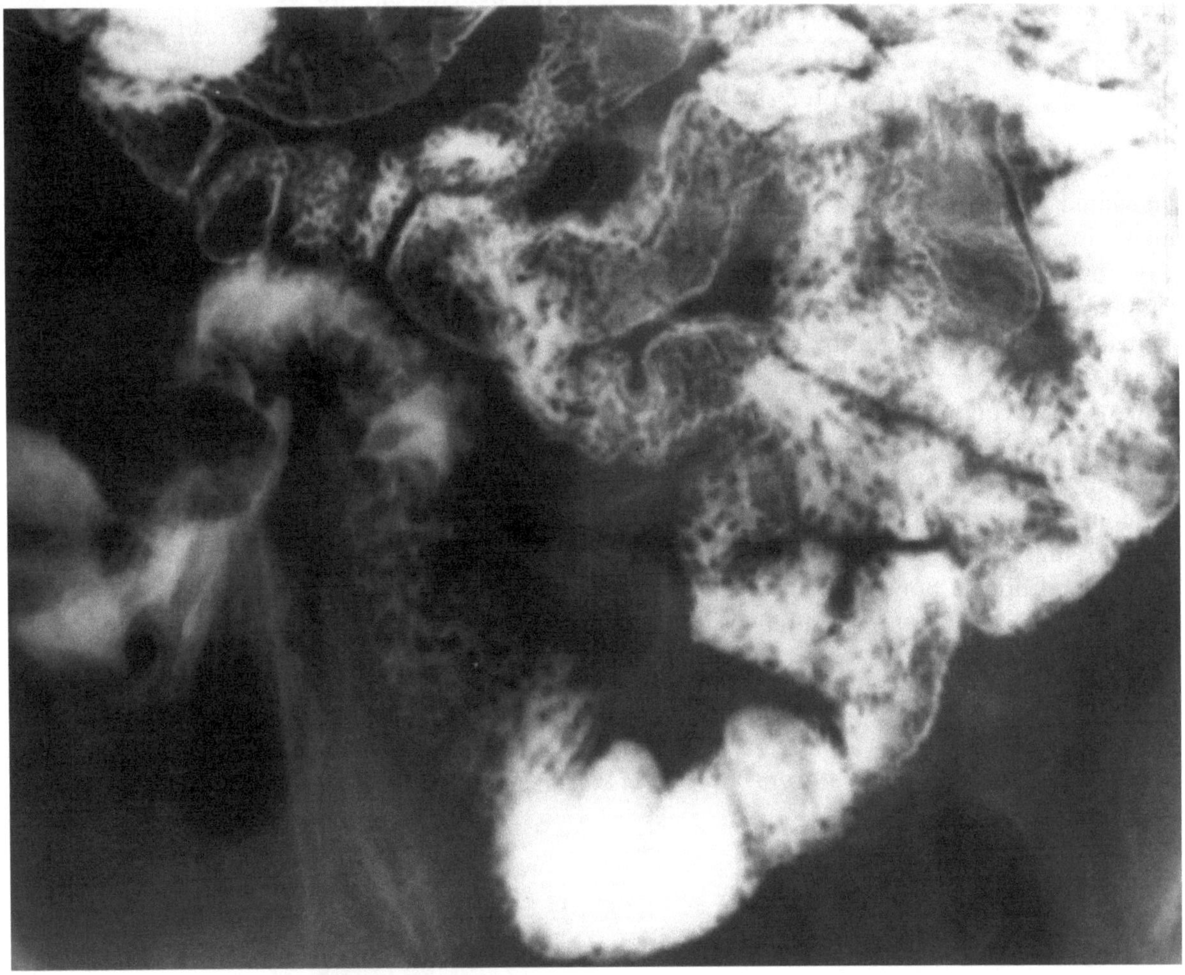

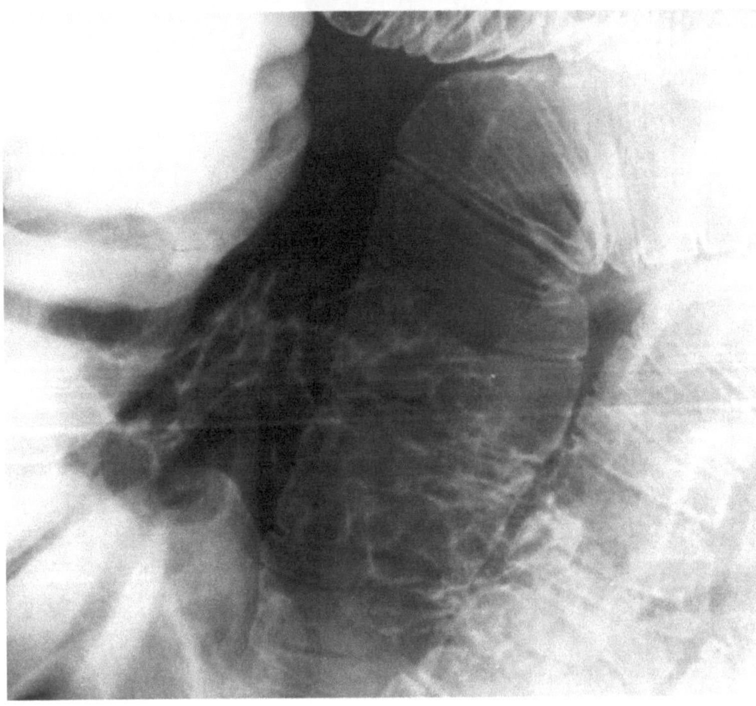

Fig. 5.2.-1. Lymphofollicular hyperplasia. Accidental finding in the entire ileum in an asymptomatic 32-year-old man

Fig. 5.2.-2. Lymphofollicular hyperplasia. Enlarged lymph follicles in the terminal ileum in a 31-year-old patient with IgA deficiency

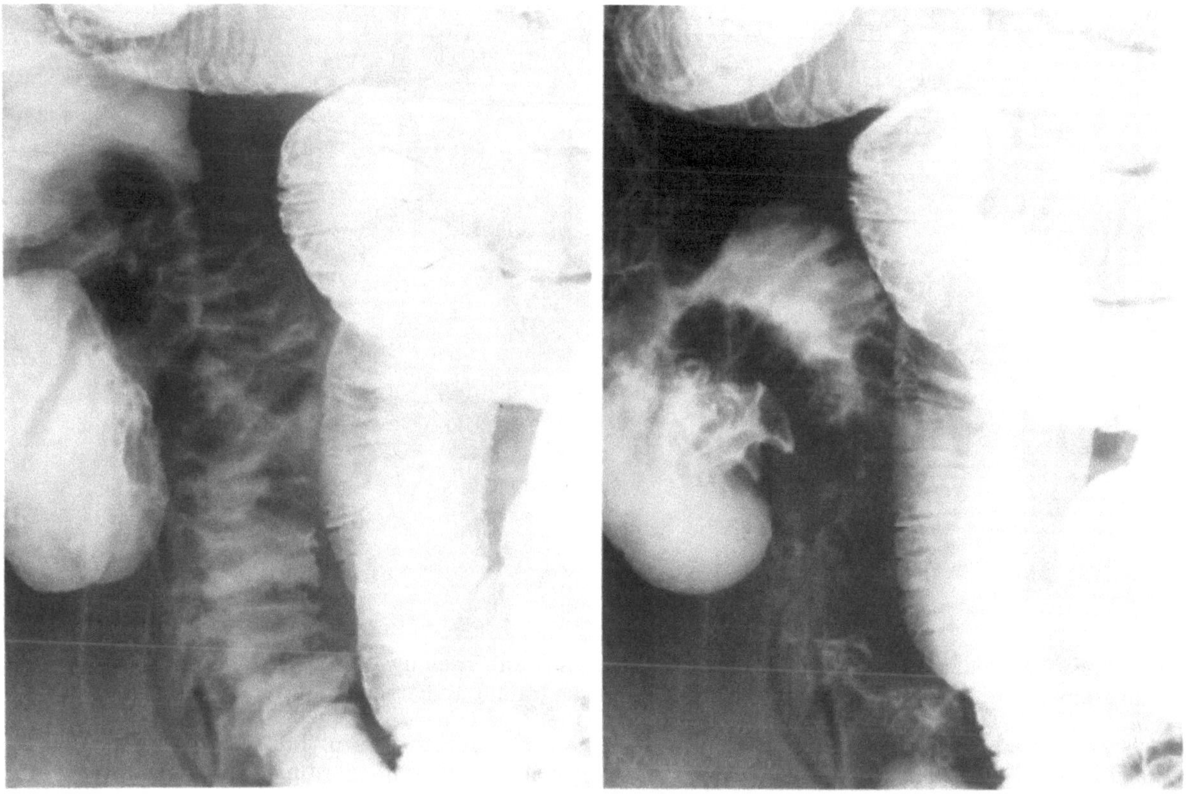

a b

Fig. 5.2.-3a and b. Yersinia enteritis. Irregularly thickened mucosal folds with reduced mucosal coating in the terminal ileum and swollen ileocecal valve (**a**). Local hyperperistalsis, but no evidence of string sign (**b**). Patient with diarrhea, crampy abdominal pain and recurrent joint pain. High titer against Yersinia enterocolica type III

Fig. 5.2.-4a and b. Yersinia enteritis. Young female with disease in the terminal ileum. Single (**a**) and double (**b**) contrast. Similar changes as in Fig. 5.2.-3

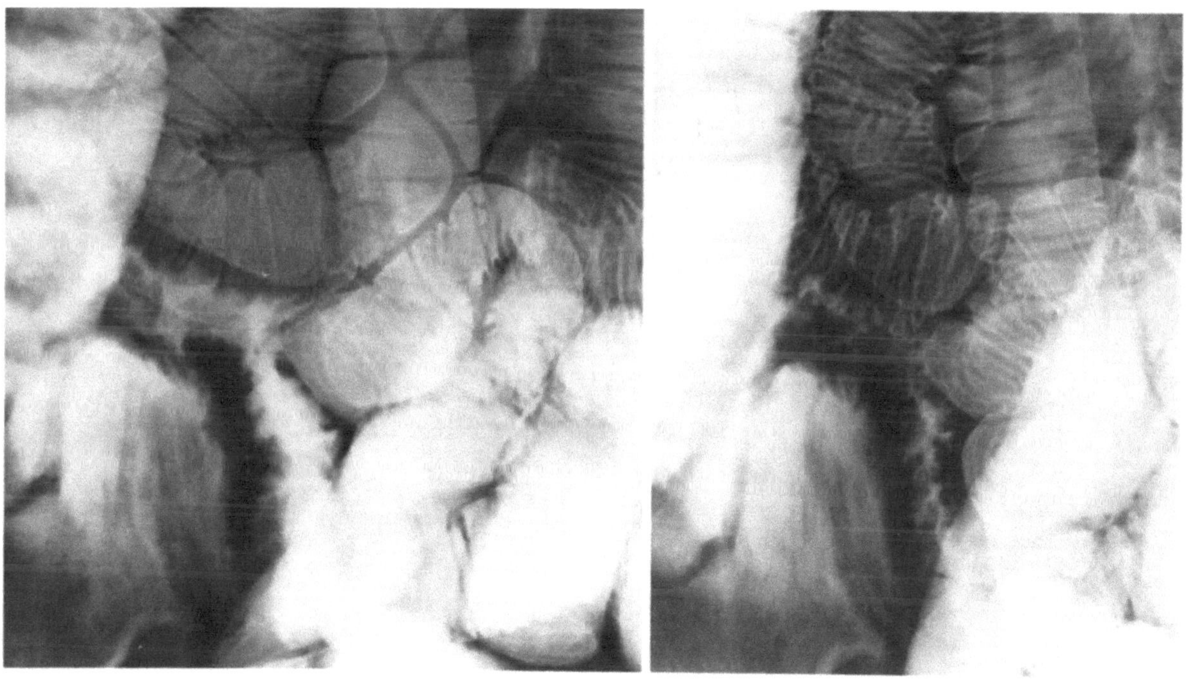

a b

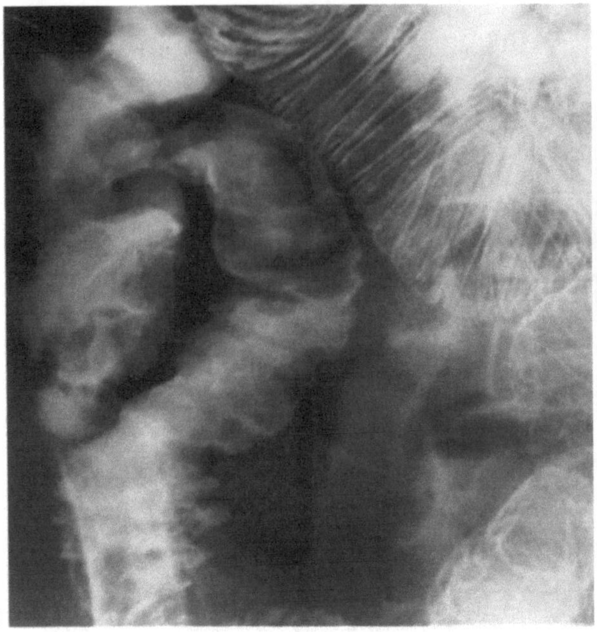

5

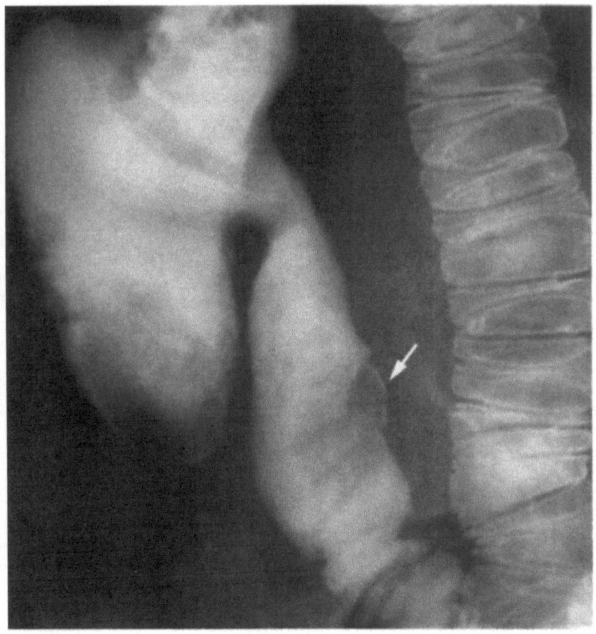

6

Fig. 5.2.-5. Yersinia enteritis. Terminal ileum with significant swelling of the folds and Peyer's patches. Young female with abdominal pain in the lower right quadrant and diarrhea of 4 weeks duration

Fig. 5.2.-6. Campylobacter enteritis, chronic. Smooth surface due to loss of folds in the terminal ileum and ulceration (→). Widened ileocecal valve. Distancing of the adjacent intestinal loops, probably due to an accompanying inflammatory reaction in the mesentery. Histologically, there was nonspecific inflammation and lymphatic hyperplasia. Significantly raised titer against Campylobacter. 44-year-old female with recurrent cramps in the right lower quadrant of 3 years duration, recently presenting with bloody diarrhea

Fig. 5.2.-7. Nonspecific ileitis. Similar picture as in Yersinia infection. Histologically and endoscopically, nonspecific ileitis. Young female with diarrhea, whose complaints disappeared after symptomatic treatment

Fig. 5.2.-8. Tuberculosis. Enlarged Peyer's patches and distorted folds. Thickened ileocecal valve. Reduced mucosal coating

7

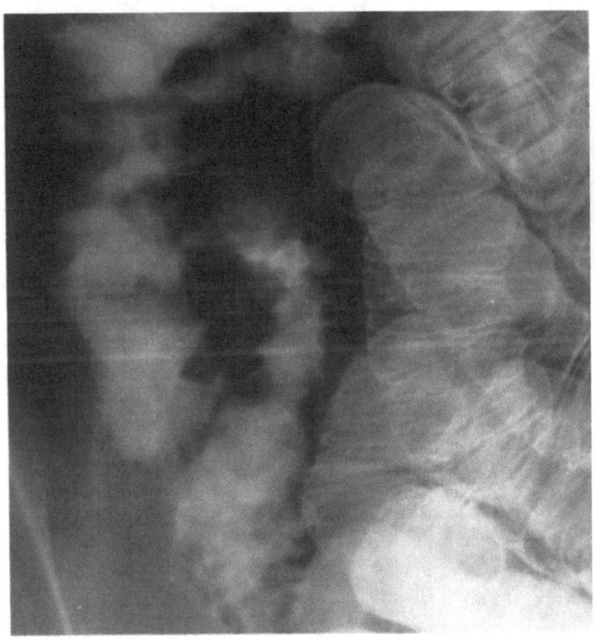

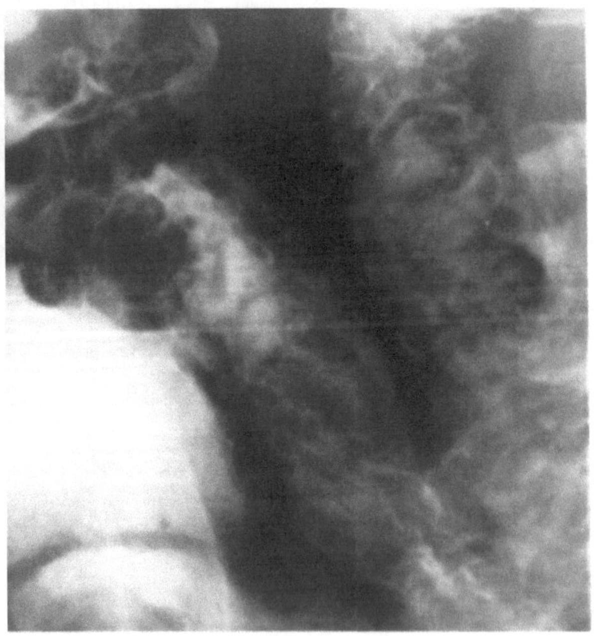

8

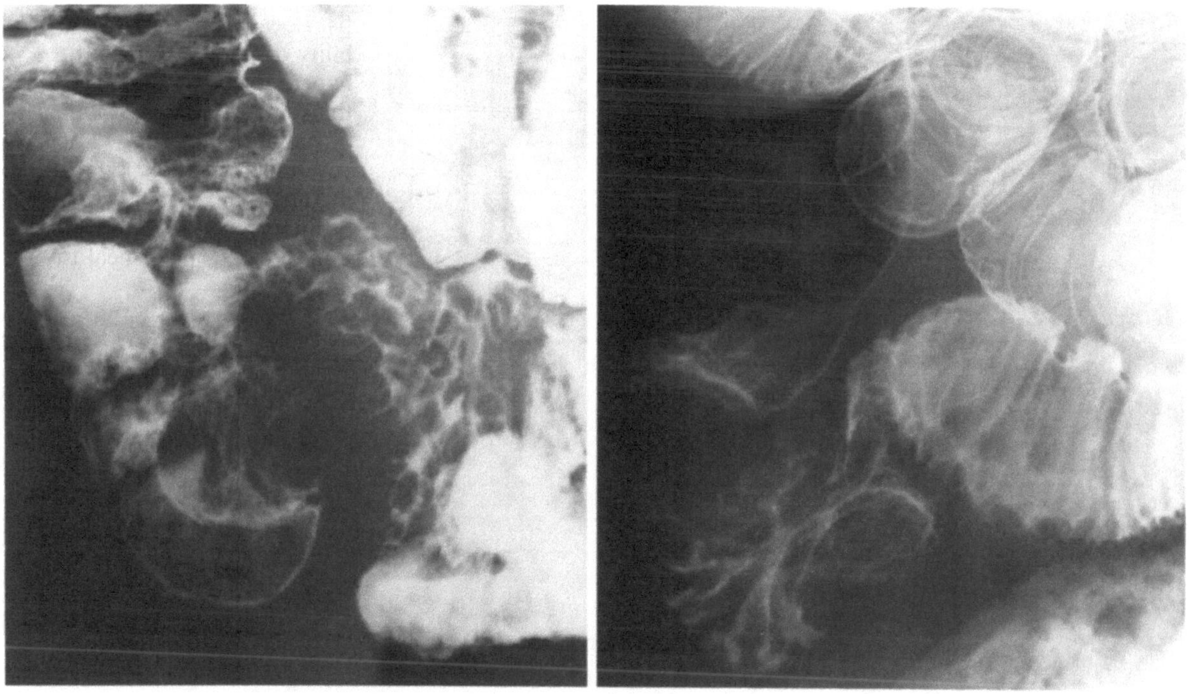

a b

Fig. 5.2.-9a and b. Tuberculosis. Cobblestone pattern in the terminal ileum and thickened ileocecal region (**a**). Normalization of the terminal ileum after tuberculostatic treatment two years later (**b**). Cicatricially shrunken cecum

Fig. 5.2.-10a and b. Tuberculosis. Ileocecal region in barium enema (**a**). Similar picture can be produced through invasion of the cecum by Crohn's disease (**b**)

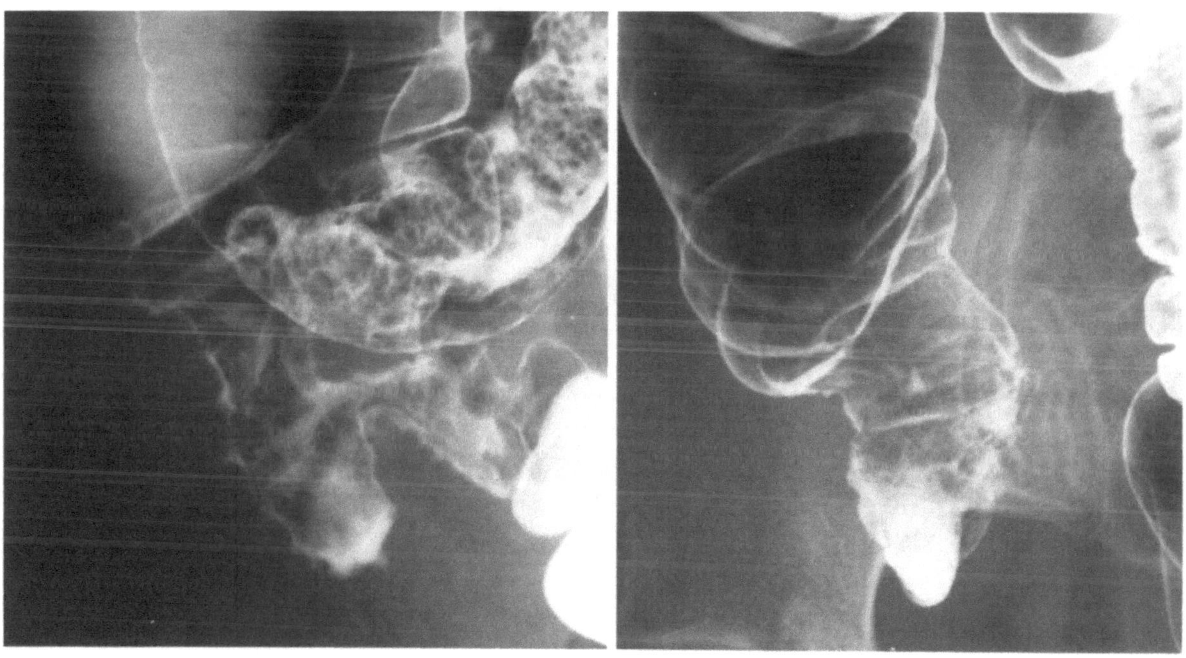

a b

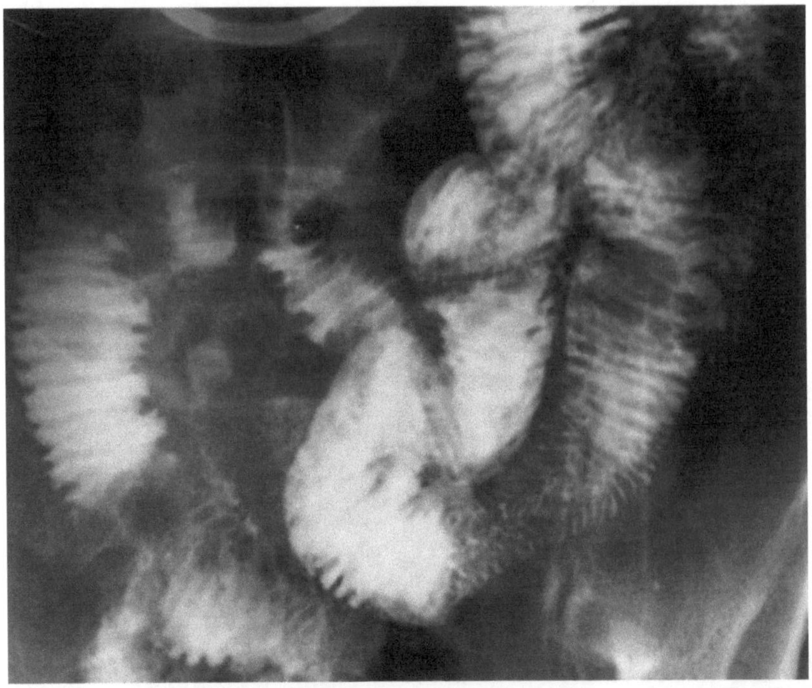

Fig. 5.2.-11. Radiation enteritis. Locally reduced distensibility of the intestine with hyperperistalsis and slight fold thickening in a less severe case of radiation enteritis. Patient with recurrent, colicky abdominal pain lasting 4 years, beginning 2 years after radiation of a retroperitoneal tumor

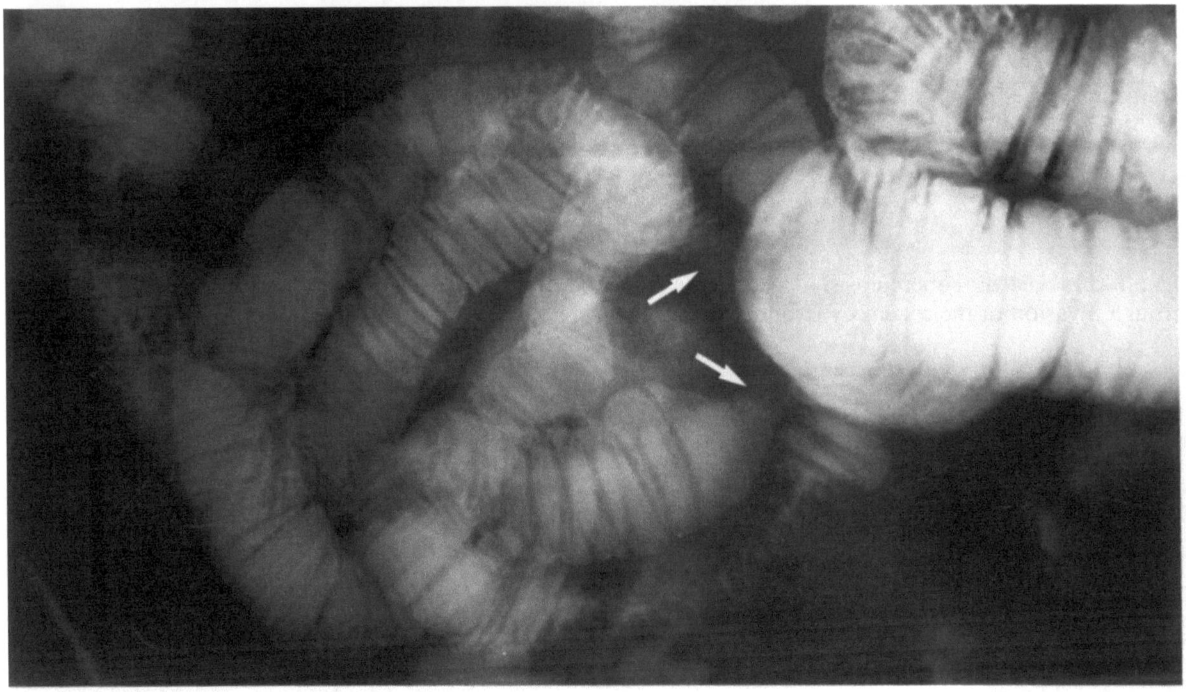

12a

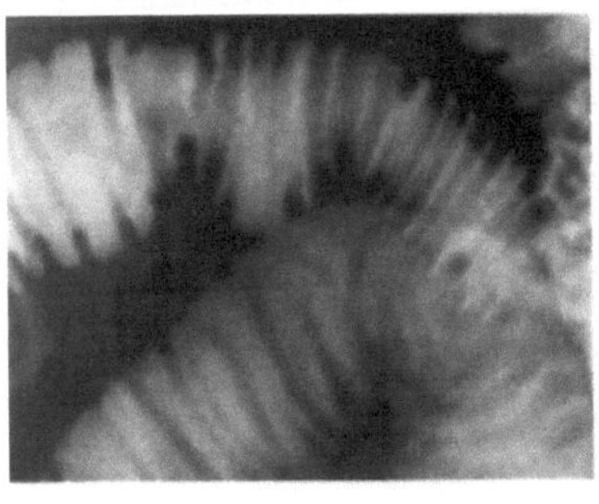

12b

Fig. 5.2.-12a and b. Radiation enteritis. Circumscribed immobile and narrowed ileal segment (→) showing irregular thickened folds with compressed interfold spaces (**b**) and a small area of fold deficiency. There is some prestenotic dilatation and spastic hyperperistalsis proximal to it. Patient with postprandial crampy pain starting 2 years after irradiation for Hodgkin's disease. A follow-through examination was negative

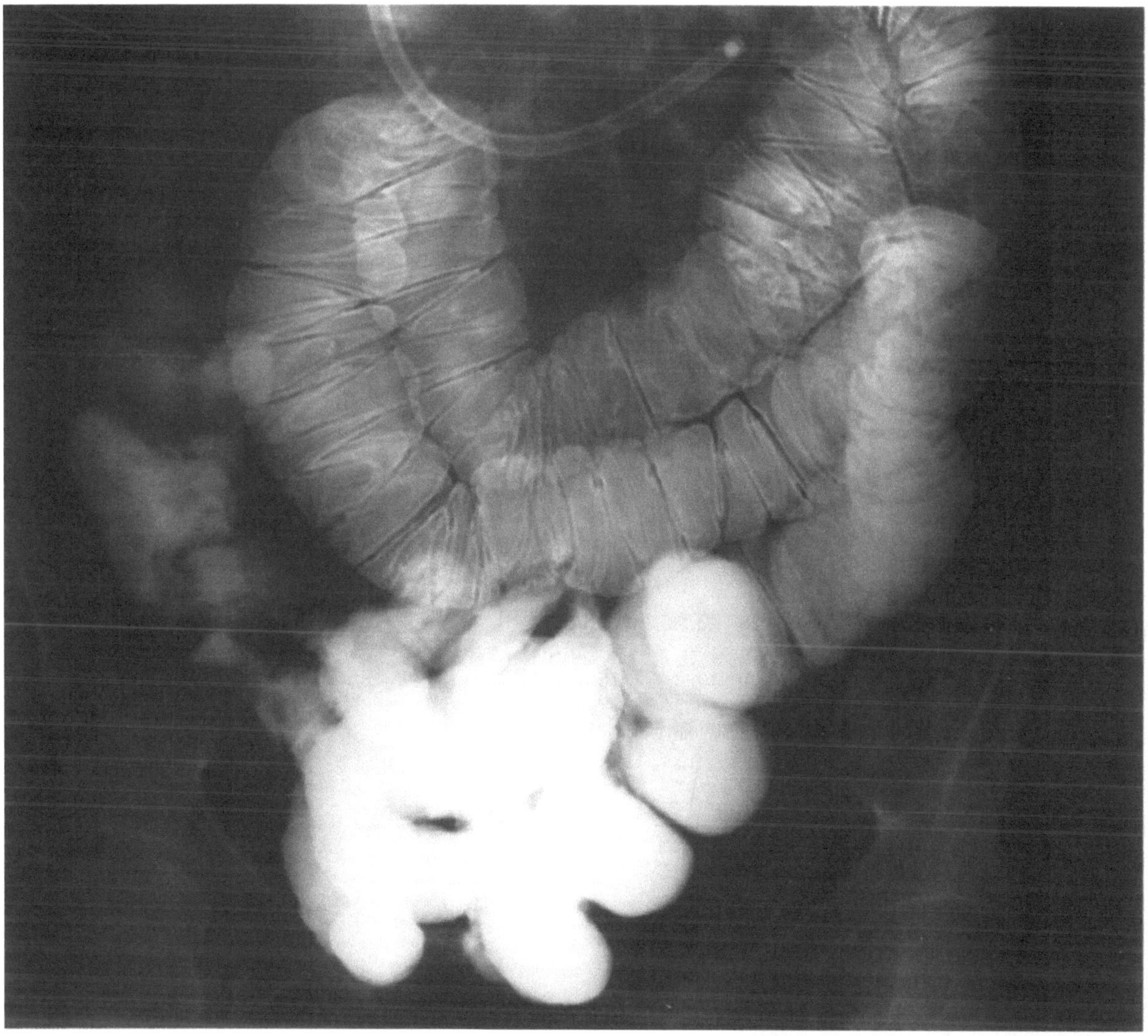

a

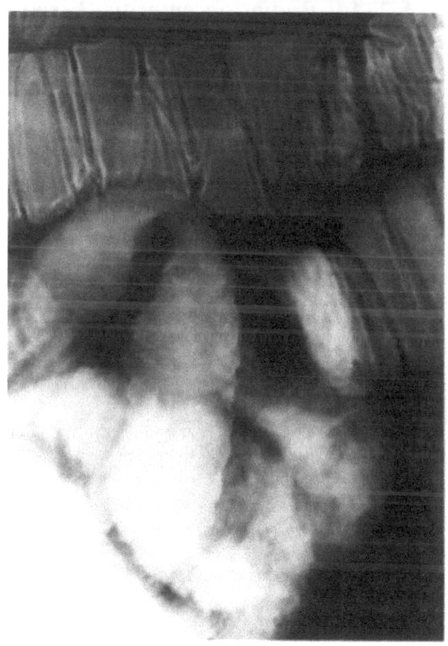

b

Fig. 5.2.-13a and b. Radiation enteritis. Localized fixed segment in the ileum with prestenotic dilatation. Gathering up of the fixed intestinal loops (**a**). In the stenosed area, the folds are thickened and flattened with reduced mucosal coating (**b**). Patient with subileus symptoms 12 years after gynecological irradiation

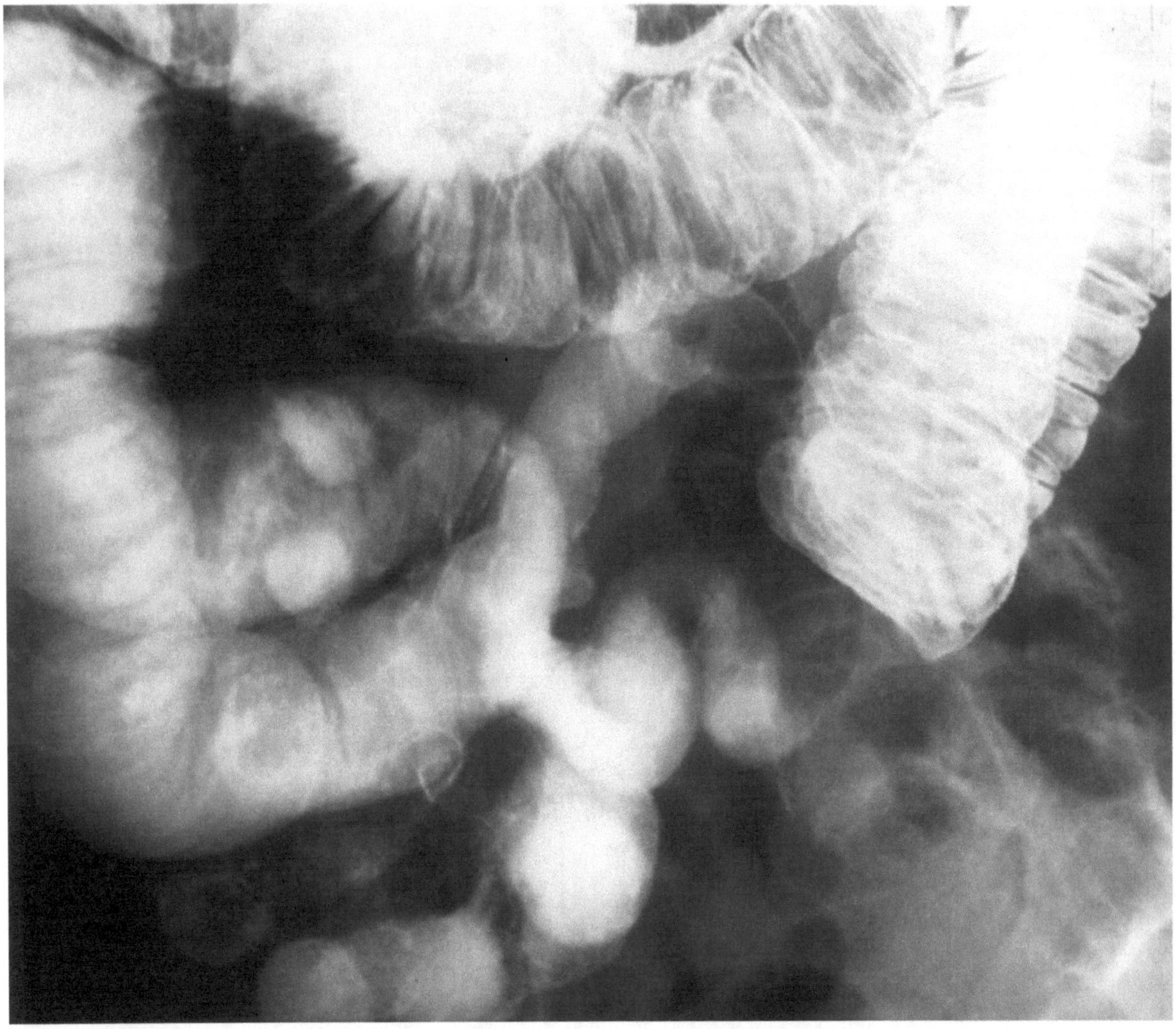

Fig. 5.2.-14. Radiation enteritis. Fixed, rigid, narrowed and foldless ileal loops with prestenotic dilatation. Reduced coating. Patient with subileus symptoms lasting several years. Irradiation for seminoma 10 years ago

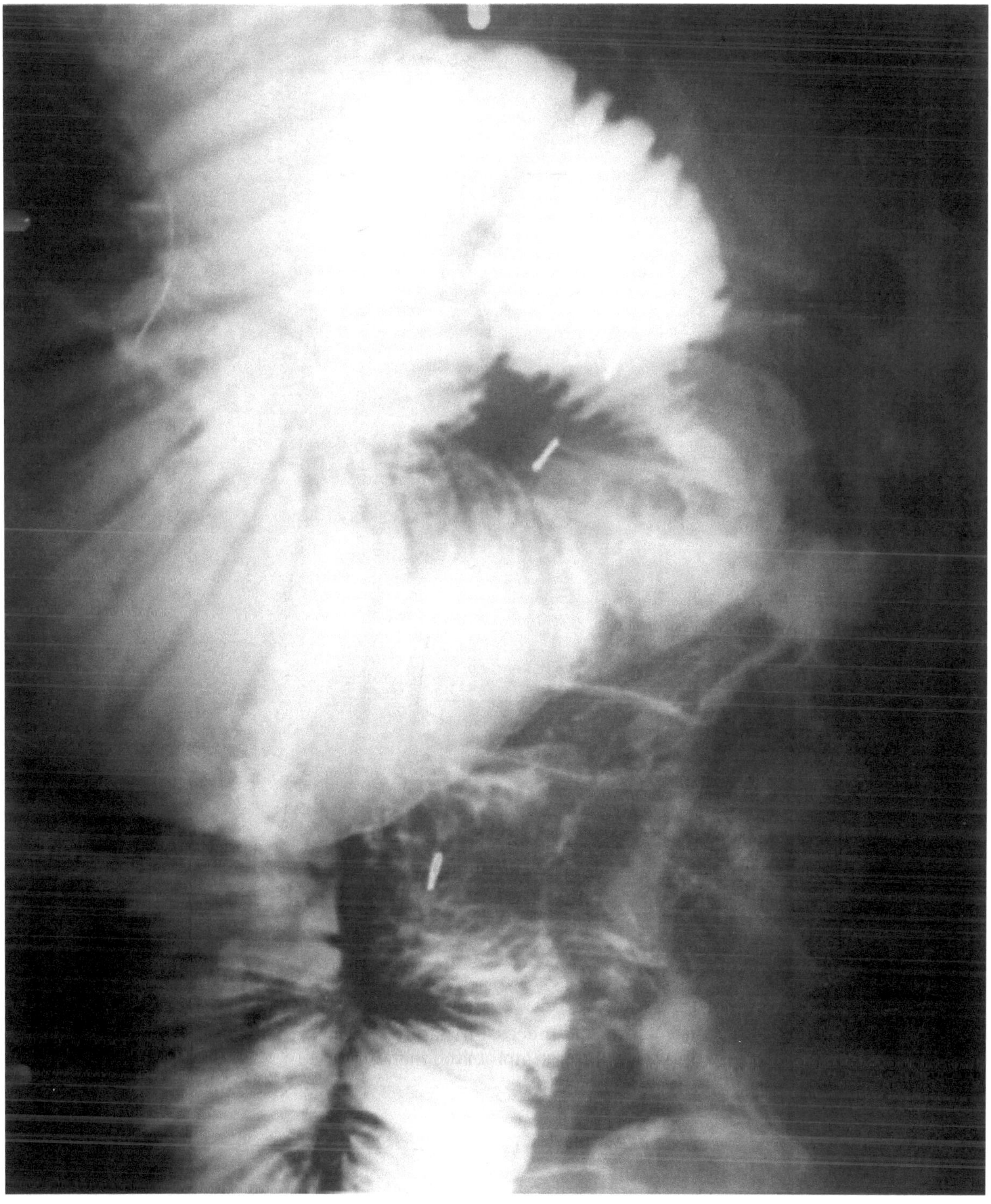

Fig. 5.2.-15. Radiation enteritis. Advanced stenosis in the jejunum after surgery and irradiation for a carcinoma of the left kidney

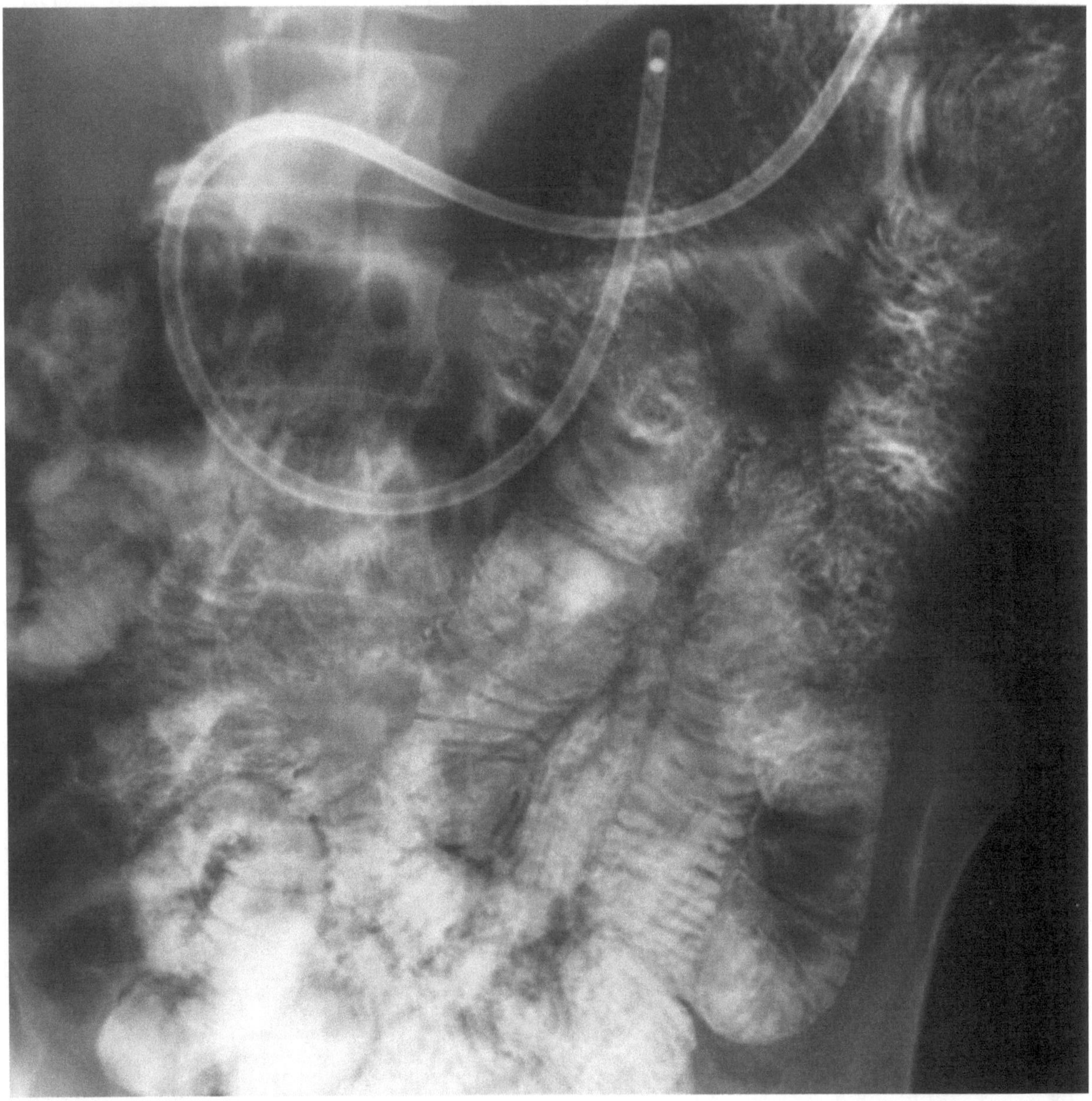

Fig. 5.2.-16. Enteritis. Nonspecific enteritis and mucosal irritation with hyperperistalsis. Patient with chronic diarrhea after a trip to Asia. Improvement after symptomatic therapy

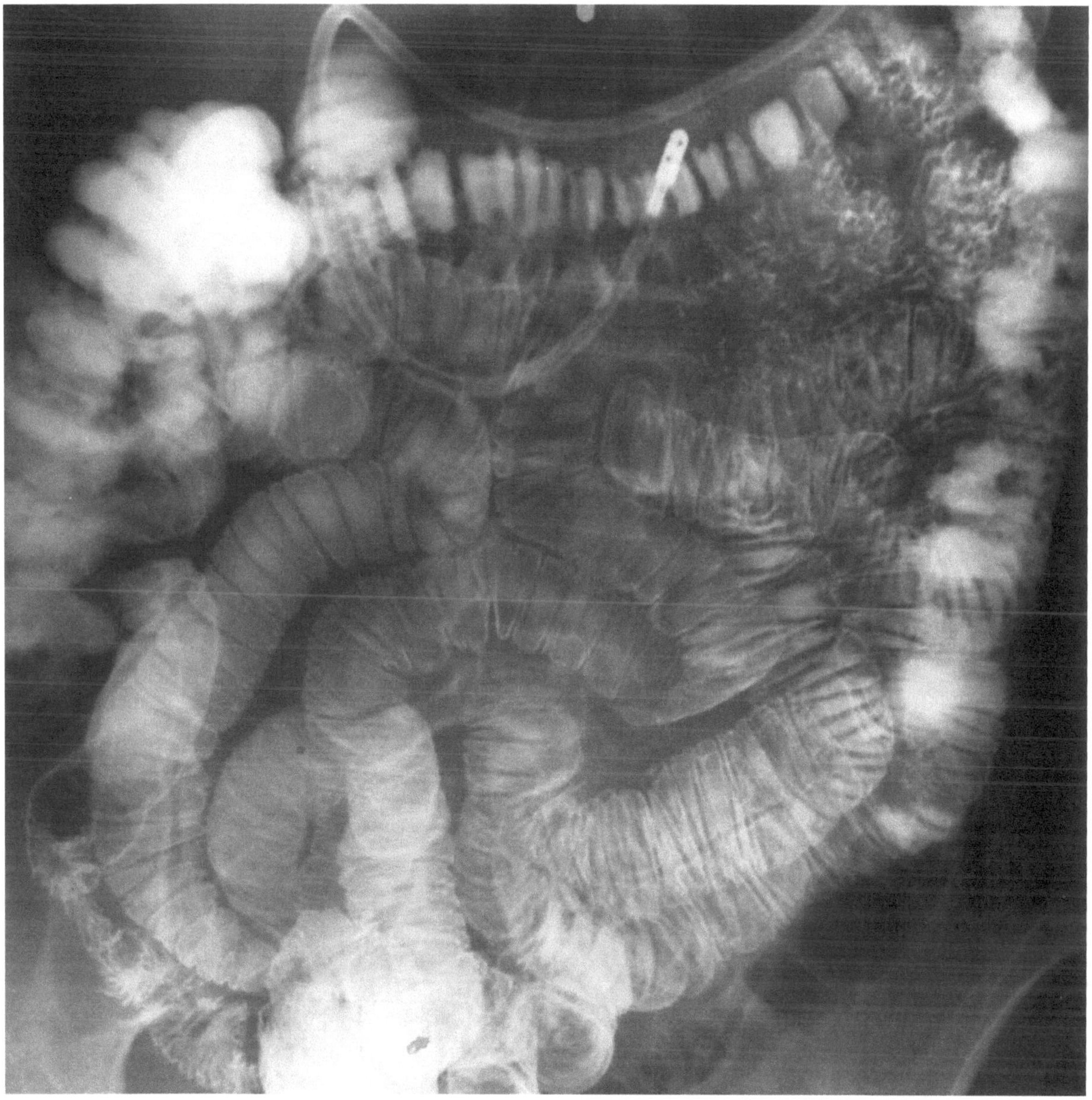

Fig. 5.2.-17. Enteritis. Local hyperperistalsis and poor coating in the jejunum (no rinsing effect). Patient with nonspecific upper abdominal complaints. Small bowel biopsy revealed an erosive mucosal defect and chronic inflammation. Bacteriology: Klebsiella pneumoniae

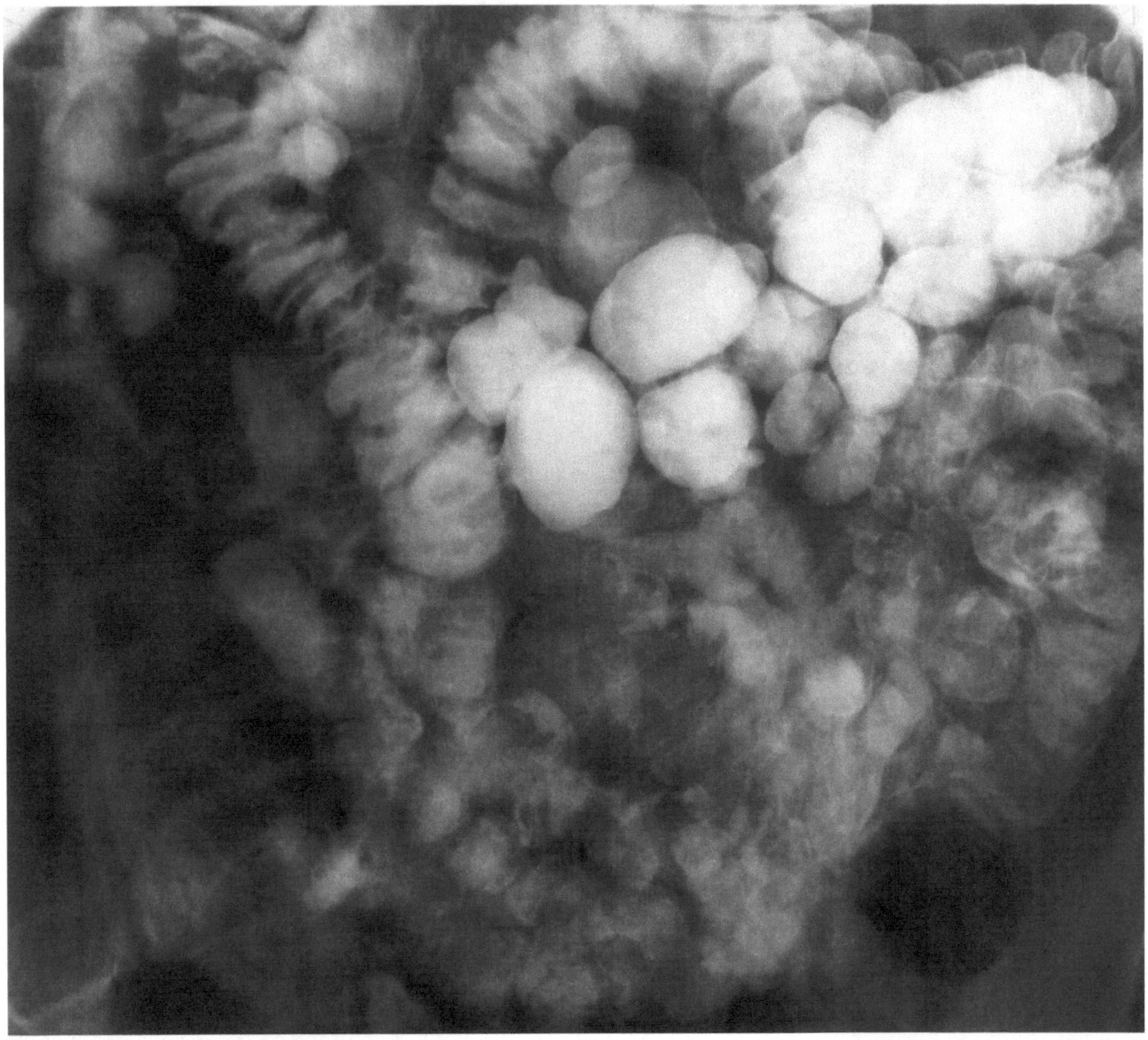

Fig. 5.2.-18. Enteritis. Due to bacterial overgrowth in small bowel diverticulosis. Nonspecific enteritis and mucosal irritation, nonpropulsive peristalsis. Patient with chronic diarrhea and malabsorption

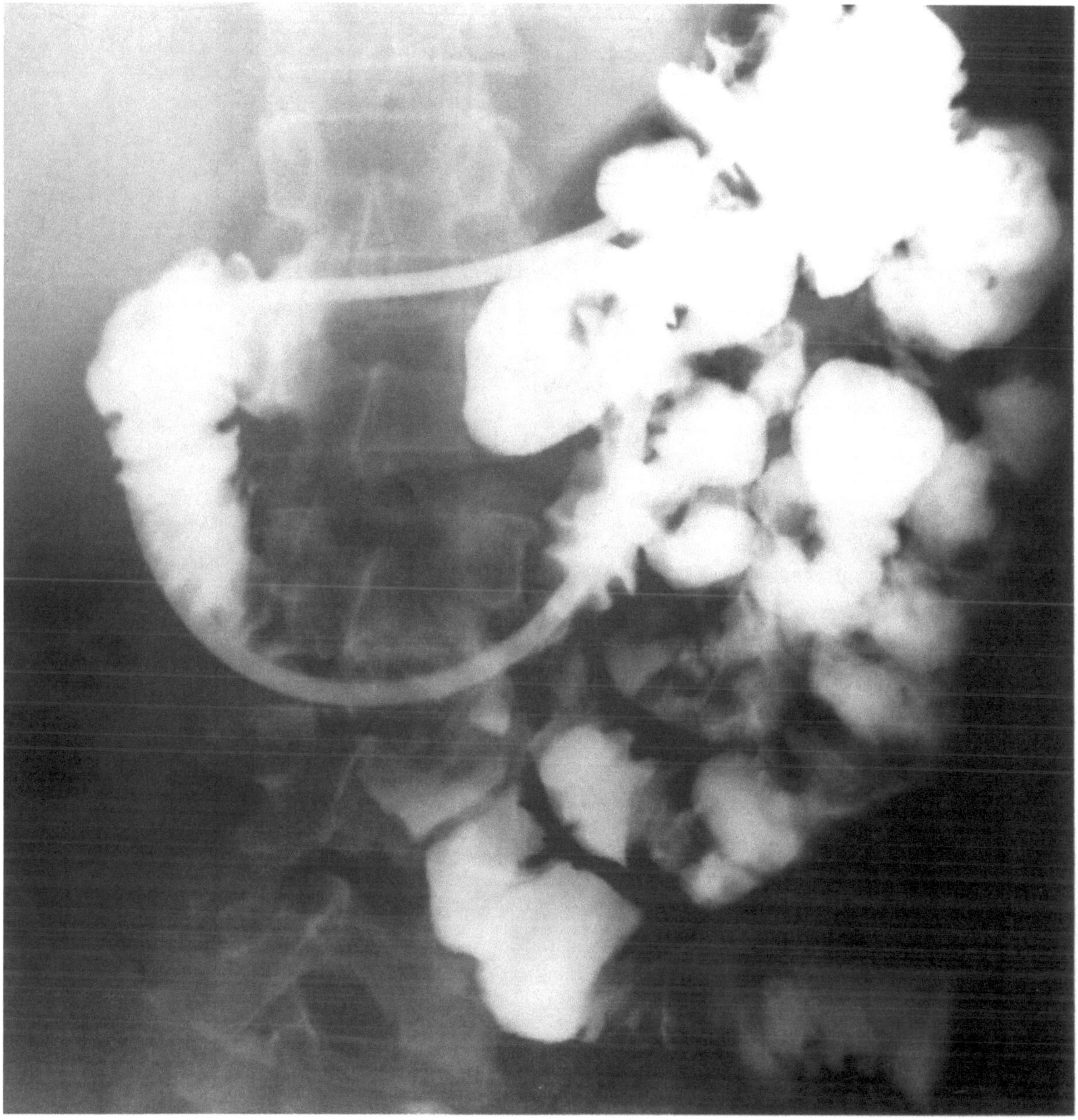

a

Fig. 5.2.-19 a to c. Eosinophilic enteritis. Thickened, distorted folds with luminal narrowing, thickening of the wall and nonspecific enteritis and mucosal irritation, nonpropulsive peristalsis. Patient with chronic diarrhea and malabsorption. Improvement on corticosteroid therapy. **a** Barium phase. **b** and **c** Methylcellulose phase

b 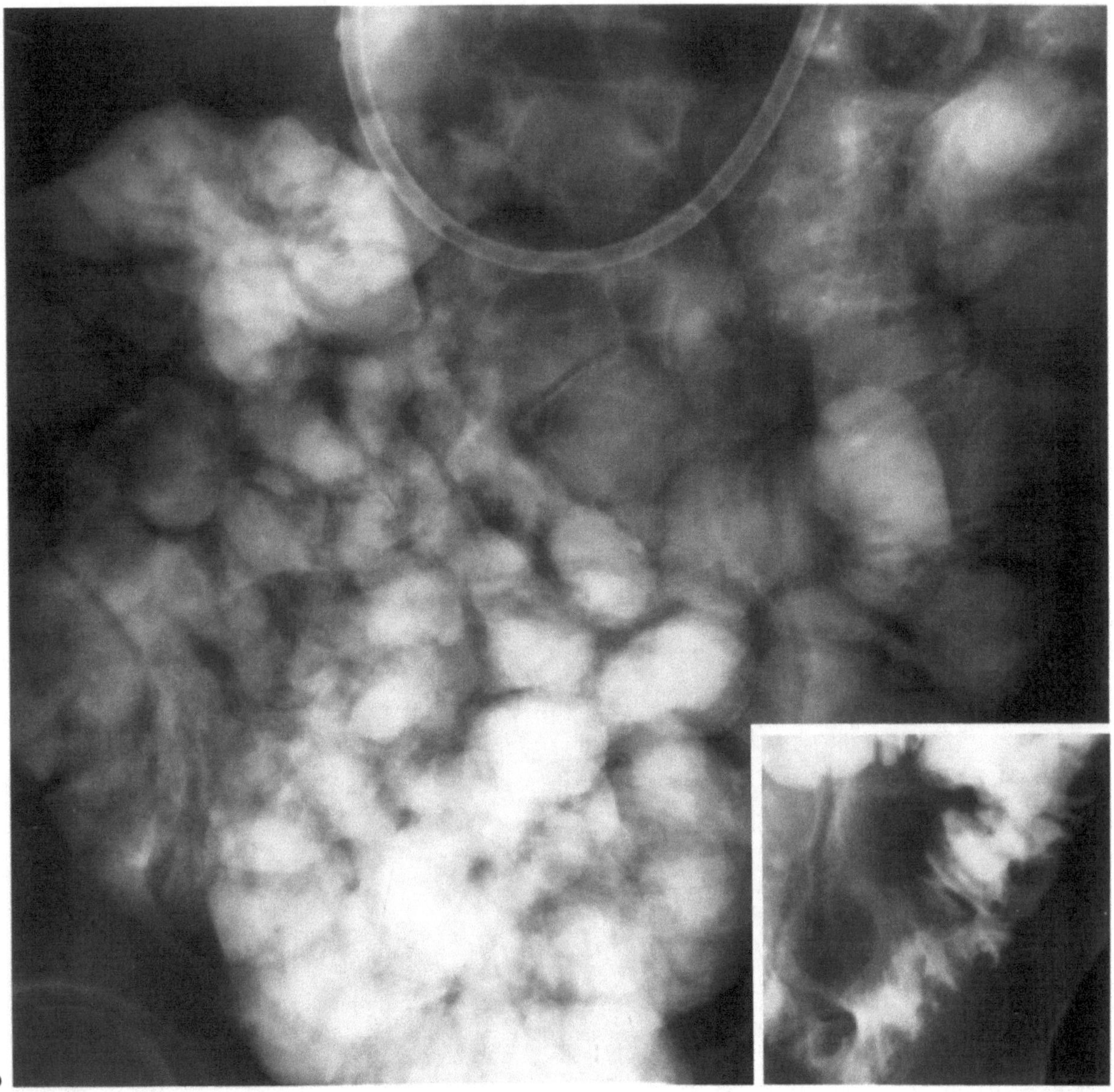 c

Fig. 5.2.-19b and c

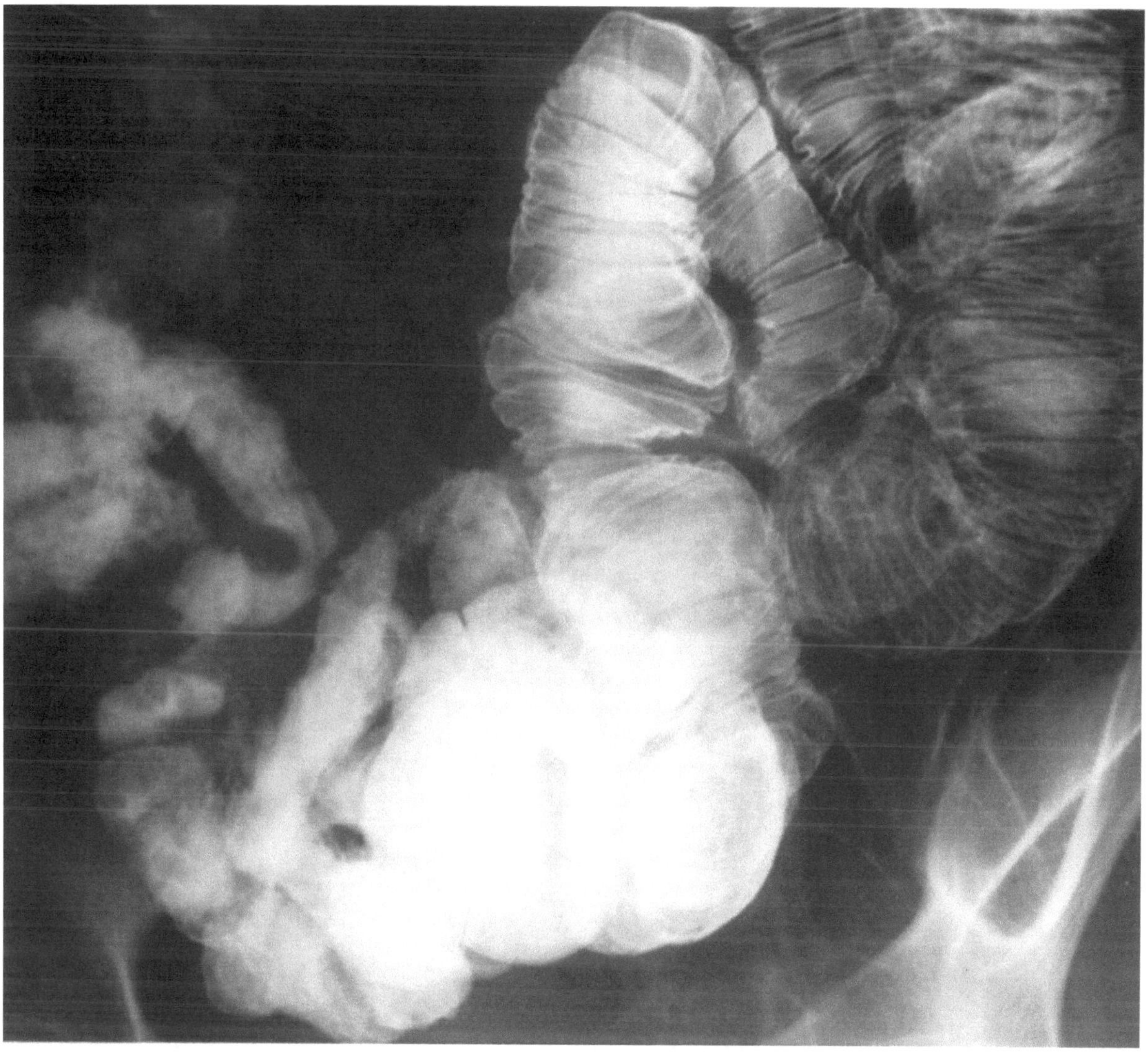

Fig. 5.2.-20. Eosinophilic enteritis. Lumen narrowing of varying degree, thickening and deformation of the folds, mainly in the ileum. 30-year-old female with persistent subileus symptoms after two small bowel segment resections due to stenoses by eosinophilic infiltrates. Blood eosinophilia. Improvement on corticosteroid therapy

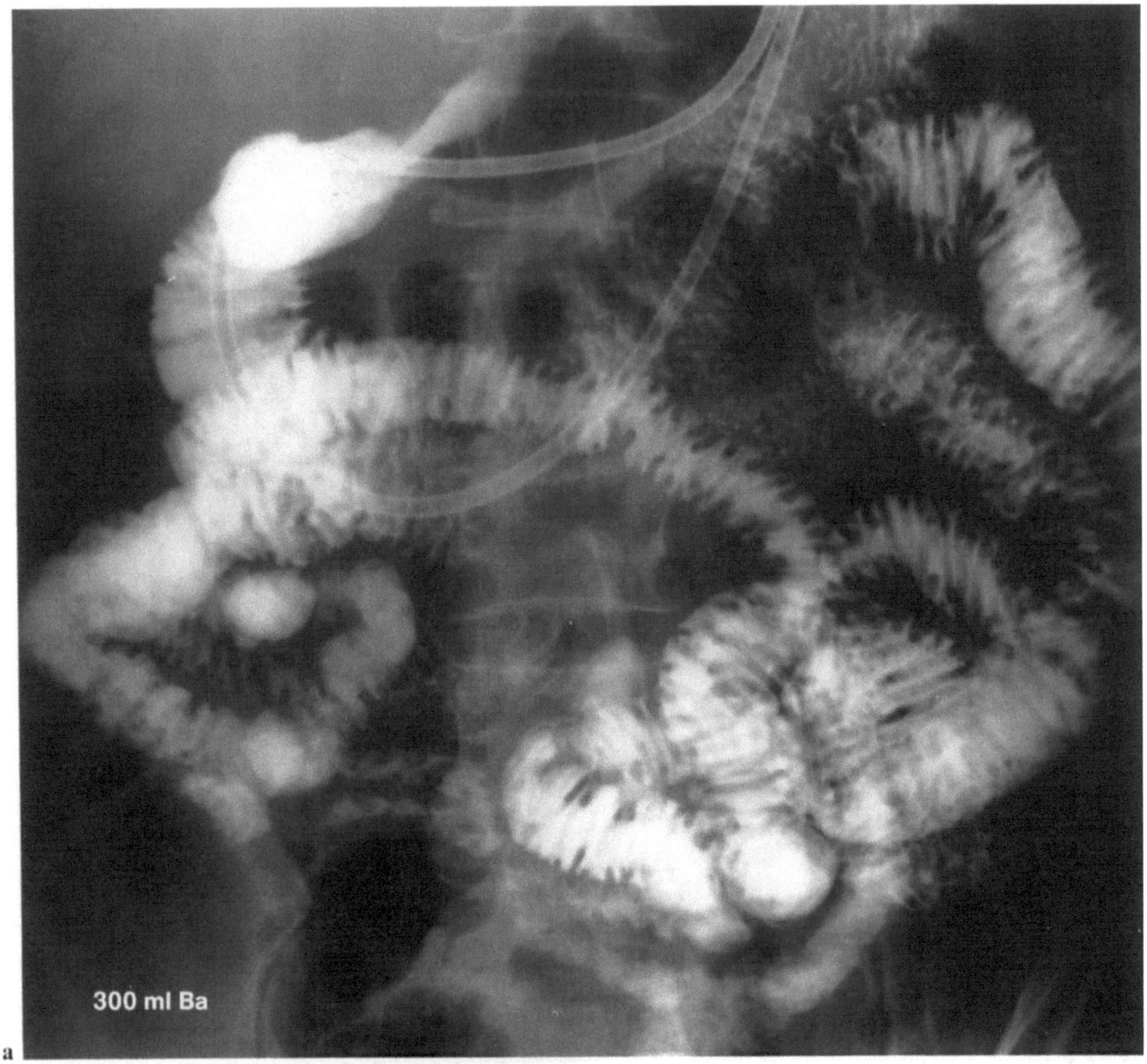

a

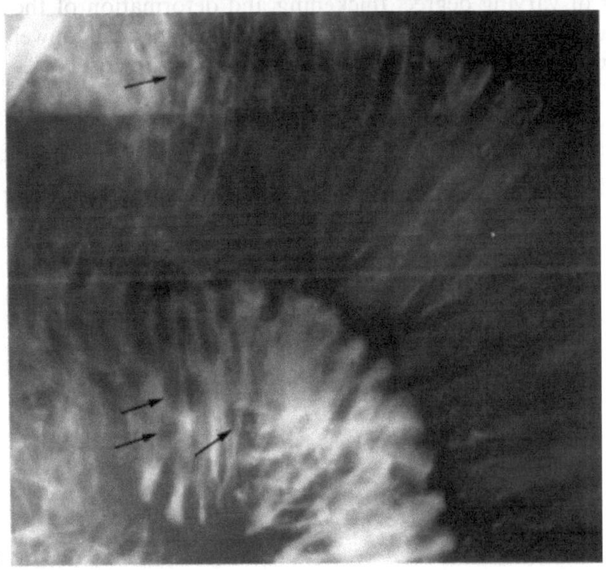

c

Fig. 5.2.-21 a to d. Whipple's disease. Hyperperistalsis in the barium phase (**a**). The methylcellulose phase shows a nonspecific enteritis and mucosal irritation, thickening of the folds (**b**). Nodular mucosal infiltrates (**c** (→) and **d**) and displacement of the terminal ileum with macronodular infiltrates by mesenteric lymph node enlargements (**b** (→) and **d**). 60-year-old male with typical clinical and histological signs of Whipple's disease

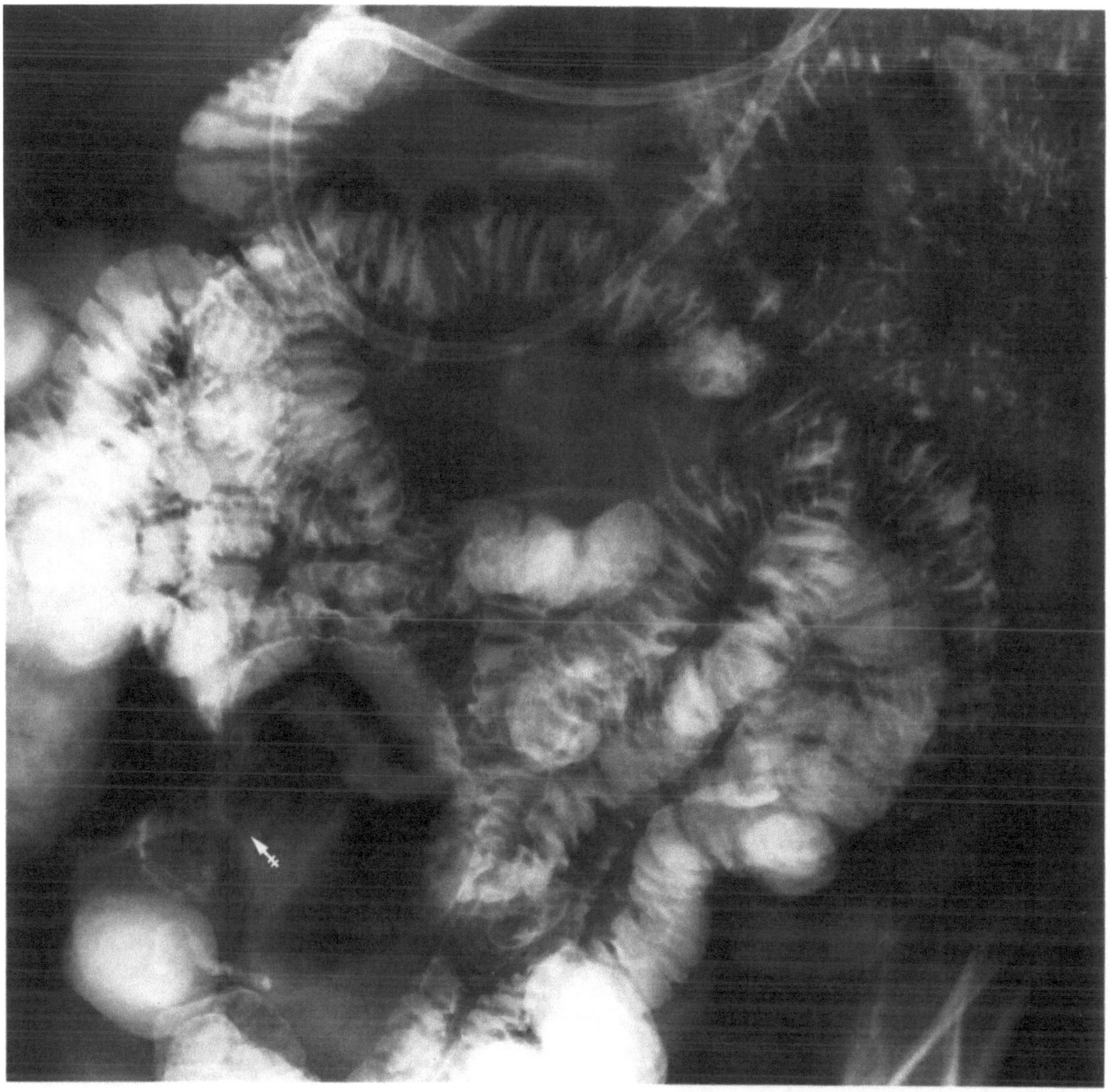

b

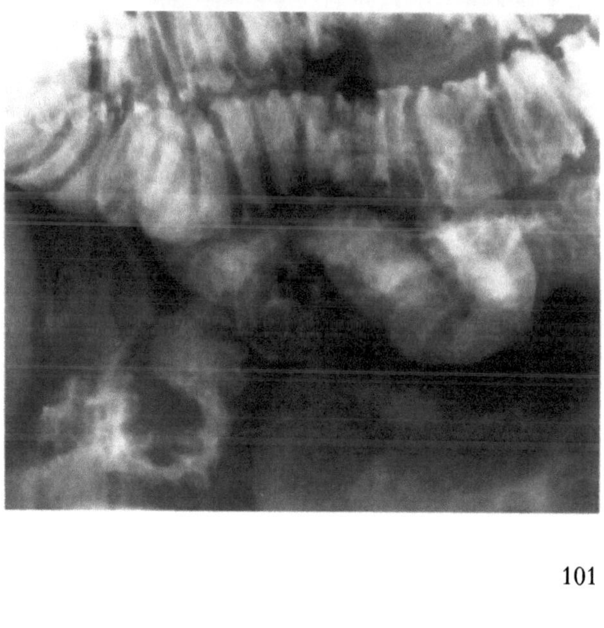

d

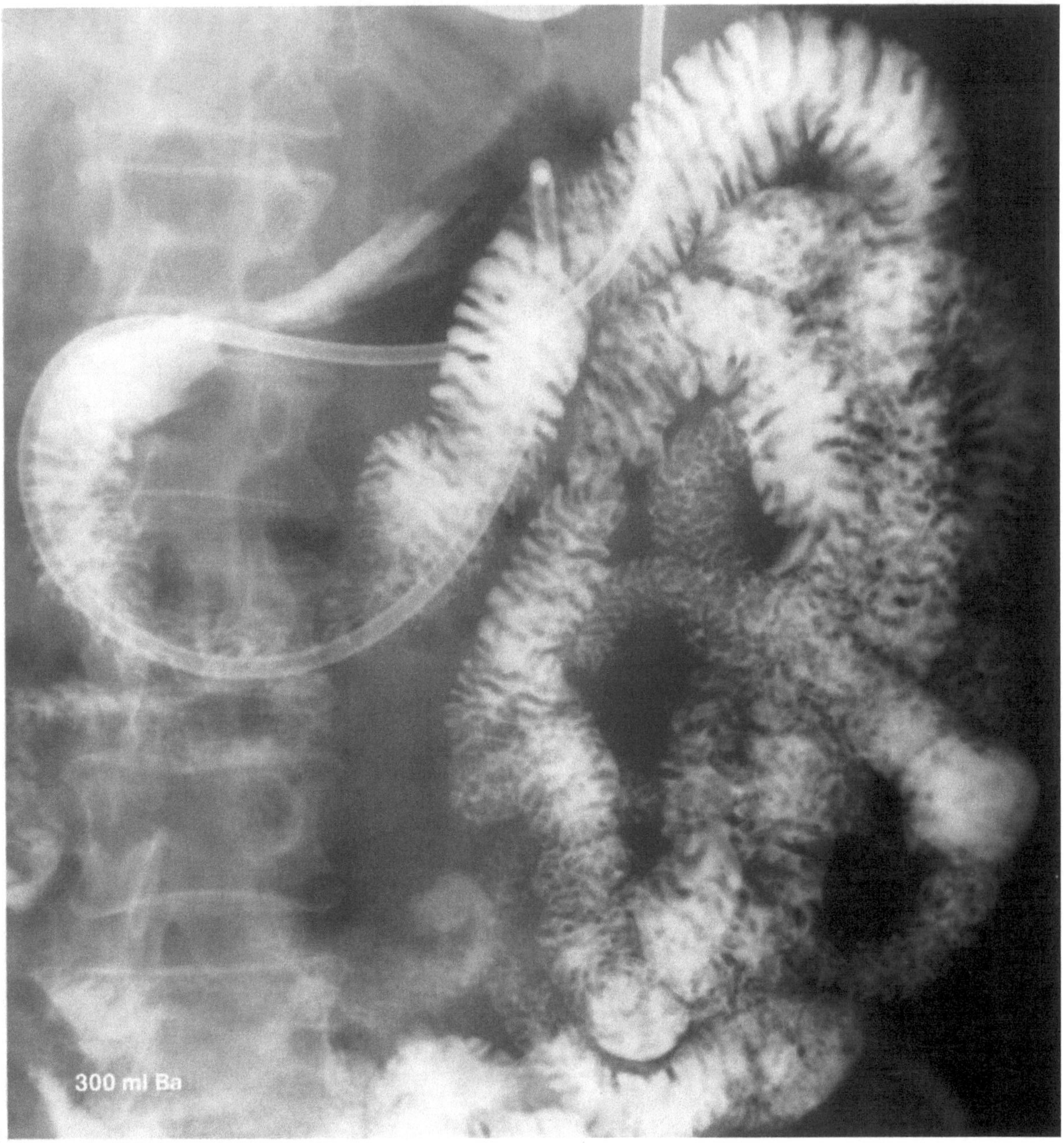

a

Fig. 5.2.-22a to c. Whipple's disease. Patient as in Fig. 5.2.-21 after antibiotic therapy and in remission. Reduction of hyperperistalsis (**a**), normalization of mucosal coating, fold configuration and position of the terminal ileum (**b**). There are still small residual infiltrates (→) in the mucosa (**c**)

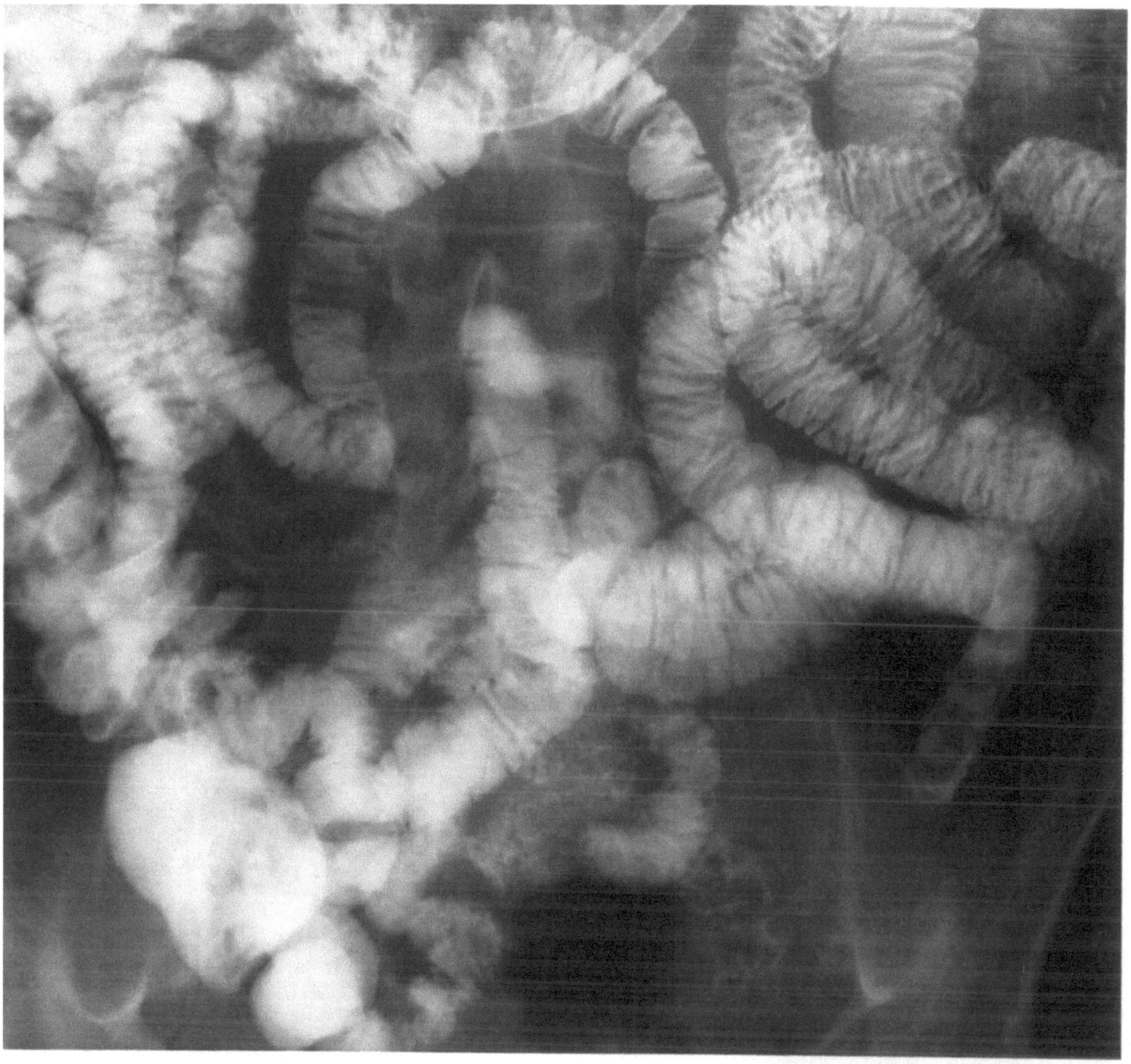

b

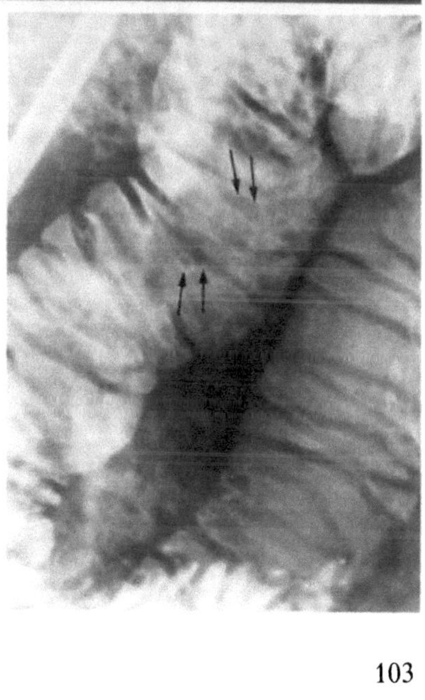

c

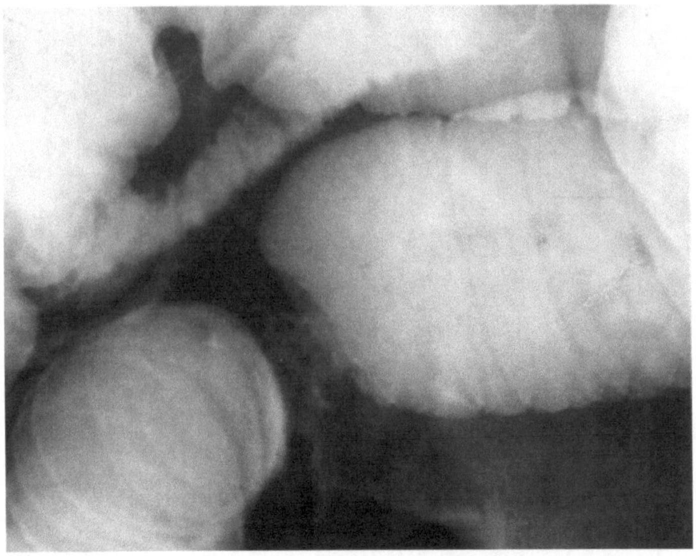

Fig. 5.2.-23. Small bowel ulcer (primary, nonspecific). Short circular stenosis in the ileum with ulceration. 69-year-old patient with diarrhea and noncharacteristic abdominal complaints

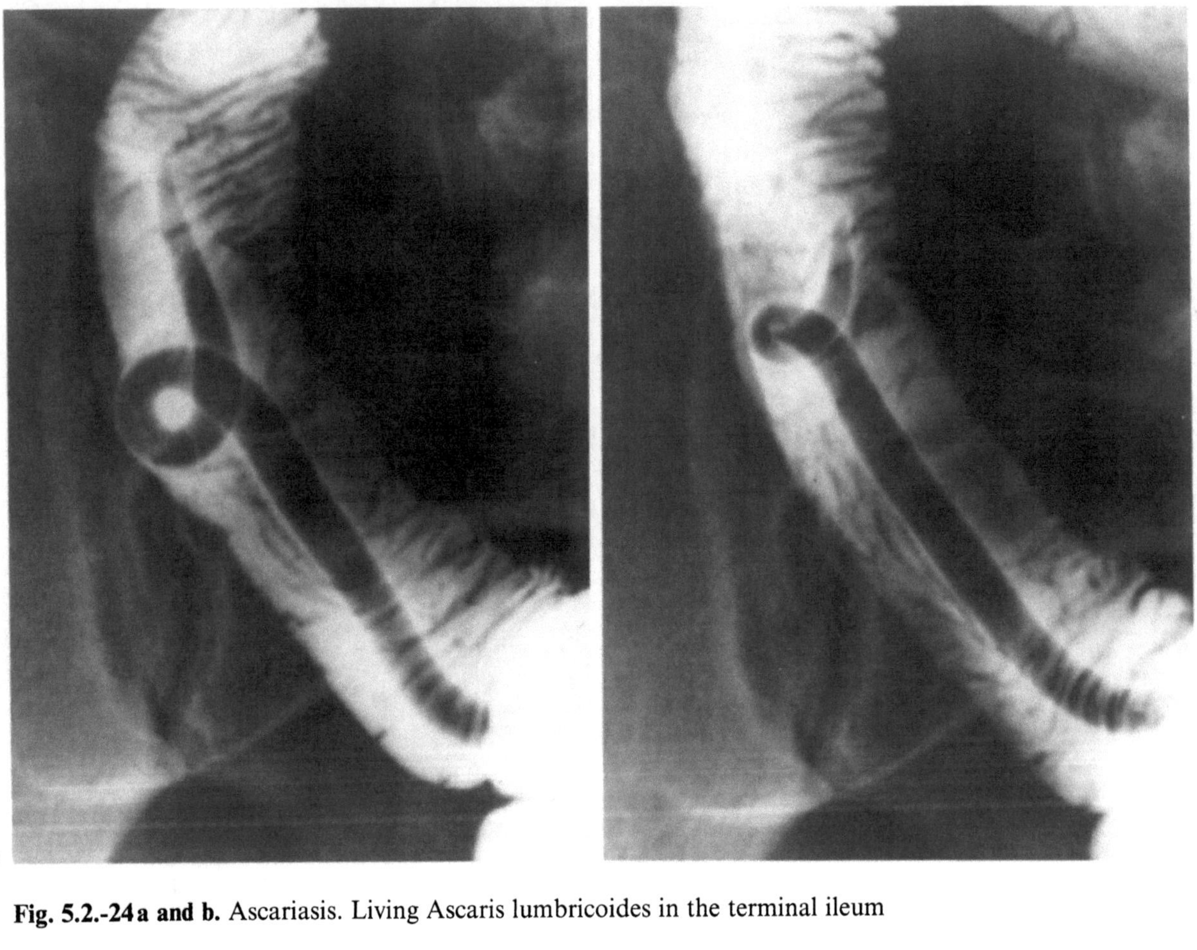

a b

Fig. 5.2.-24 a and b. Ascariasis. Living Ascaris lumbricoides in the terminal ileum

a
b

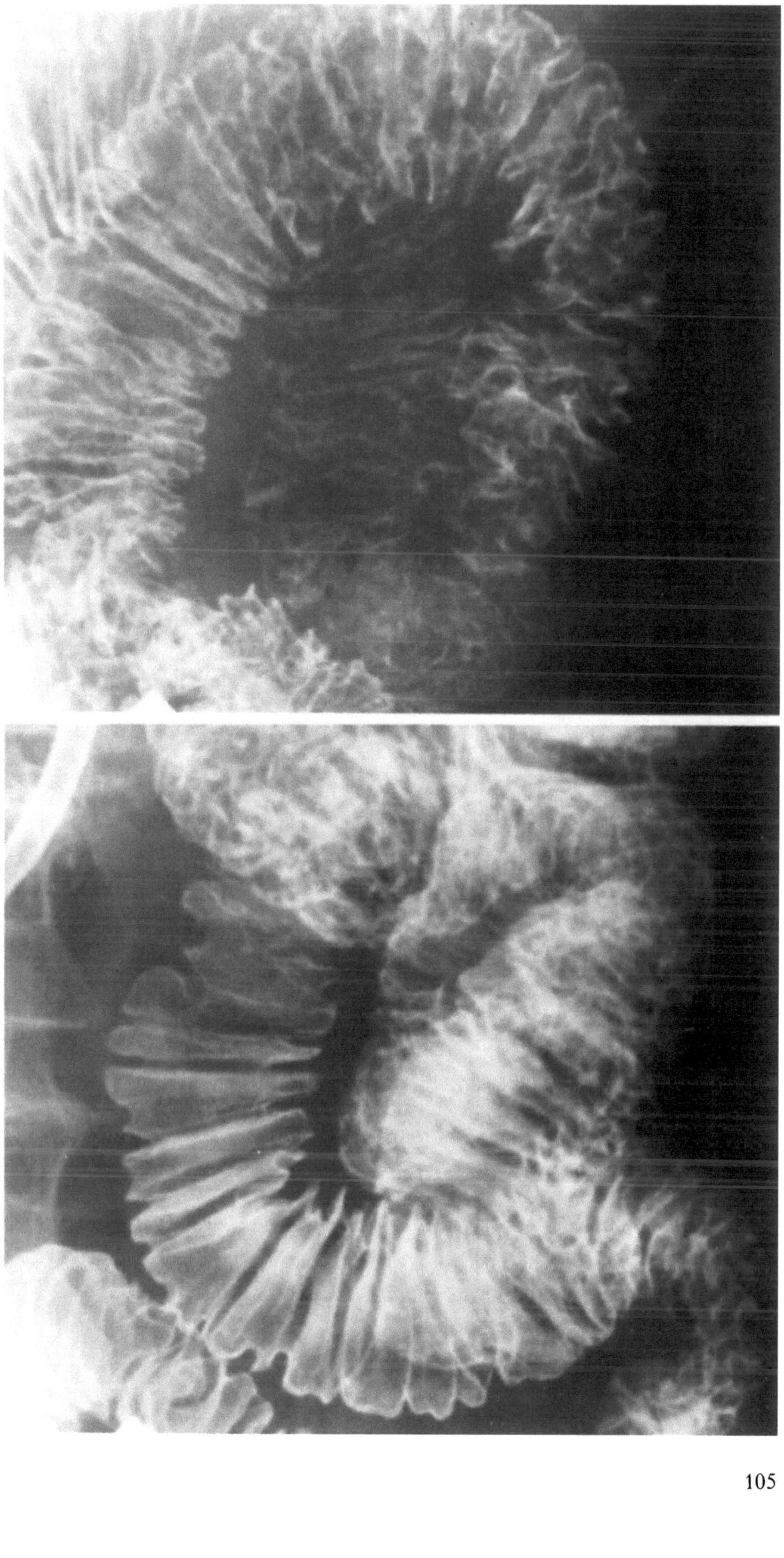

Fig. 5.2.-25 a and b. Giardiasis (lambliasis). Nonspecific enteritis and mucosal irritation prior to treatment in a patient with abdominal complaints. Giardia lamblia were found in the duodenal aspirate (**a**). After treatment, significant improvement. Folds, however, are still slightly thickened (**b**), normal mucosal coating

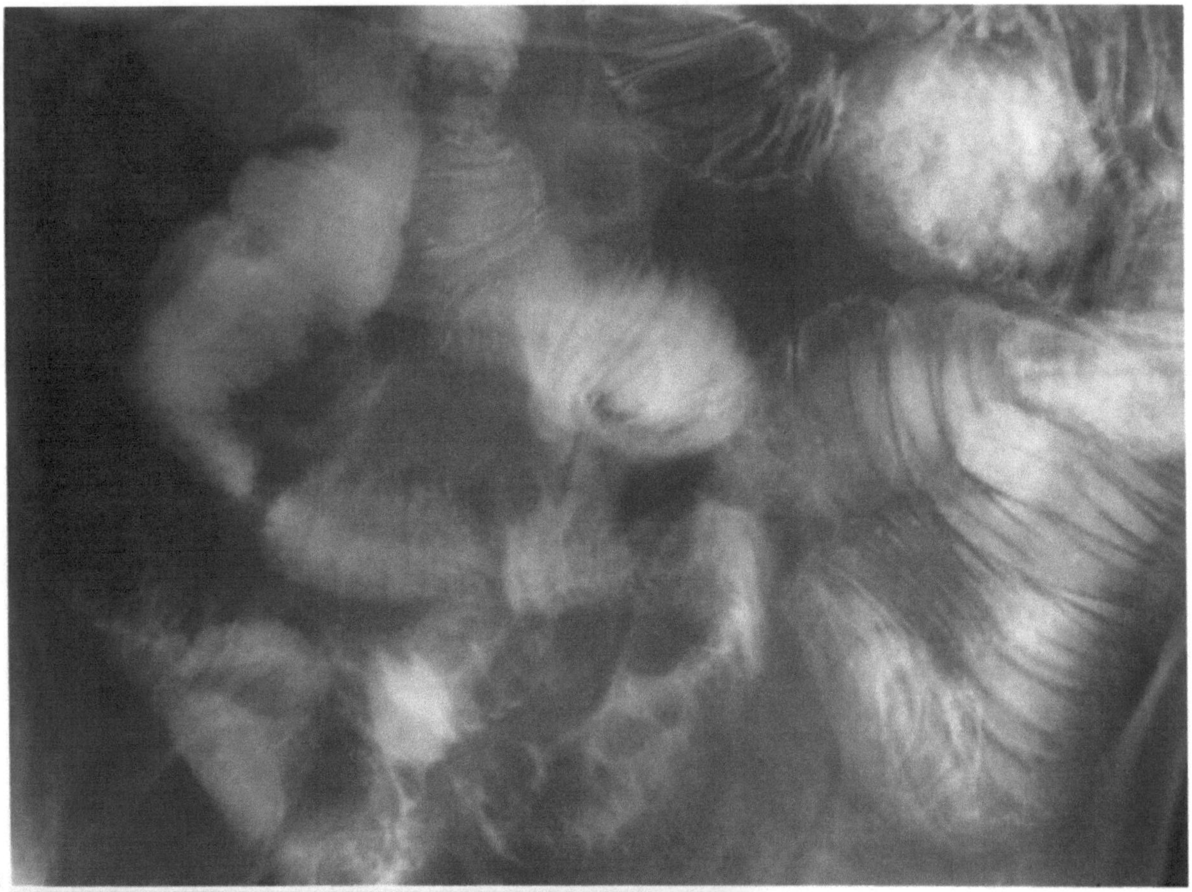

a

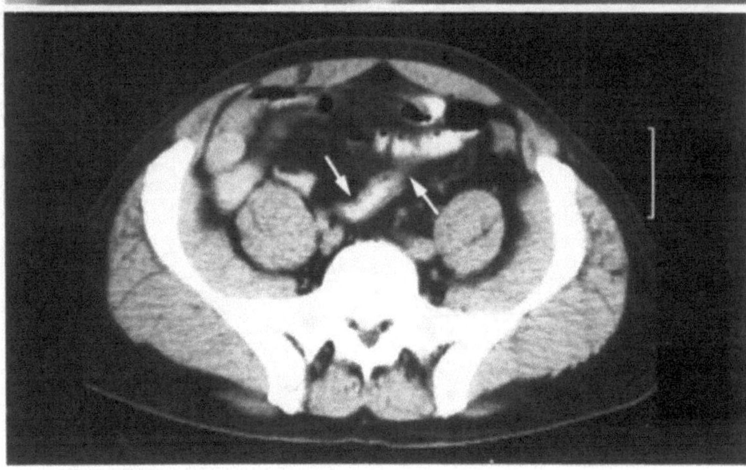

b

Fig. 5.2.-26 a and b. Accompanying inflammatory macronodular infiltration of ileal loops with fixation and slight prestenotic dilatation due to inflammatory reaction in diverticulitis of the sigmoid colon close to a sealed perforation (**a**). The CT examination for suspected lymphoma shows the significantly thickened intestinal wall (→) of the adherent ileal loops (**b**)

5.3 Tumors

Small bowel tumors are rare. The frequency of primary malignant small bowel tumors is probably around 1.6% of all gastrointestinal tumors (Barclay and Schapira 1983). They account for up to 60% of all neoplasms of the small bowel (Morson and Dawson 1979). Because of the rarity of small bowel tumors, the long-lasting asymptomatic clinical appearance and due to insufficient investigational techniques, diagnosis is frequently delayed. Since the introduction of enteroclysis technique, radiological accuracy in the diagnosis of the small bowel tumors has been greatly improved. Even small and asymptomatic tumors can be detected more frequently.

Increasing tumor size can lead to partial or total obstruction of the intestinal lumen causing the clinical signs of an ileus. The obstruction, frequently intermittent, is the most common manifestation of small bowel tumors (ca. 25%). Another 25% of patients suffer from chronic gastrointestinal bleeding. In such cases, enteroclysis in addition to angiography obtains the best diagnostic results. However a specific diagnosis of malignancy is rarely possible by enteroclysis alone. Only carcinoid and adenocarcinoma may have characteristic signs (Ekberg and Ekholm 1980). Differentiation between primary and secondary tumors is also often impossible.

5.3.1 Benign Tumors

Enteroclysis can detect even very small mucosal *polyps* (e.g. Gardner syndrome, Cronkhite-Canada syndrome) (Fig. 5.3.-1). These adenomatous polyps can become malignant, rarely also the Peutz-Jeghers polyps. These are hamartomas emerging from the muscularis mucosae which mostly grow into the intestinal lumen. They can reach a considerable size (Fig. 5.3.-2). The differential diagnosis of superficial polypoid lesions is dealt with in chapter 4.3 (see also Meschan 1984).

Most benign small bowel tumors originate from the deeper intestinal layers. These are *leiomyomas, fibromas, lipomas, angiomas and neurinomas* (Figs. 5.3.-3; 5.3.-4, 5.5.-8, p. 173) as well as a combination of these (e.g. in neurofibromatosis). Growing intramurally, they narrow the intestinal lumen only slightly and can be diagnosed by enteroclysis only by showing a submucosal mass effect. They rarely cause ileus symptoms except in a case of intussusception (see chapter 5.5). Arrosion of the mucosa may cause bleeding. In gastrointestinal bleeding, angiography and/or nuclear medicine studies are indicated if endoscopy and enteroclysis are negative (Fig. 5.3.-3). In the case of massive hemorrhage, angiography should be the first investigation.

In the diagnosis of carcinoid tumors, too, angiography is often mandatory (Fig. 5.3.-8) (Boijsen et al. 1974).

5.3.2 Primary Malignant Tumors

The *carcinoid* is found in the entire gastrointestinal tract but mostly in the appendix (Fig. 5.3.-5) and in the distal ileum (Clements et al. 1984). Carcinoid of the appendix is almost always benign whilst the small bowel carcinoid is malignant with only few exceptions. In the polypoid form – often detected by chance –, the carcinoid may not be differentiated from other polypoid tumors (Fig. 5.3.-6). Many small intestinal carcinoids have already metastasized by the time of their diagnosis (Morson and Dawson 1979). Fibrotic changes caused by the tumor are typical for carcinoids (fibro- or desmoplastic reaction, Bancks et al. 1975). This fibrosis results in shrinking of the tissues causing kinking of the bowel, irregular distortion and thickening of the folds of Kerckring with formation of spiculae and diverticula. In the presence of these alterations, the radiologic picture is relatively characteristic. In most cases this is already an advanced stage (Figs. 5.3.-7 and 8). The tumor can extensively infiltrate the intestinal wall and mesentery. The bowel lumen becomes constricted and the loops are separated. The primary tumor is then often no longer visible. Serotonin secretion and tumor infiltration result in a striking local hyperperistalsis. There are morphological similarities to peritoneal carcinomatosis, adhesions, Crohn's disease, radiation enteritis and endometriosis (Figs. 5.3.-24 to 26; 5.5.-17, p. 180).

Apart from carcinoids, adenocarcinoma, leiomyosarcoma, and malignant lymphoma are the most frequent malignant primary tumors of the small bowel. In our radiological records non-Hodgkin lymphoma are twice as frequent as adenocarcinoma and leiomyosarcoma together. An involvement of the gastrointestinal tract by Hodgkin's disease is a rarity (Sartoris et al. 1984). A primary manifestation has not yet been reported (Castellino 1986).

Adenocarcinomas are primarily found in the duodenum, proximal jejunum and distal ileum. Obstruction and blood loss are typical manifestations, rarely intussusception. Characteristic pictures are described in the radiological literature (Marshak and Lindner 1976; Ekberg and Ekholm 1980; Meschan 1984): a short annular stricture with overhanging edges or napkin ring form (Fig. 5.3.-9). Diffuse infiltrative or polypoid growth is just as frequent in our patients (Figs. 5.3.-10 to 12).

In contrast to the carcinoma, the *leiomyosarcoma* growing in the intestinal wall mostly remains symptomless until it ulcerates the mucosa and causes bleeding. Often it appears as a palpable mass and/or by abdominal pain (Bruneton et al. 1981). Only large leiomyosarcoma will narrow the lumen or cause intussusception (Figs. 5.3.-13 and 5.5.-7, p. 173).

Radiomorphology of the *malignant lymphomas* (Figs. 5.3.-14 to 17) is variable and often similar to Crohn's disease. Both diseases can present with aphthous and fissural ulcerations, polypoid infiltrates – sometimes with deeper necrotic ulcerations (bull's eye sign) –, cobblestoning, thickening or loss of folds, (so-called aneurysmatic) dilatation and strictures. Clinical presentation and predominant localization in the distal ileum can be alike (Sartoris et al. 1984). Progressive infiltration of bowel wall and mesentery will lead to separation of intestinal loops, fistula formation, perforation, cavitation and rarely to obstruction or intussusception.

The *malignant histiocytosis* reveals similar pictures (Figs. 5.3.-18 and 19).

5.3.3 Secondary Tumors

The most frequent *tumors spreading from the adjacent organs* to the small bowel are carcinomas of the colon, pancreas and stomach. The infiltrates are mostly undifferentiable from primary small bowel tumors.

This is frequently true also for solitary *metastases* (Fig. 5.3.-20). By contrast, the nodular growth of multiple metastases is often evident (Figs. 5.3.-21 to 23). Melanoma is the most common tumor with small bowel metastases (Figs. 5.3.-22, 23) (Smith et al. 1977). Carcinomas of kidney, lung, uterus, ovary, breast, pancreas and esophagus (Sellink and Miller 1982), stomach and colon may also metastasize to the small intestine. As in all other intramural small bowel tumors, intussusception can occur (Fig. 5.3.-22).

The *peritoneal carcinomatosis* (Figs. 5.3.-24 to 26) can infiltrate the small bowel and mesentery causing distortion of the folds and kinking of the intestinal wall. Differential diagnosis is referred to in the description of carcinoid tumors.

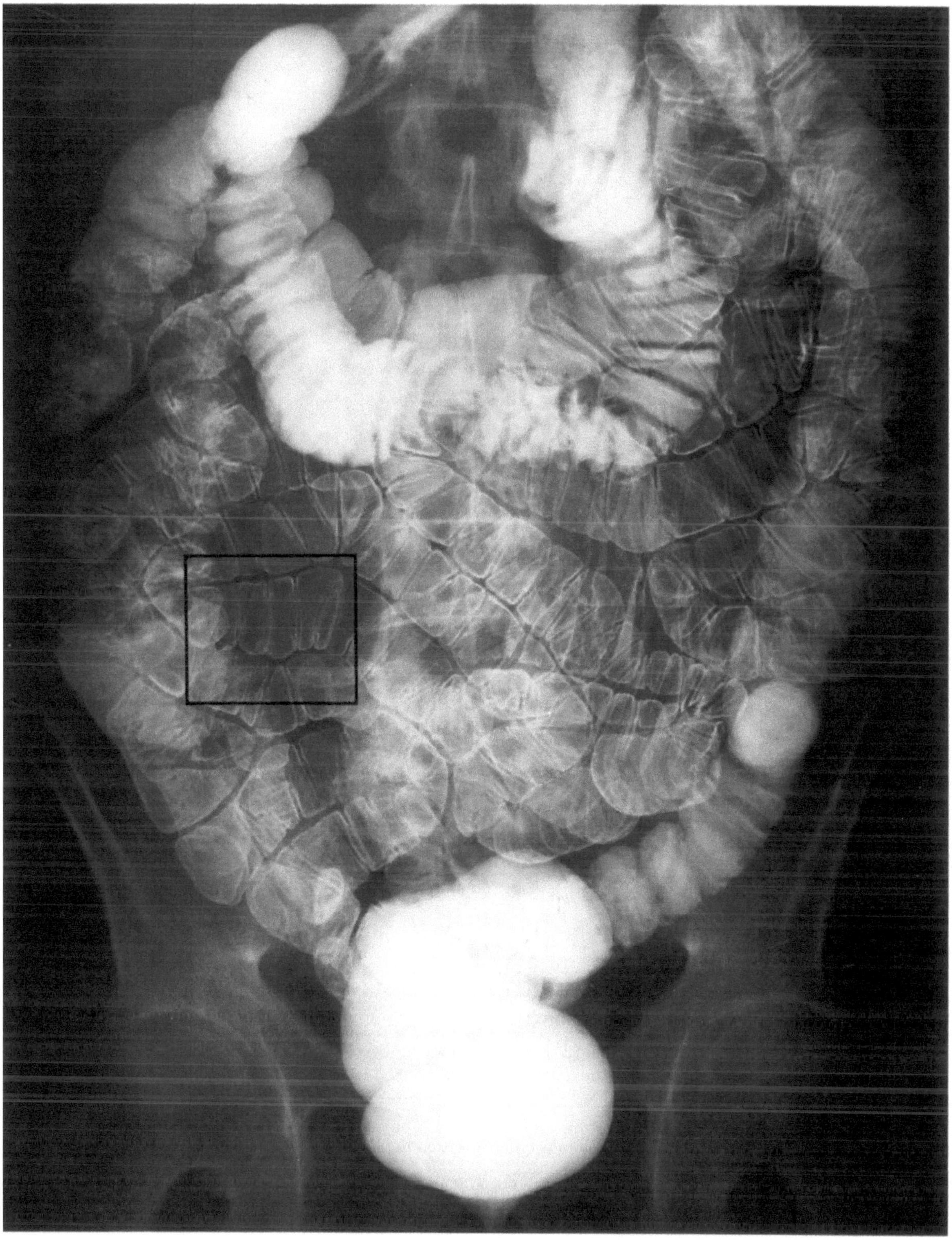

a

Fig. 5.3.-1 a and b. Adenomatous polyp in the ileum. The picture (**a**) demonstrates that with careful viewing, the smallest tumors may be detected. Detailed view p. 110 (**b**). The polyp is 6 mm in diameter

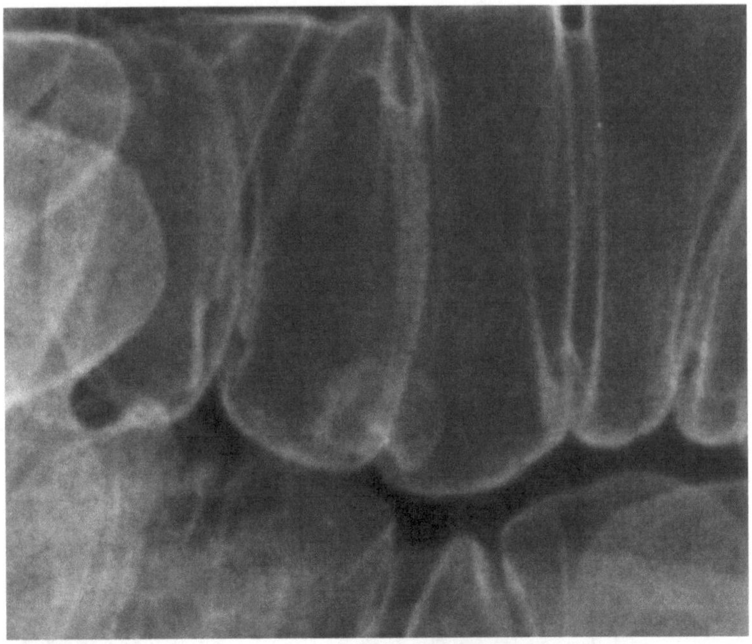

Fig. 5.3.-1 b. Adenomatous polyp (detail from p. 109)

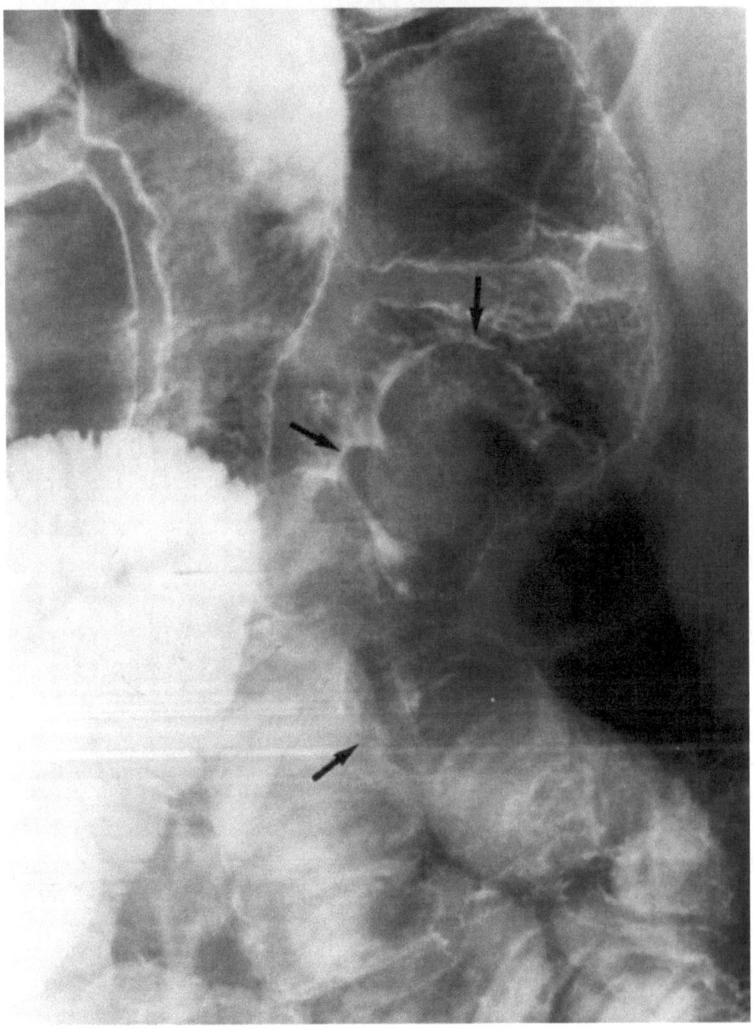

Fig. 5.3.-2. Peutz-Jeghers polyps. The partially lobulated polyps caused intermittent obstruction

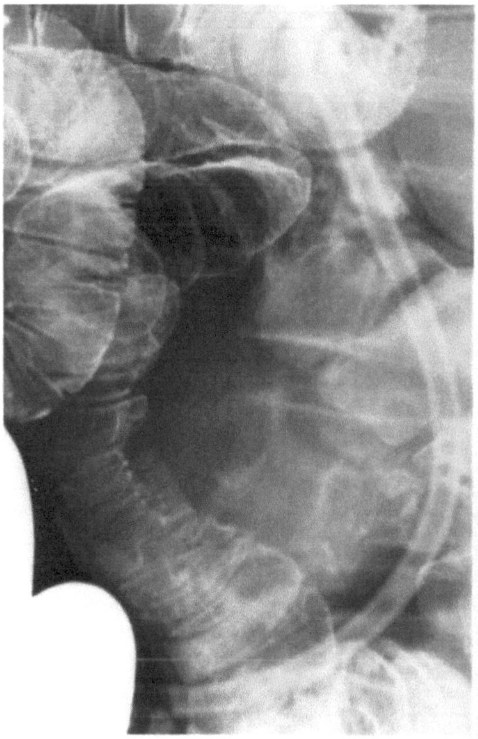

a

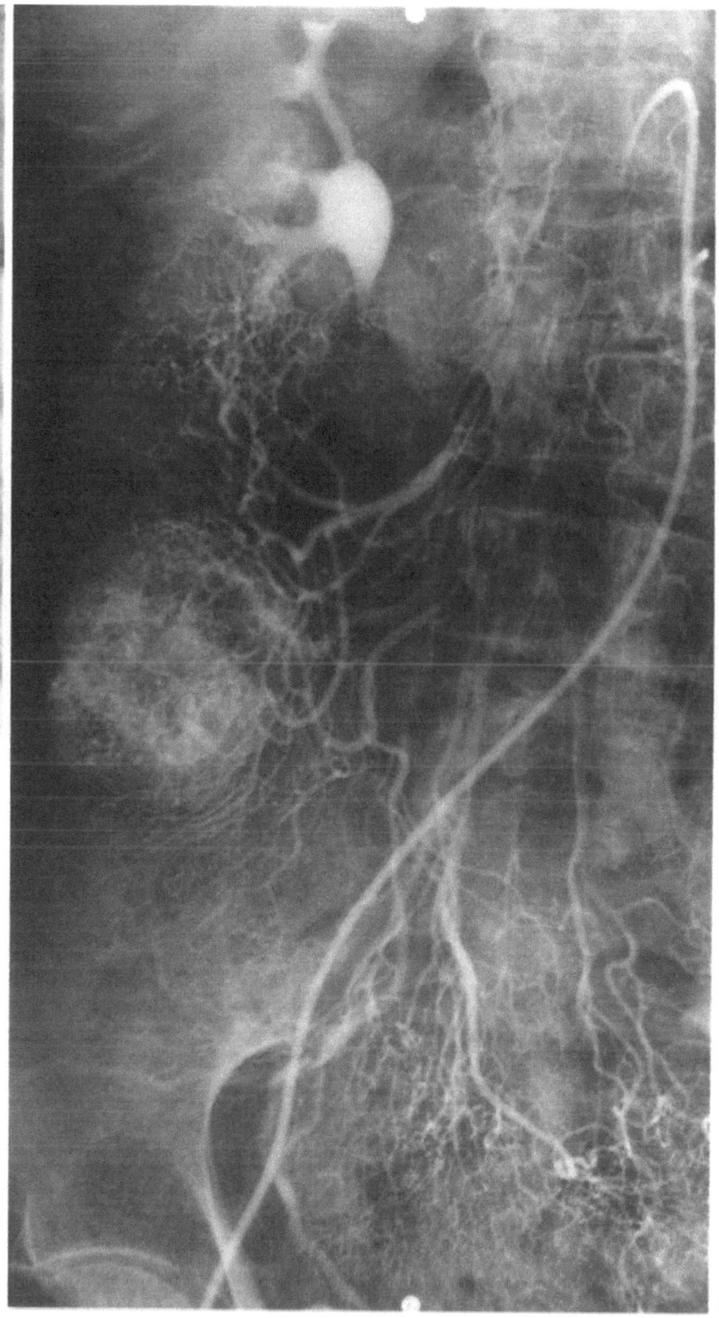

b

Fig. 5.3.-3a and b. Bleeding leiomyoma of the small bowel. Mass effect on the intestinal lumen by a submucosal mass (**a**). Differential diagnosis: extrinsic process. Angiography of superior mesenteric artery shows a 7 cm large vascular tumor (**b**). (Courtesy of Dr. V. Hufen, Dept. of Radiology, Municipal Hospital Munich-Schwabing, Germany)

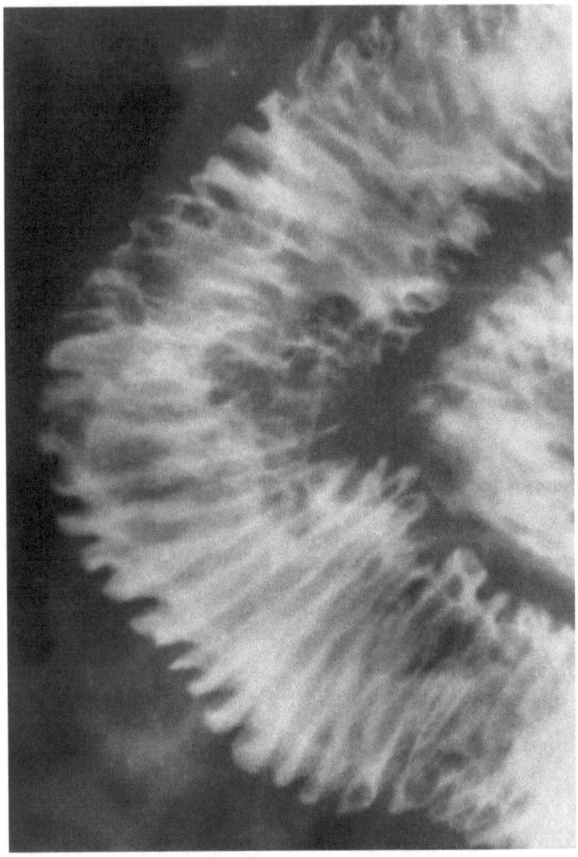

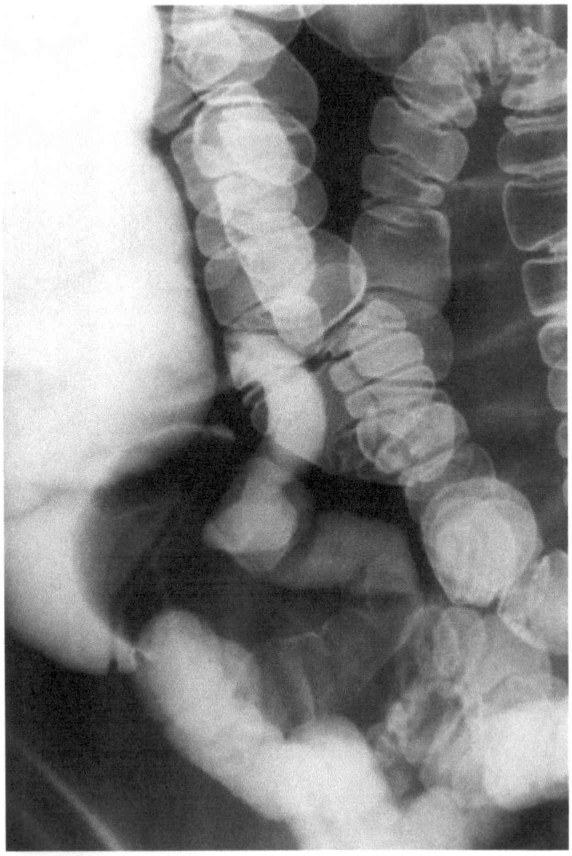

Fig. 5.3.-4. Angiodysplasia. Tiny polypoid lesions representing angiomas distributed over the entire small bowel. Patient with chronic blood loss

Fig. 5.3.-5. Mucocele of the appendix caused by carcinoid tumor of the appendix. Smooth wall impression of the cecum from medial due to a tumor (diameter 5 cm). Normal terminal ileum. Please observe: The examination of the cecum is a constituent of enteroclysis

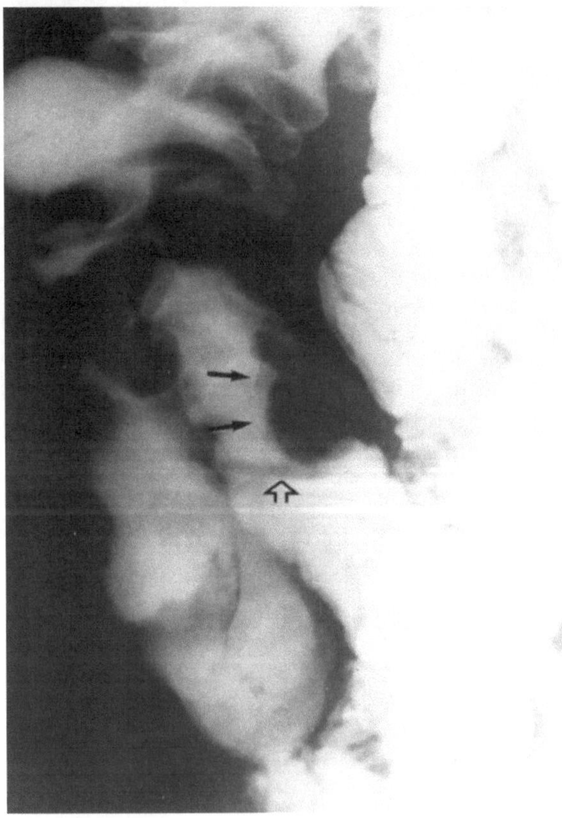

Fig. 5.3.-6. Carcinoid tumor in the terminal ileum. Polypoid submucosal tumor with mass effect (→). Fibrous band due to desmoplastic reaction in the intestinal wall (⇒)

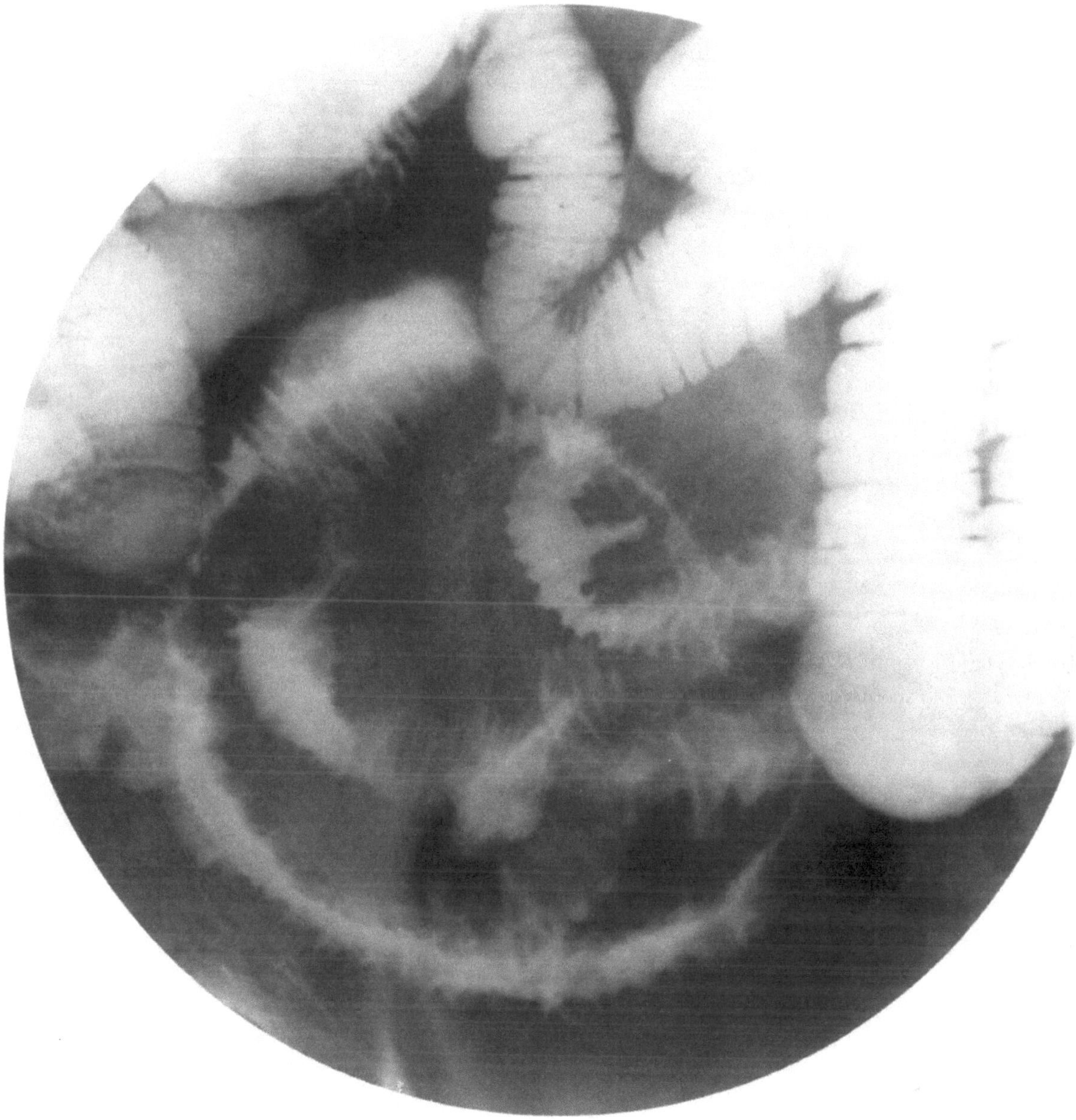

Fig. 5.3.-7. Metastatic carcinoid of the ileum. Extensive involvement of the intestine and mesentery with constriction and separation of the intestinal loops. Thickening of the folds with formation of spiculae. The primary tumor is no longer visible. Marked local hyperperistalsis. Partial obstruction with prestenotic dilatation. (Courtesy of Prof. K.J. Pfeifer, Dept. of Radiology and Surgery, University Hospital Munich-Innenstadt, Germany)

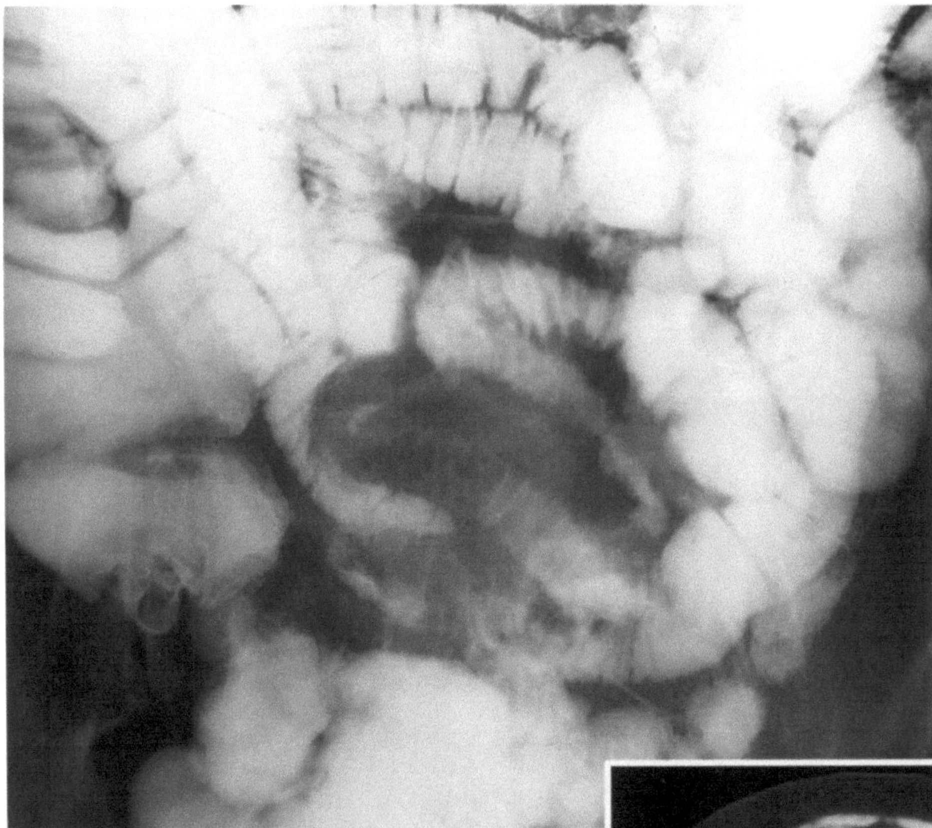

a

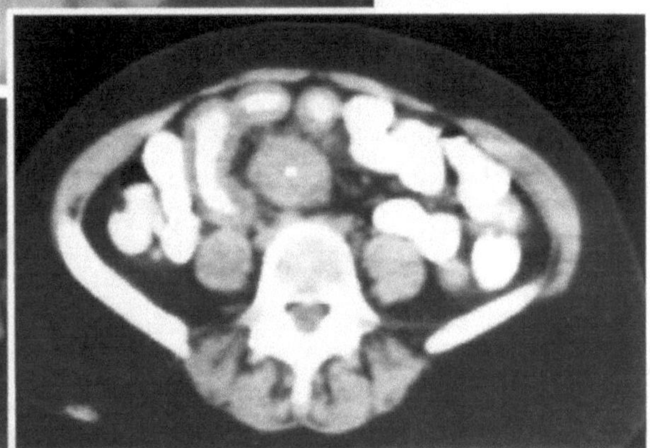

b

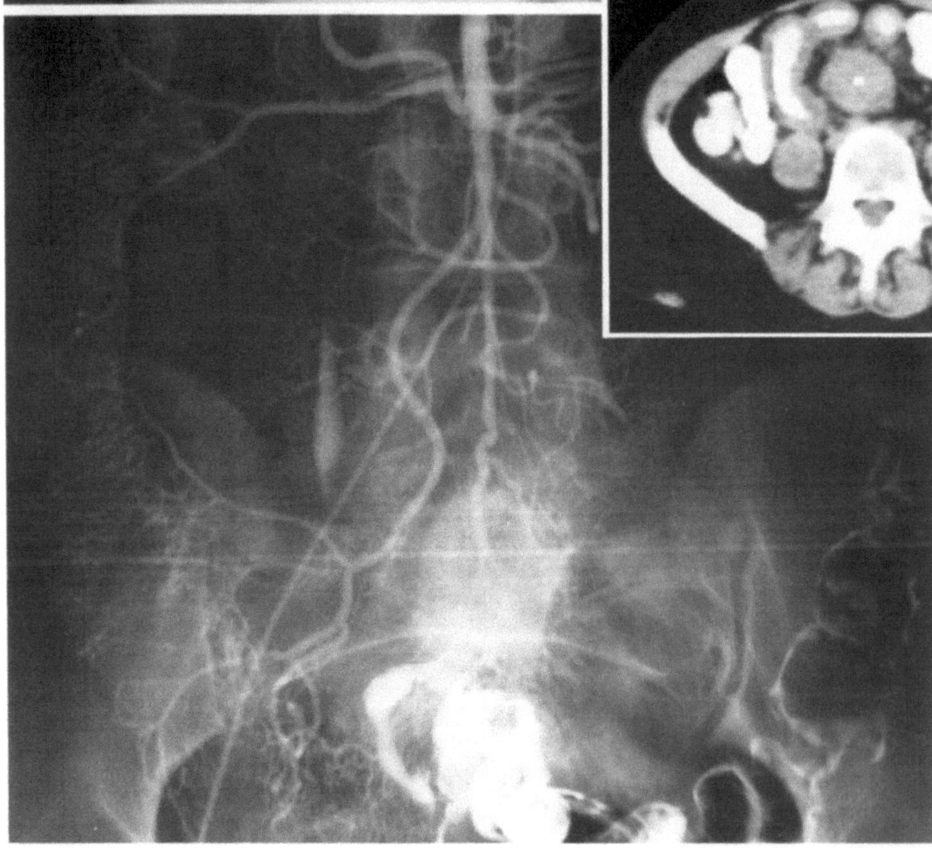

c

Fig. 5.3.-8a to c. Carcinoid. Typical mass in the mesentery and thickened bowel walls, first detected by CT **(b)**. Diagnosis confirmed by enteroclysis **(a)** and angiography **(c)**. Female with subileus and flush symptoms. Liver metastases

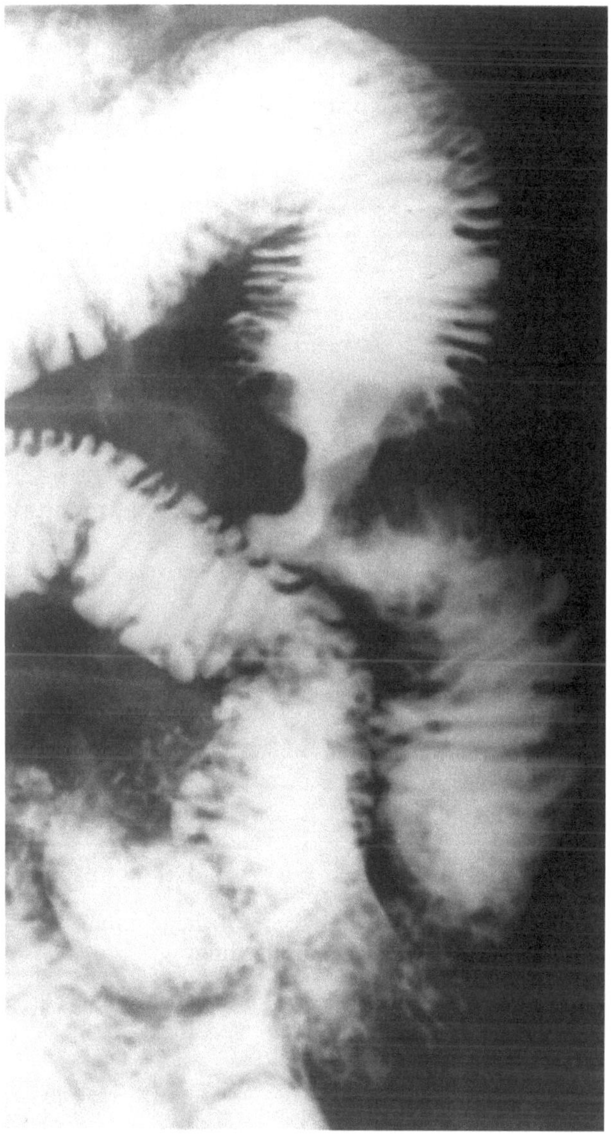

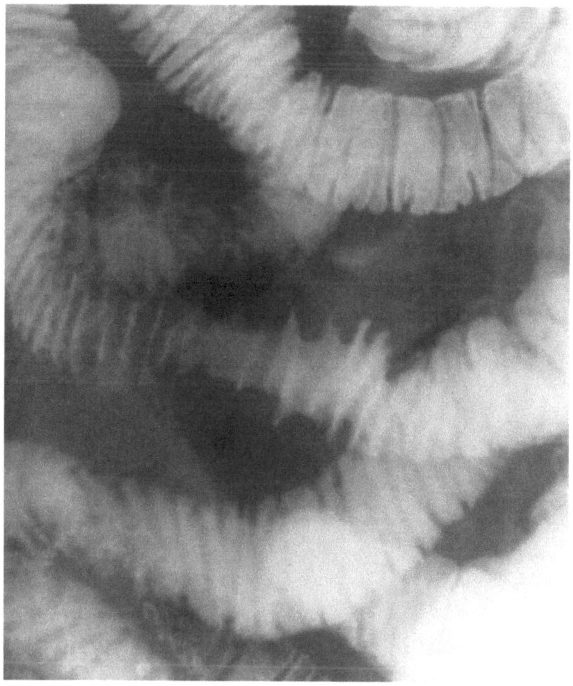

Fig. 5.3.-10. Adenocarcinoma of the ileum. Irregular thickening of the folds due to diffuse infiltration. Similar picture to that of chronic radiation enteritis

Fig. 5.3.-9. Adenocarcinoma of the jejunum. Annular stenosis with kinking and polypoid mucosal surface

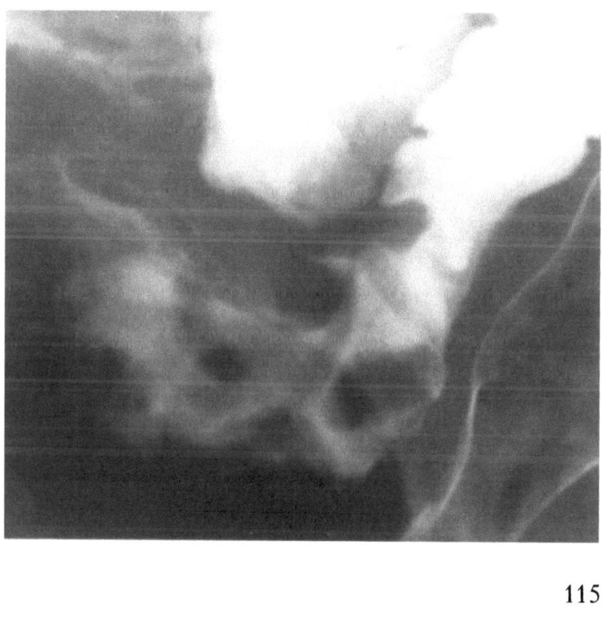

Fig. 5.3.-11. Adenocarcinoma of the ileum. Cauliflower-like growing tumor

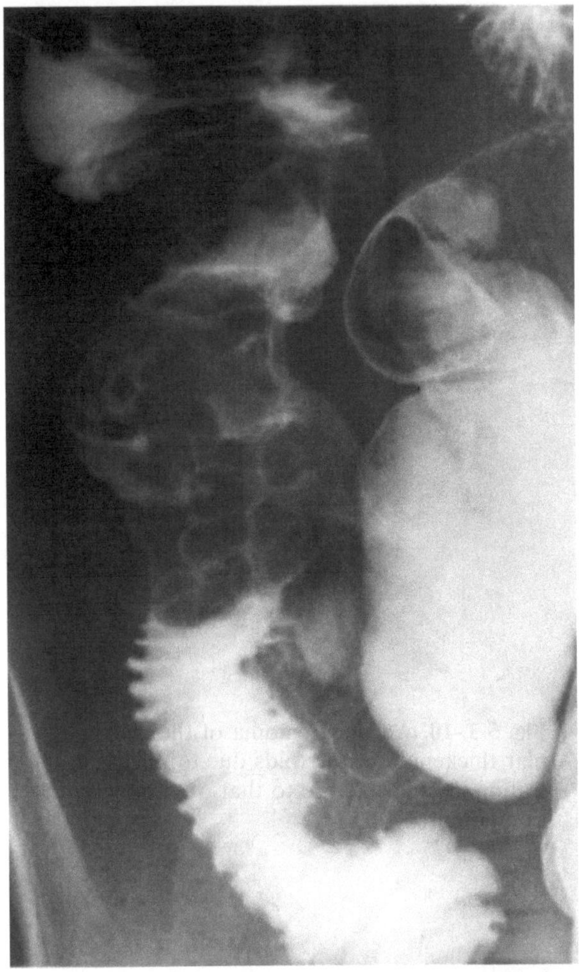

Fig. 5.3.-12. Adenocarcinoma at the ileocecal junction. Involvement of the terminal ileum and cecum with ileocecal valve. Cobblestoning due to polypoid tumor growth. Difficult to differentiate from Crohn's disease. No string sign

Fig. 5.3.-13. Leiomyosarcoma of the jejunum. Patient with gastrointestinal bleeding

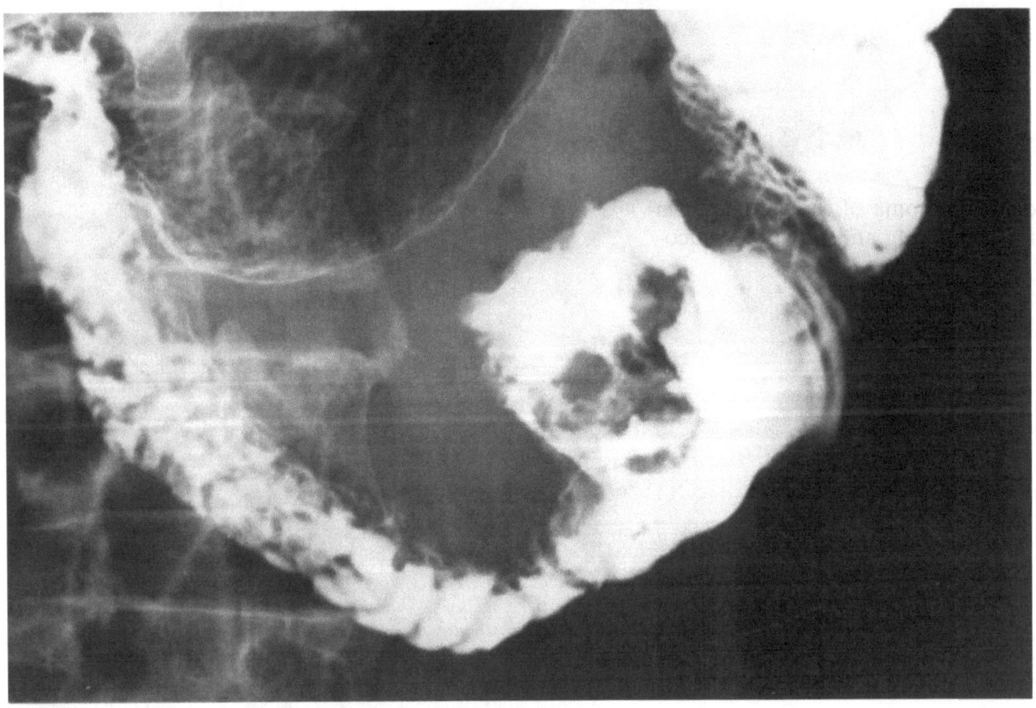

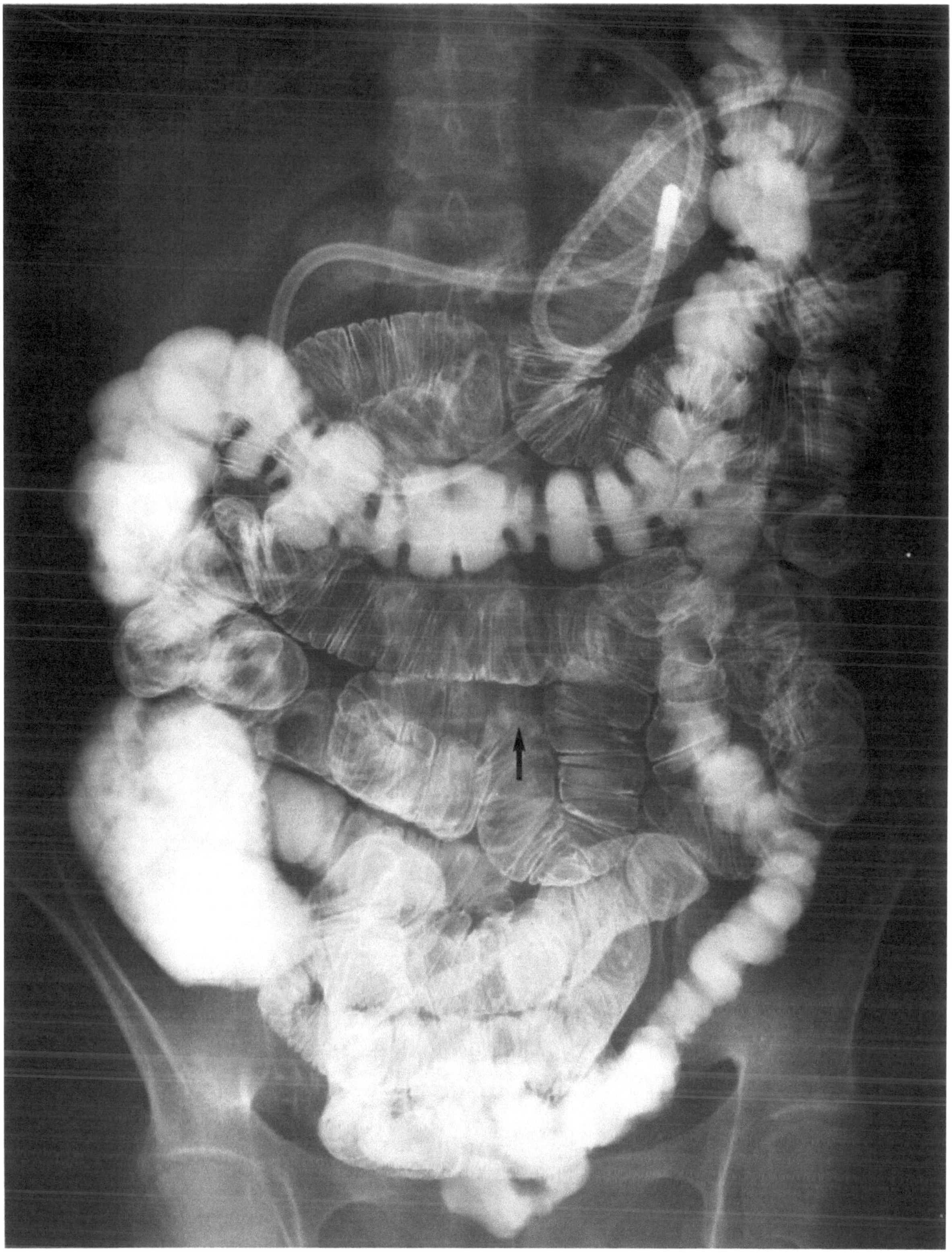

Fig. 5.3.-14. Non-Hodgkin lymphoma of the small bowel. Isolated mural defect of a small bowel loop. The findings were originally overlooked, although present in the center of the picture (→). Perforation ensued several days later

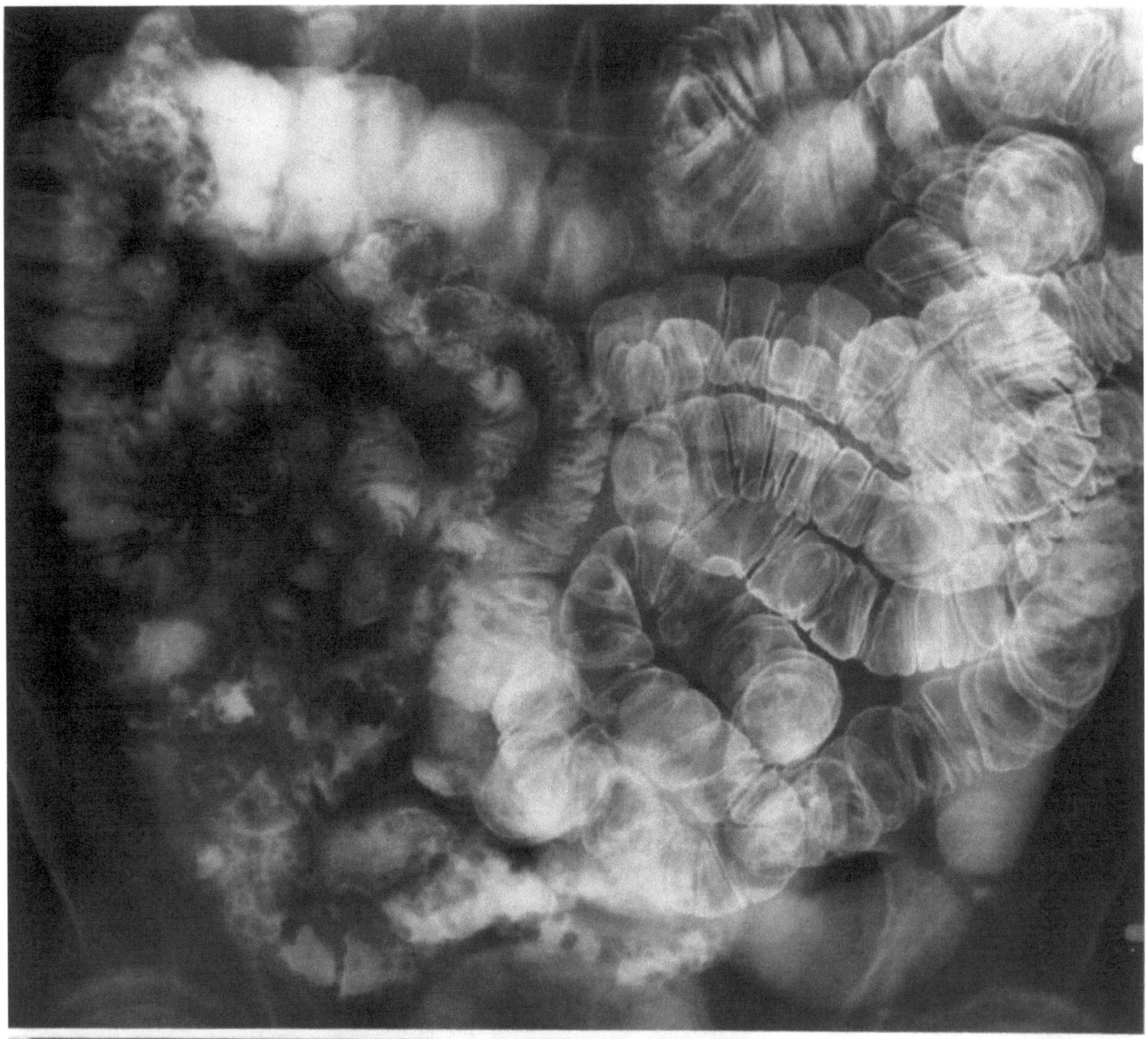

b

a

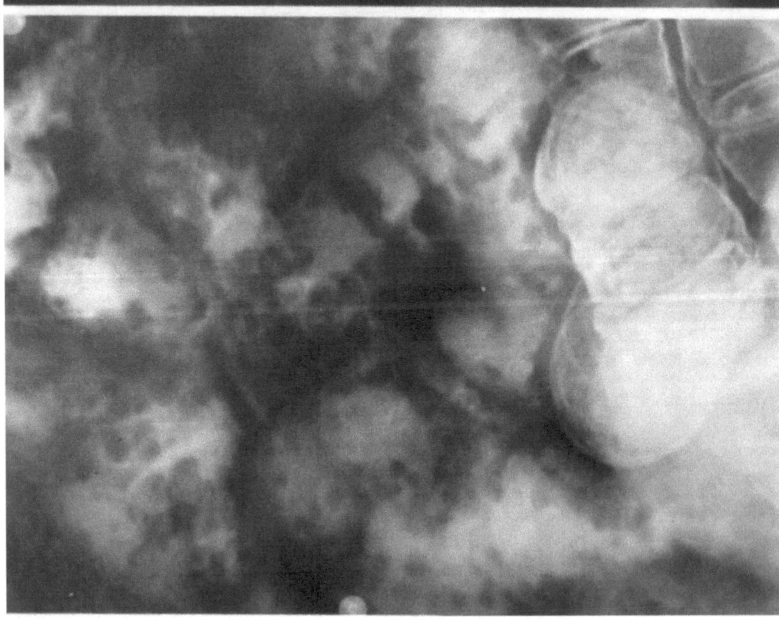

Fig. 5.3.-15a and b. Primary gastrointestinal non-Hodgkin lymphoma. Multiple nodular tumor infiltrates. Nonspecific irritation with poor mucosal coating and hypermotility of the involved bowel (**a**). Detail (**b**)

Fig. 5.3.-16. Non-Hodgkin lymphoma of the small bowel. Irregular, nodular and destructing infiltrates causing stenosis

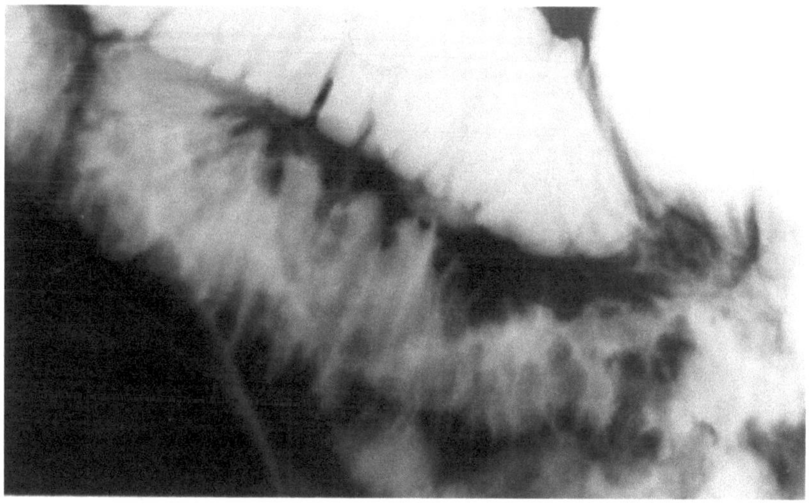

Fig. 5.3.-17. Non-Hodgkin lymphoma of the ileum. Annular stenosis of the preterminal ileum with obstruction. Diffuse infiltration of the terminal ileum with involvement of the mesentery (→)

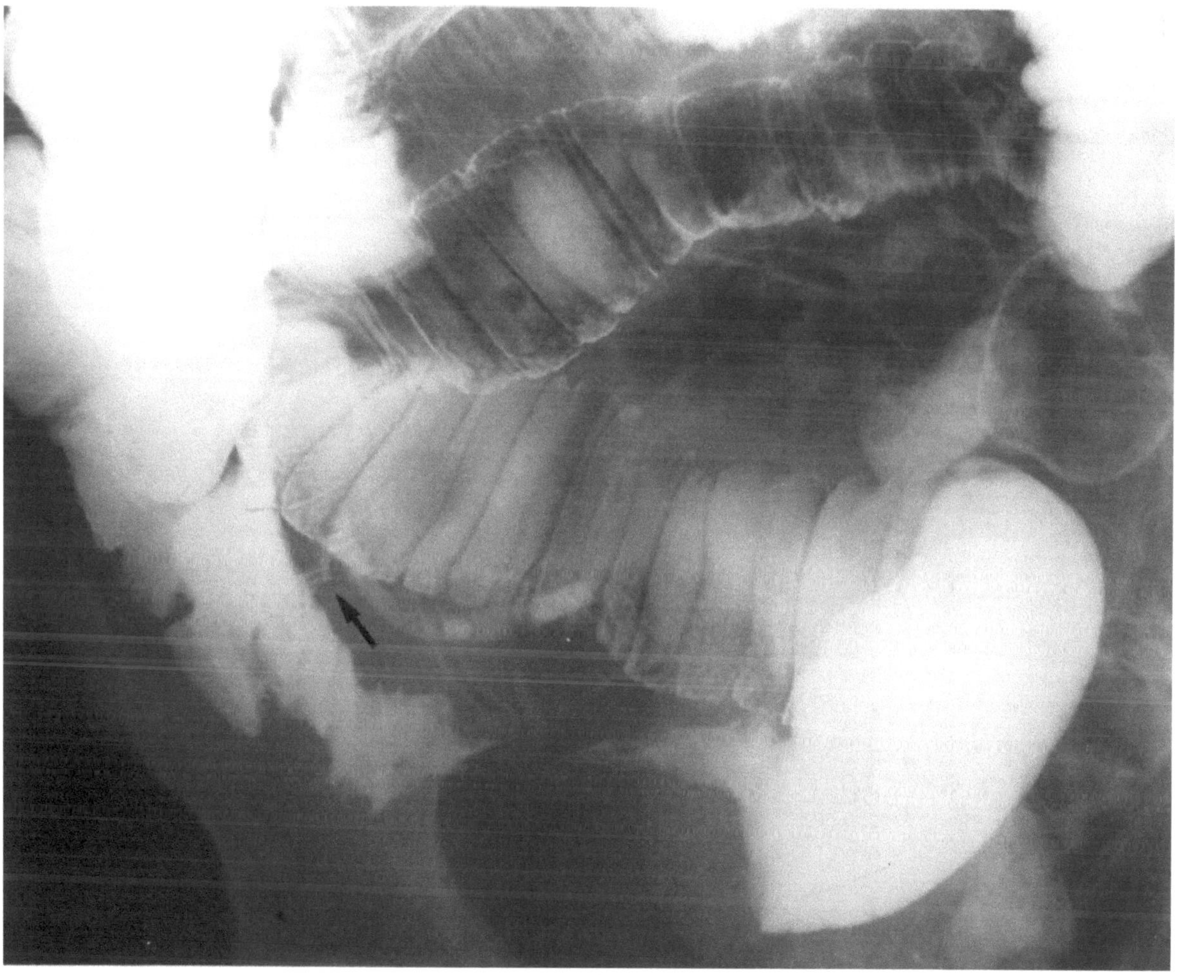

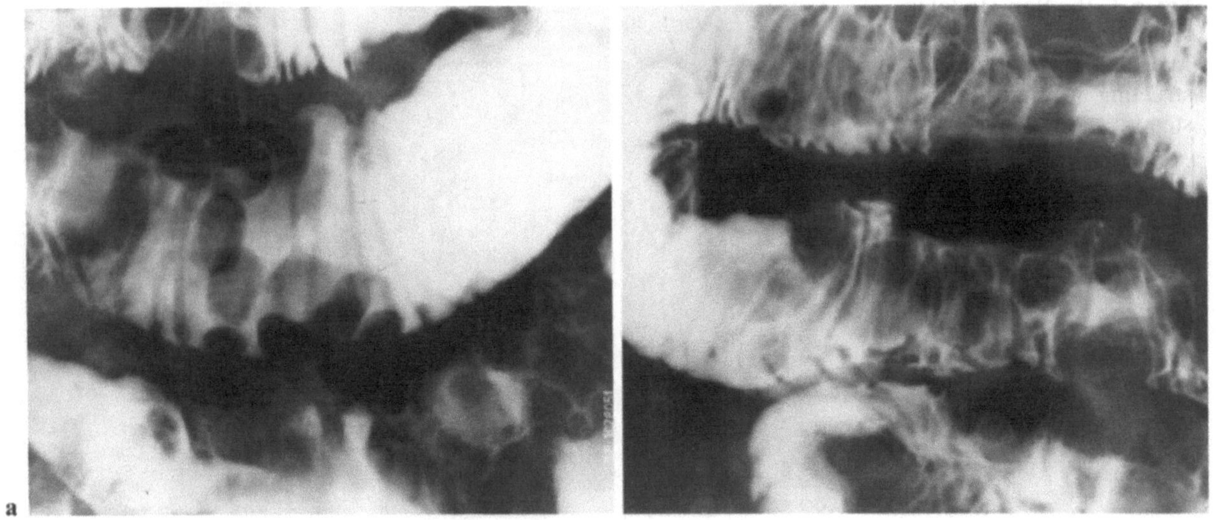

Fig. 5.3.-18a and b. Malignant histiocytosis of the small bowel. Multiple polypoidal infiltrates (spot films)

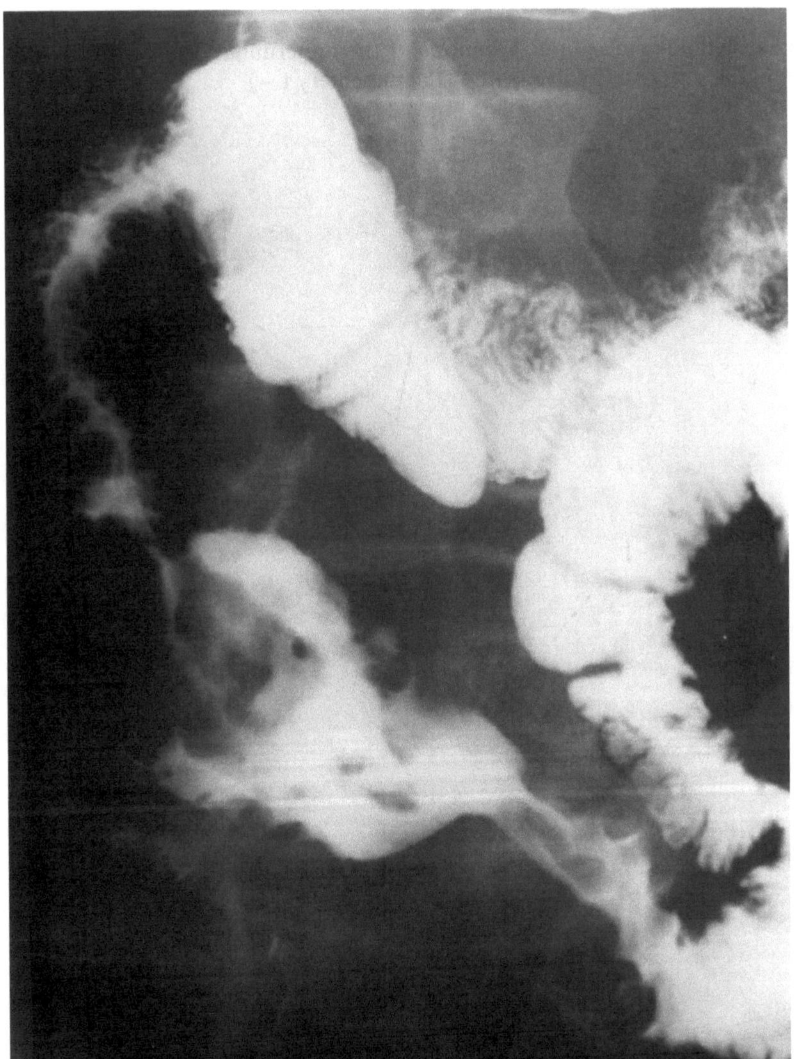

Fig. 5.3.-19. Malignant histiocy tosis of the small intestine. Partial polypoidal, partial diffuse infiltration of the terminal ileum and the ascending colon. Stenosis and cavitation by tumor destruction

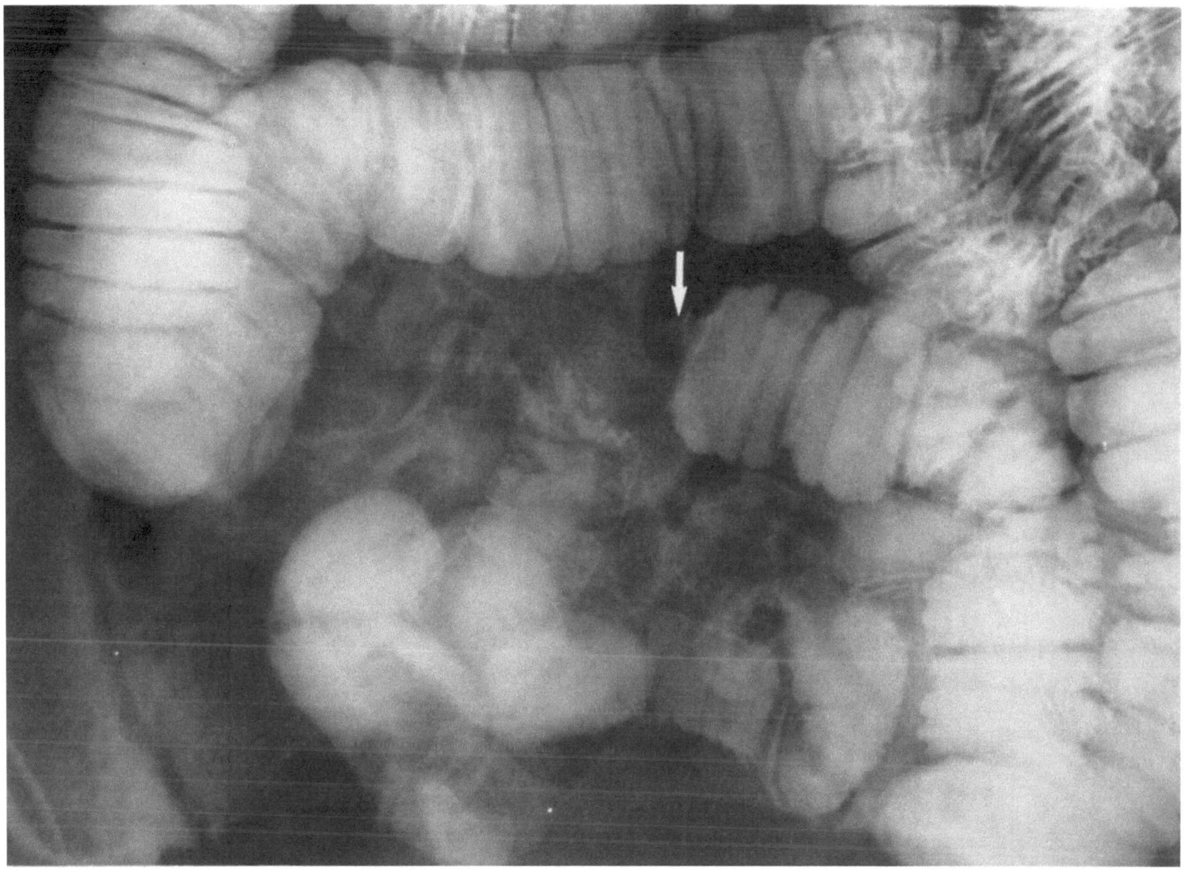

Fig. 5.3.-20. Metastasis from a pancreatic carcinoma causing a short filiform stenosis (→)

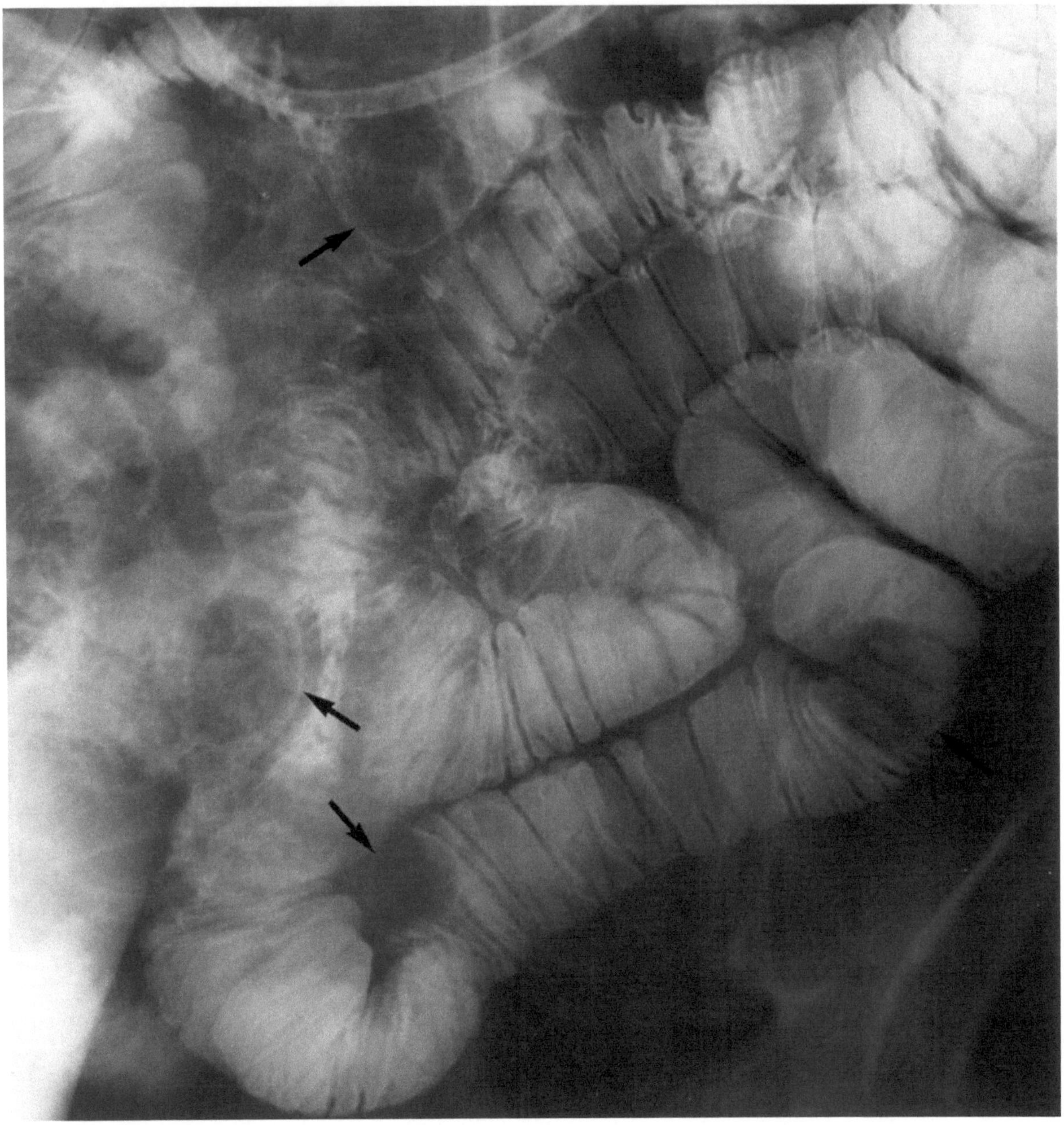

Fig. 5.3.-21. Multiple metastases of a colon carcinoma. Partial lumen compression by metastases (→) without significant obstruction

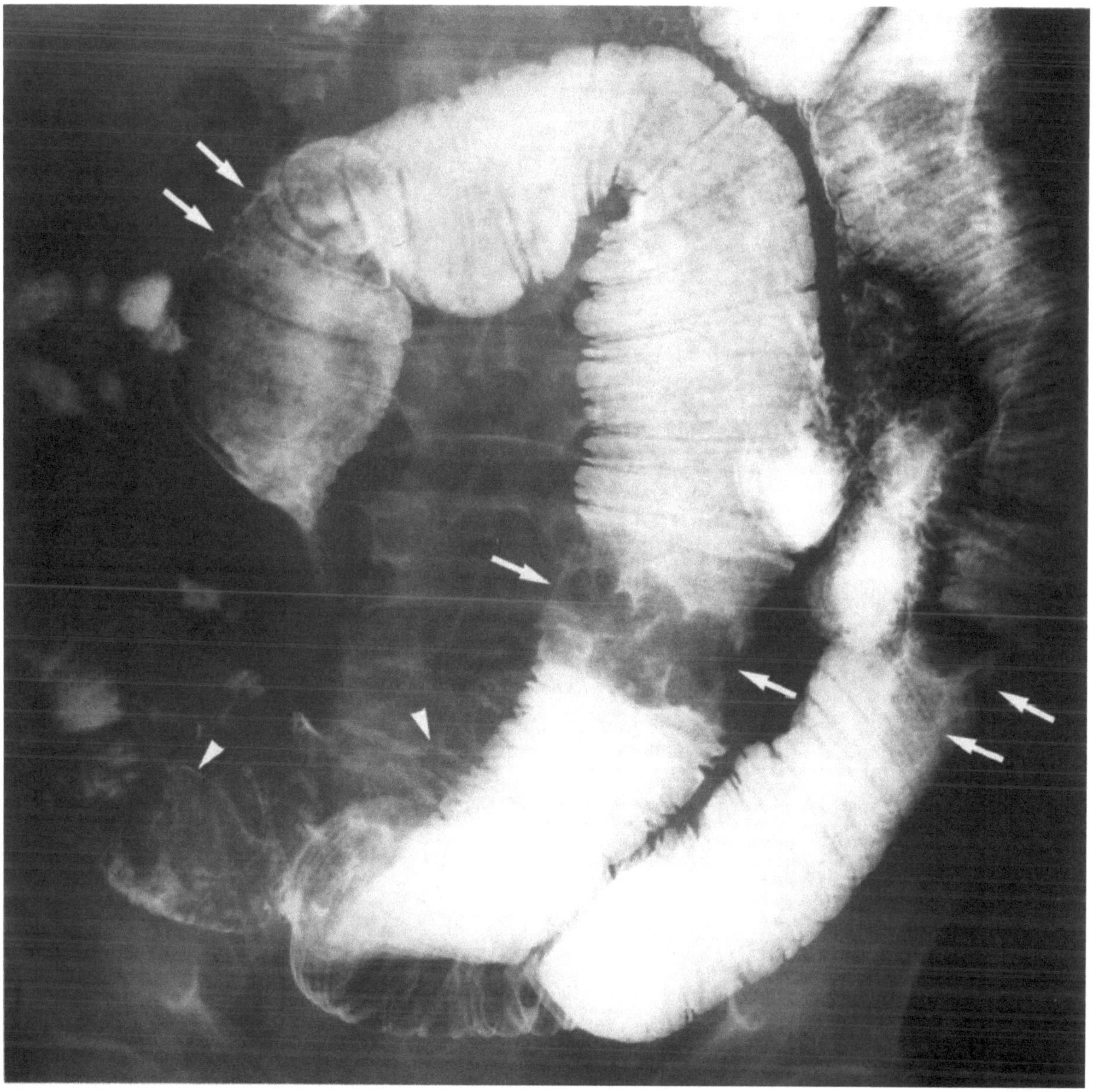

Fig. 5.3.-22. Multiple metastases of a melanoma with intussusception. The long distance intussusception (►) is caused by one of the metastases (→)

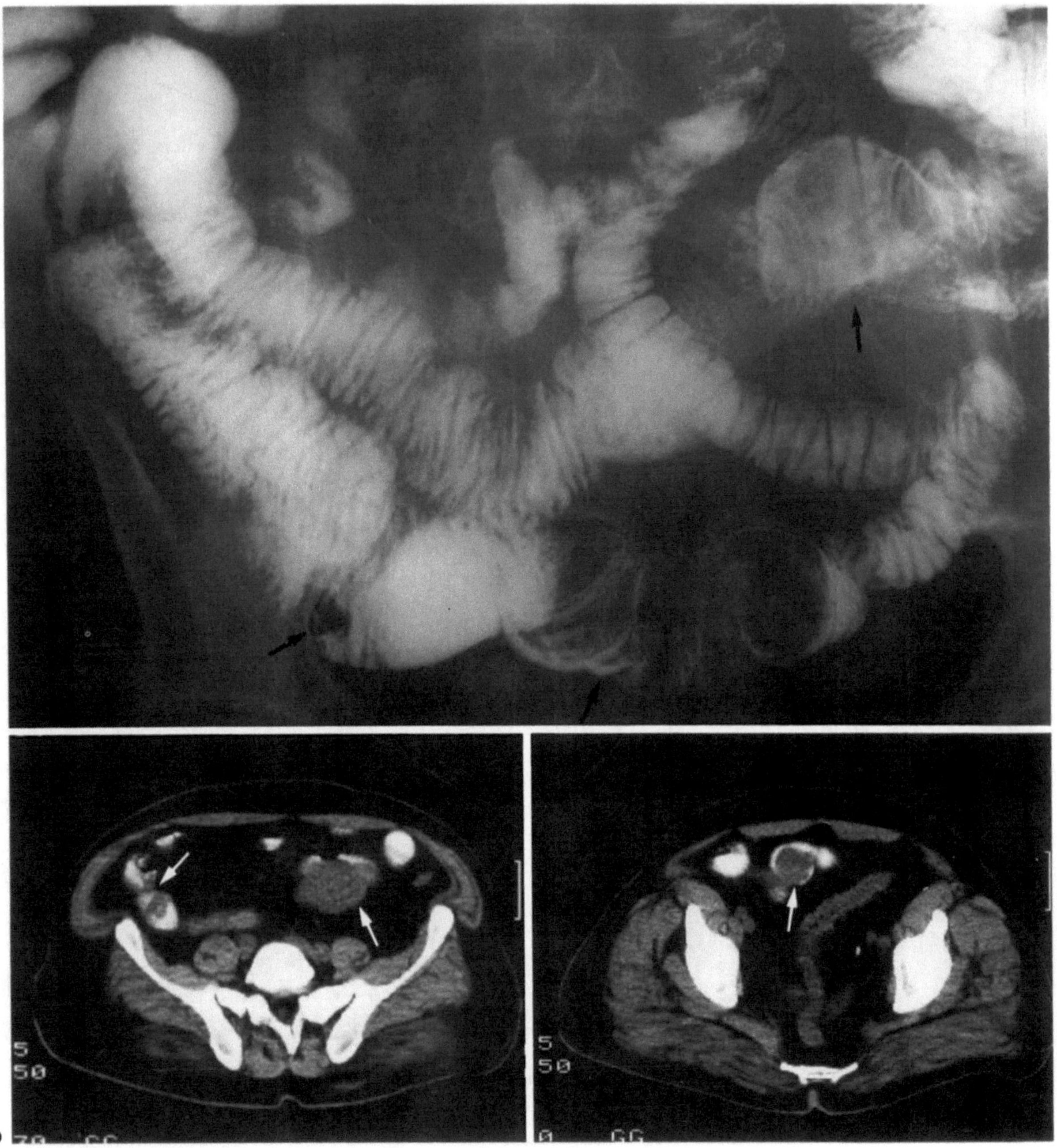

a

b

c

Fig. 5.3.-23a to c. Metastases of malignant melanoma (→) (**a**). In CT, several nodules (→) along the small bowel (**b** and **c**). Patient with anemia due to gastrointestinal blood loss. Gastroscopy and ileocolonoscopy were normal. Primary tumor site was first unknown, retrospectively it was found on the right shoulder

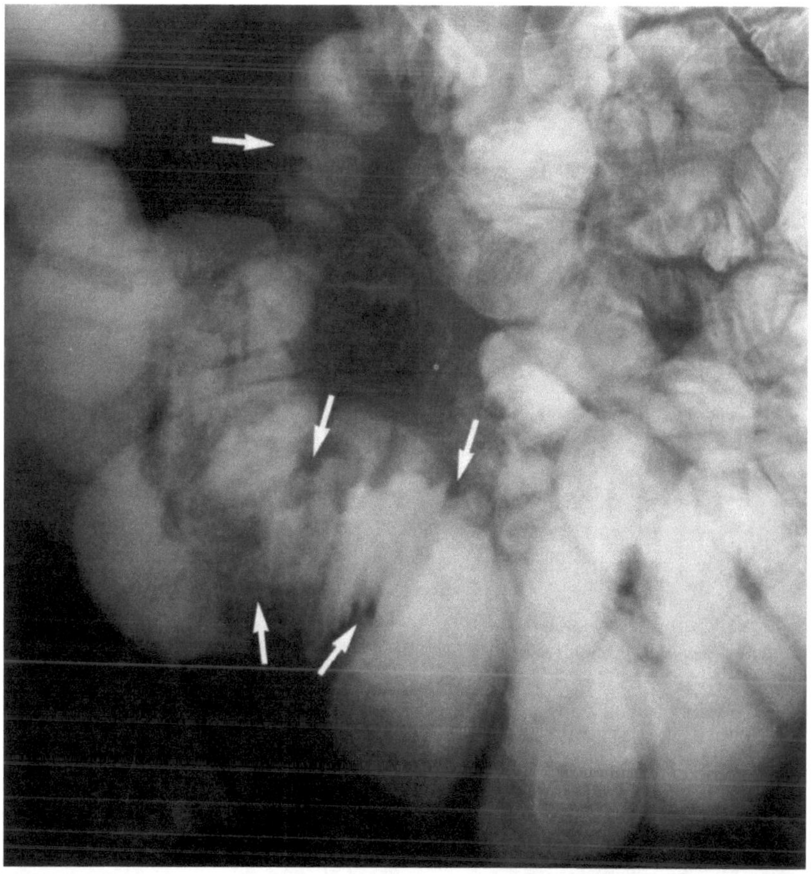

Fig. 5.3.-24. Peritoneal carcinomatosis in pancreatic carcinoma. Transverse stretching and kinking of the intestine by tumor infiltration. The picture simulates fibrous bands

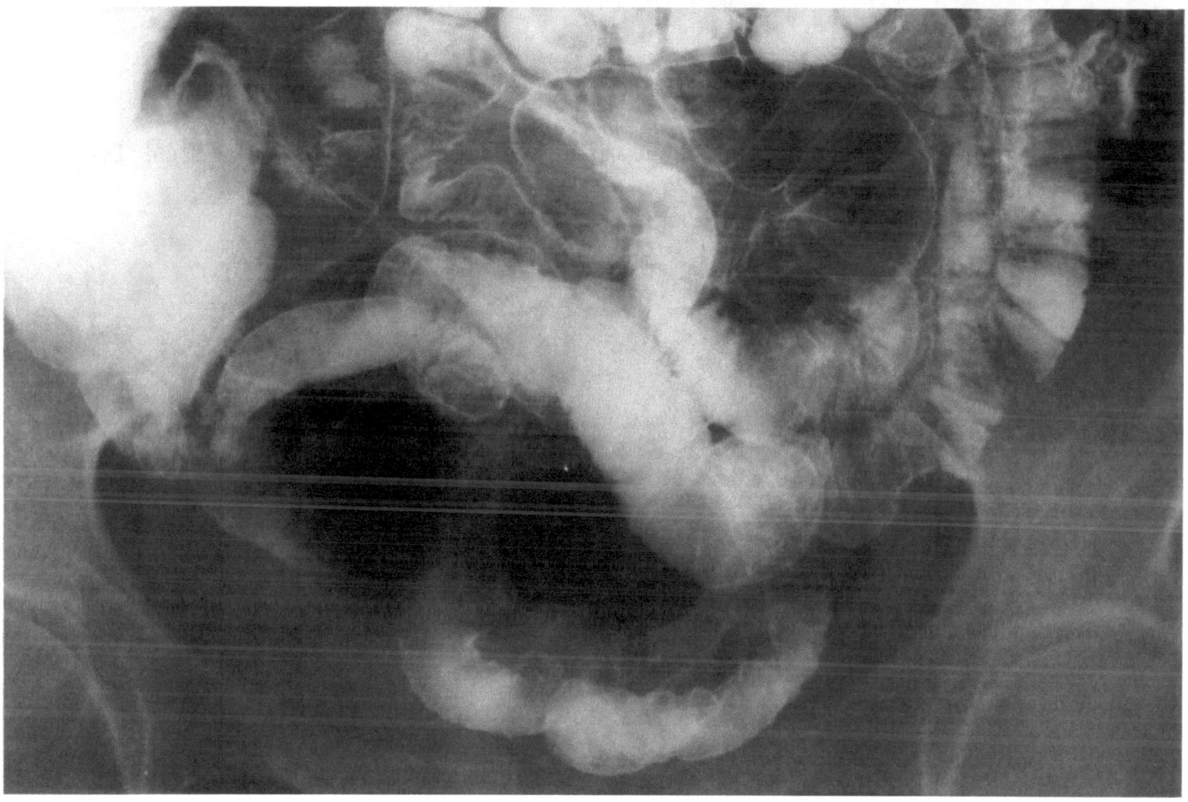

Fig. 5.3.-25. Peritoneal carcinomatosis in ovarian carcinoma. Diffuse infiltration of the ileum with separation and effacement of the folds. Fixation of the intestinal loops by tumor growth in the intestinal wall and mesentery

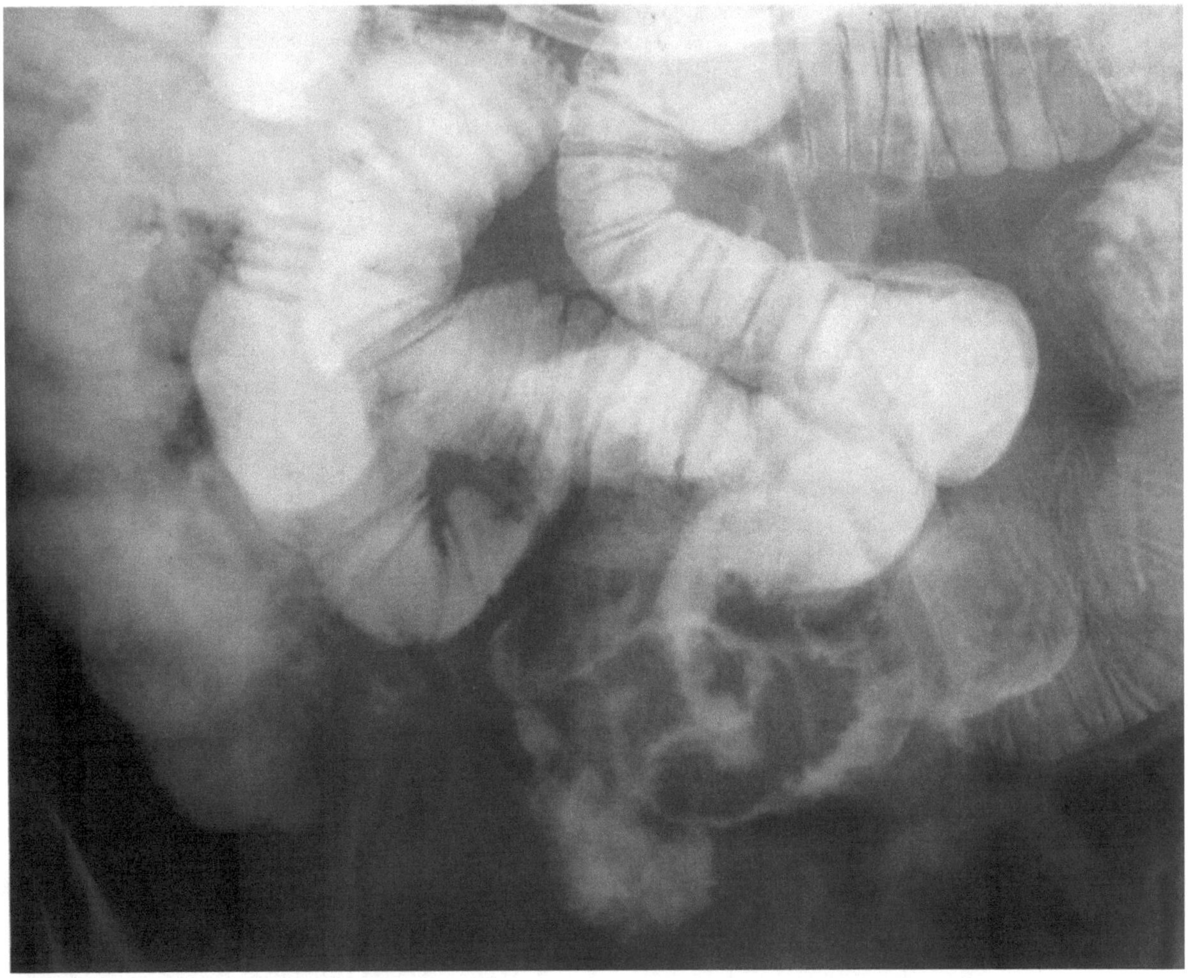

Fig. 5.3.-26. Peritoneal carcinomatosis in colonic carcinoma. Infiltration of the distal ileum. Differential diagnosis: carcinoid, Crohn's disease

5.4 Motility Disorders

The complex process of the small bowel motility is not yet completely understood. Regulation of the motor actions ensues by means of the musculature as myoelectrical activity, by the intrinsic nervous system, humoral factors and blood supply (Wienbeck 1980). The migrating motor complex plays an important role in the regulation of bowel motility. This myoelectrical activity complex moves from the stomach to the distal small bowel. It consists of three phases which run through a cycle. Each phase is composed of slow waves and spike potentials of different extent (Wienbeck and Erckenbrecht 1983; Erckenbrecht and Wienbeck 1984). Changes in these regulative mechanisms or diseases generate local or general motility disorders (Sellink 1976; Cornell 1982). Enteroclysis allows for selective investigation of the small bowel, whereby factors such as a too rapid or too slow emptying of the stomach, which could produce a false picture of the small bowel motility, are ruled out. Constant examination conditions expose the gut to a kind of test and its behavior can be recorded. The possibility of pursuing the contrast medium bolus under intermittent fluoroscopy allows for better evaluation of local changes of the motility than in conventional methods.

According to the regulation processes and causes of disease, motility disorders may be divided into four main groups:

- neurogenic and humoral factors,
- malabsorption,
- diseases of the intestinal wall,
- vascular changes.

In each of these groups, hyper- or hypomotility – either local or general – may occur. Combinations of the above are also possible. The pattern of motility disorder can change. Diseases initially associated with hyperperistalsis (e.g. sprue or amyloidosis) may show a marked hypomotility in the later stages if the innervation, blood supply and musculature of the deeper layers have been damaged.

Overlapping with pathologic pictures shown in chapters 5.1–5.3 and 5.5 is inevitable, since both locally and generally disturbed motility may also occur in those entities. This chapter deals mainly with general motility disturbances. Local disorders, e.g. string sign, local hyperperistalsis in the presence of fibrous bands or radiation enteritis, are dealt with in the appropriate chapters.

The etiology of motility disorders is summarized in Tables 5.4.-1 and 5.4.-2.

5.4.1 Neurogenic and Humoral Factors

The influence of the *thyroid hormones* on small bowel activity has been known for a long time. Hyperthyroidism causes hypermotility and diarrhea whilst hypothyroidism causes constipation.

General hyperperistalsis is also caused by *psychogenic and emotional factors* (Figs. 5.4.-1 and 2). These patients complain of symptoms referred to as the "irritable bowel syndrome" which manifests itself in uncharacteristic abdominal pain, the spectrum of which ranges from discomfort to agonizing pain and colic-like pictures. Flatulence, meteorism, borborygmi, bloating and stool irregularities, e.g. diarrhea or frequent bowel movements with small portions or constipation, often alternating, bother the patients. The colon is mostly affected. When the small bowel is involved, the hyperperistalsis can be so marked that it results in *intestinal hurry*. Since the mucosa is intact in this functional disorder, there is no premature flocculation of the contrast medium. Naturally, due to the strong bowel movement, the coating cannot be maintained for as long as usual, but it is quickly restored with additional doses of barium and methylcellulose. The hyperperistalsis also persists in the methylcellulose phase. The flow rate sometimes has to be increased to 100–150 ml/min in the case of hyperperistalsis, so that adequate filling and distension of the bowel are achieved.

Rare, *hormone producing tumors* (vipoma), e.g. glucagonoma and gastrinoma (Zollinger-Ellison syndrome) cause massive hyperperistalsis with watery diarrhea which is partially due

Table 5.4.-1. Hyperperistalsis

	General, propulsive	*Nonpropulsive (pendular) peristalsis*	*Local*
Normal or narrowed lumen	Psychogenic, emotional factors Hyperthyroidism Allergies Lactose intolerance Dermatitis herpetiformis Mastocytosis Intestinal lymphangiectasia Intestinal nodular lymphatic hyperplasia Giardiasis (lambliasis) Enteritis (bacterial, viral) Zollinger-Ellison syndrome Vagotomy Whipple's disease Celiac disease (sprue) Amyloidosis Gastrointestinal bleeding Carcinoid	Ischemia in diabetes arteriosclerosis vasculitis thrombosis Eosinophilic enteritis Bacterial overgrowth Hypoalbuminemia	Carcinoid Ulcer Segmental ischemia Radiation enteritis Adhesions Fibrous bands Hernia Amyloidosis Crohn's disease (e.g. string sign) Tumors Adjacent inflammation Parasites
Normal or increased lumen	Celiac disease ("colonization") (also hypoperistalsis)	Chronic pancreatic insufficiency Naish syndrome (also hypoperistalsis) Diabetes	

Table 5.4.-2. Hypoperistalsis

General		*Local*
Chronic abuse of laxatives tranquilizers and sedatives antipsychotic drugs spasmolytics pain killers vincristin Hypothyroidism Scleroderma and other collagen diseases Amyloidosis Diabetic neuro- and angiopathy Chronic alcoholism Amyotrophic lateral sclerosis Hypercalcemia Hypokalemia Sepsis Peritonitis Severe abdominal pain Lymphedema Uremia	Chronic lead poisoning Pregnancy Prolonged fasting Congenital (idiopathic intestinal pseudoobstruction) Advanced celiac disease or sprue	Mechanical obstruction Celiac disease Ischemia e.g. in trauma hematoma Amyloidosis

to malabsorption. Therefore nonspecific enteritis or mucosal irritation may be observed. The serotonin producing carcinoid causes local and/or general hyperperistalsis (see Fig. 5.3.-7, p. 113). After vagotomy, the hyperperistalsis and diarrhea are probably brought about by changes in the migrating motor complex.

Chronic *drug* abuse (e.g. laxatives, tranquilizers, sedatives, antipsychotic drugs, spasmolytics and pain killers) can result in a general hypoperistalsis (Figs. 5.4.-3 to 5). The clinical symptoms are subileus and ileus but without signs of peritonitis (Fig. 5.4.-3).

It is particularly important to know the effect of these drugs on the bowel, otherwise patients are subjected to unnecessary operations. It is also important to differentiate hypoperistalsis from dilatation in prolonged mechanical obstructions (see chapter 4.5). Since there are no signs of enteritis, the folds are normal and the mucosal coating remains intact.

The *idiopathic intestinal pseudoobstruction* also manifests itself in recurring, ileus-like attacks without evidence of a mechanical obstruction. The etiology of this rare disease is probably a disturbance of the slow waves of myoelectric activity. Enteroclysis reveals, like in drug-induced hypoperistalsis, dilatation and hypomotility of the jejunum as far as the ileojejunal junction. Afterwards, the contrast medium flows undisturbed in the undilated ileum, which may show even increased peristalsis (Figs. 5.4.-5 to 6). The jejunal peristalsis can also return to normal during the examination (Fig. 5.4.-6).

Naish syndrome is a rare disease (Naish et al. 1960). It is characterized by recurring episodes of colics with abdominal distension and diarrhea due to intestinal pseudoobstruction with steatorrhea. The cause is a considerable hypertrophic thickening of the intestinal wall, mainly of the inner muscular layer. Enteroclysis reveals dilated bowel loops, especially in the jejunum, with nonpropulsive hyperperistalsis (pendular peristalsis) and poor mucosal coating due to residual and partially undigested bowel contents (Fig. 5.4.-7). The final diagnosis can be established only by means of medical history and biopsy of the small intestinal musculature. Since elevated prostaglandin E level was found in these patients, therapy with indomethacin may be successful.

Other factors causing a general hypoperistalsis in this group are electrolyte imbalances (hypokalemia, hypercalcemia), neurological diseases, diabetes, uremia, chronic lead poisoning, severe abdominal pain, pregnancy, sepsis, peritonitis, and prolonged fasting (Franken et al. 1980).

5.4.2 Malabsorption

The causes of malabsorption are manifold. In this chapter, we will discuss the clinical pictures with special reference to motility disorders. These are partially pathological processes having a secondary effect on the small bowel, and partially primary diseases of the small bowel. Motility disorders are a result of changes in the mucosa, submucosa or in the structures of the deeper mural layers. A frequent symptom is chronic diarrhea with steatorrhea. The partially digested food results in a disturbed "intestinal milieu" which leads to the radiological appearance of a *nonspecific enteritis or mucosal irritation.*

This picture, associated with a nonpropulsive hyperperistalsis, is found in marked *exocrine pancreatic insufficiency*, the causes of which may be manifold. The intestinal wall and folds are thickened because of the often associated hypoalbuminemia and/or lymphedema. This intestinal wall edema is a further cause for a disturbed motility (Figs. 5.4.-8 and 21).

Allergic reactions on the gut may cause hyperperistalsis. This is mostly observed only in the presence of an allergen acting on the mucosa during the examination. This is why abnormality is rarely detected in the small bowel, when hypersensitivity to certain foods (milk protein, sea foods, citrus fruits etc.) is known from history. The same goes for lactose intolerance which is quite common in many parts of the world. If lactose is added to the contrast medium, a hyperperistalsis with poor mucosal coating may be observed (Gupta 1984). We do not perform this test. In marked disaccharidase deficiency, we observed this phenomenon without lactose additive (Fig. 5.4.-9). Allergic reactions with general or local hyperperistalsis can also be caused by the Schönlein-Henoch allergic vasculitis, ascaris and other worms as well as by giardiasis (see Fig. 4.5.-2, pp. 48–51). *Celiac disease* (sprue) is defined as intolerance against gluten, mostly found in wheat. It belongs to the most frequent causes of malabsorption in childhood (Shmerling et al. 1972). The term celiac disease is a specific disease whereas the term sprue syndrome (often occurring in adulthood) embraces various malabsorption conditions with similar symptoms which often respond to gluten-free foods but which are not gluten-induced. Synonyms of celiac disease are idiopathic steatorrhea, nontropical sprue, gluten-induced enteropathy. The clinical symptoms are chronic diarrhea (can be absent in ca. 10%), anorexia, underweight, retarded growth, muscle atrophy, osteomalacia and psychological alterations.

In most cases, the radiological picture is characteristic (Figs. 5.4.-10 to 13). In celiac disease, the average number of folds in the proximal jejunum is reduced to 2.88/2.5 cm (0–5 folds) in comparison with 4.88/2.5 cm (3–7) in normal individuals. Sprue leads to an increase of folds in the ileum on the average of 4.76/2.5 cm (4–6 folds) against 3.15/2.5 cm (2–4) in normal controls. Demonstration of five or more folds in the jejunum and/or three or fewer folds in the ileum are evidence against a diagnosis of celiac disease (Herlinger and Maglinte 1986). In order to assess the pathological changes, the flow rate of the contrast medium has to be raised, to ensure adequate filling of the bowel. Corresponding to the mucosal atrophy in the duodenum and jejunum, there is a loss of folds, so that the well-filled small bowel shows a colon-like haustration ("colonization" of the jejunum). This picture is also known as "moulage sign". The intestinal lumen may be considerably dilated (Fig. 5.4.-12). This is associated with local hypoperistalsis. In the ileum, there is a resulting increase of folds ("jejunization" of the ileum) and reactive hyperperistalsis. This process may be conceived as a compensatory response to the loss of mucosal surface in the jejunum. In active disease manifestation there is reduced mucosal coating due to malabsorption and inflammation (Figs. 5.4.-10 and 11). In adult sprue, the morphological fold changes do not disappear with appropriate treatment whereas the mucosal irritation will subside (Fig. 5.4.-13). However, in a small percentage there are only slight or even no radiological changes in spite of a positive biopsy. One should bear in mind that a gastrointestinal lymphoma or carcinoma can develop on the basis of celiac disease. Follow-up examinations are therefore indicated.

Other diseases which are accompanied by malabsorption and disturbed motility include Whipple's disease (Fig. 5.2.-21, pp. 100–101), eosinophilic enteritis (Fig. 5.2.-19, pp. 97–98), bacterial overgrowth (Fig. 5.2.-18, p. 96), viral and bacterial enteritis (Figs. 5.2.-16, 17, pp. 94–95), Crohn's disease, mastocytosis, dermatitis herpetiformis and intestinal lymphangiectasis (Figs. 5.4.-21 and 22).

5.4.3 Diseases of the Intestinal Wall

Infiltration, inflammation or other pathological changes of the intestinal wall structures can result in motility disorders. In *scleroderma*, the esophagus and small bowel are mostly involved. Fibrin deposits in the vessels lead to ischemic necroses and atrophy of the musculature and replacement by connective tissue. This results in hypoperistalsis, dilatation and sometimes stenoses. The duodenum and proximal jejunum are mostly involved (Olmsted and Madewell 1976). Further typical changes are broad-based diverticula and the *hide-bound sign* (Horowitz and Meyers 1973), i.e. crowding of folds in a distended intestinal segment (Fig. 5.4.-14).

Other diseases pertaining to the collagenoses are *periarteritis nodosa, systemic lupus erythematosus* and *dermatomyositis*. In these diseases, vascular changes are the most conspicuous. The consequences are mostly nonpropulsive hyperperistalsis, ulceration, wall infiltration, and bleeding.

In both primary and secondary *amyloidosis*, amyloid deposits may appear locally or diffuse in all the intestinal wall layers throughout the digestive tract. The infiltrations are sometimes impossible to differentiate from diffuse malignant lymphoma (Fig. 5.4.-15). In involvement of the ileum with atrophy of the mucosa and thickening of the wall, it is impossible to differentiate between Crohn's disease or backwash ileitis in ulcerative colitis (Fig. 5.4.-16). The motility disturbances and symptoms depend on the degree and localization of amyloidosis. The spectrum extends from general hyperperistalsis to local or general hypoperistalsis with the picture of pseudoobstruction. In some cases, celiac disease may be difficult to differentiate.

5.4.4 Vascular Changes

Ischemia is the cause of many small bowel diseases, since the intramural ganglia react sensitively to oxygen deficiency. This leads to changes in the bowel motility. Some of the ischemia-induced diseases are dealt with elsewhere (e.g. radiation vasculitis, collagen diseases, allergic vasculitis, amyloid and obstructions).

Arteriosclerosis of the superior mesenteric artery is the most frequent and important reason for ischemic disorder. Other causes are the various forms of vasculitis. Since in arteriosclerosis collateral vessels have already developed, small vessel occlusion is clinically and angiographically difficult to diagnose. However, the circulation may be locally so compromised that ischemic stenoses develop (see Fig. 2.8.-3, p. 19).

A mild *ischemia* causes a general or local hyperperistalsis. The bowel lumen is narrowed, the mucosal coating is normal. In more pronounced stages, e.g. in diabetic microangiopathy which is frequently associated with neuropathy, the picture changes from a nonpropulsive hyperperistalsis to hypoperistalsis. In additional malabsorption, the mucosal coating may be reduced (Fig. 5.4.-18). This dysfunction and a subsequent bacterial overgrowth are considered as causes of diabetogenous diarrhea.

The acute *occlusion of the superior mesenteric artery* is no indication for investigation of the small bowel. In partial occlusion due to embolism or thrombosis with a protracted course, there is nevertheless damage of long bowel sections with necroses of the mucosa, wall edema and submucosal hemorrhage. Radiological findings reveal signs of a nonspecific enteritis or mucosal irritation with nonpropulsive peristalsis, possible hypoperistalsis and lumen dilatation (Fig. 5.4.-19). The intramural edema and bleeding produce a so-called thumb-printing picture which may be seen on a plain film of the abdomen.

Intramural hematomas are caused by trauma, anticoagulation therapy, hemophilia and thrombocytopenia. The affected bowel loops are hypoperistaltic or spastically narrowed. The wall and the folds are thickened and the interfold spaces are compressed showing the stacked coin sign as well as the thumb-print sign.

Mechanical obstructions caused by fibrous bands, volvulus, malrotation, internal hernias and adjacent inflammations can also influence the arterial and venous blood supply. The latter leads to a local ischemia with pseudoobstruction (Fig. 5.4.-17).

The intestinal circulation may also be influenced by low cardiac output and portal hypertension.

Blood in the intestinal lumen in itself causes a reactive hyperperistalsis with reduced mucosal coating (Fig. 5.4.-20).

Vascular diseases also include changes in the *lymphatic vessels*. The rare disease of *intestinal lymphangiectasia* is mostly a congenital malformation of the intestinal lymphatics (Shimkin et al. 1970). The patients suffer from protein loss into the intestine, which leads to hypoproteinemia. The folds are thickened and nodular. The mucosal coating is significantly reduced and the bowel is hypermotile, sometimes nonpropulsive (Figs. 5.4.-21 and 22). Similar changes are also seen in lymphatic block due to malignant diseases.

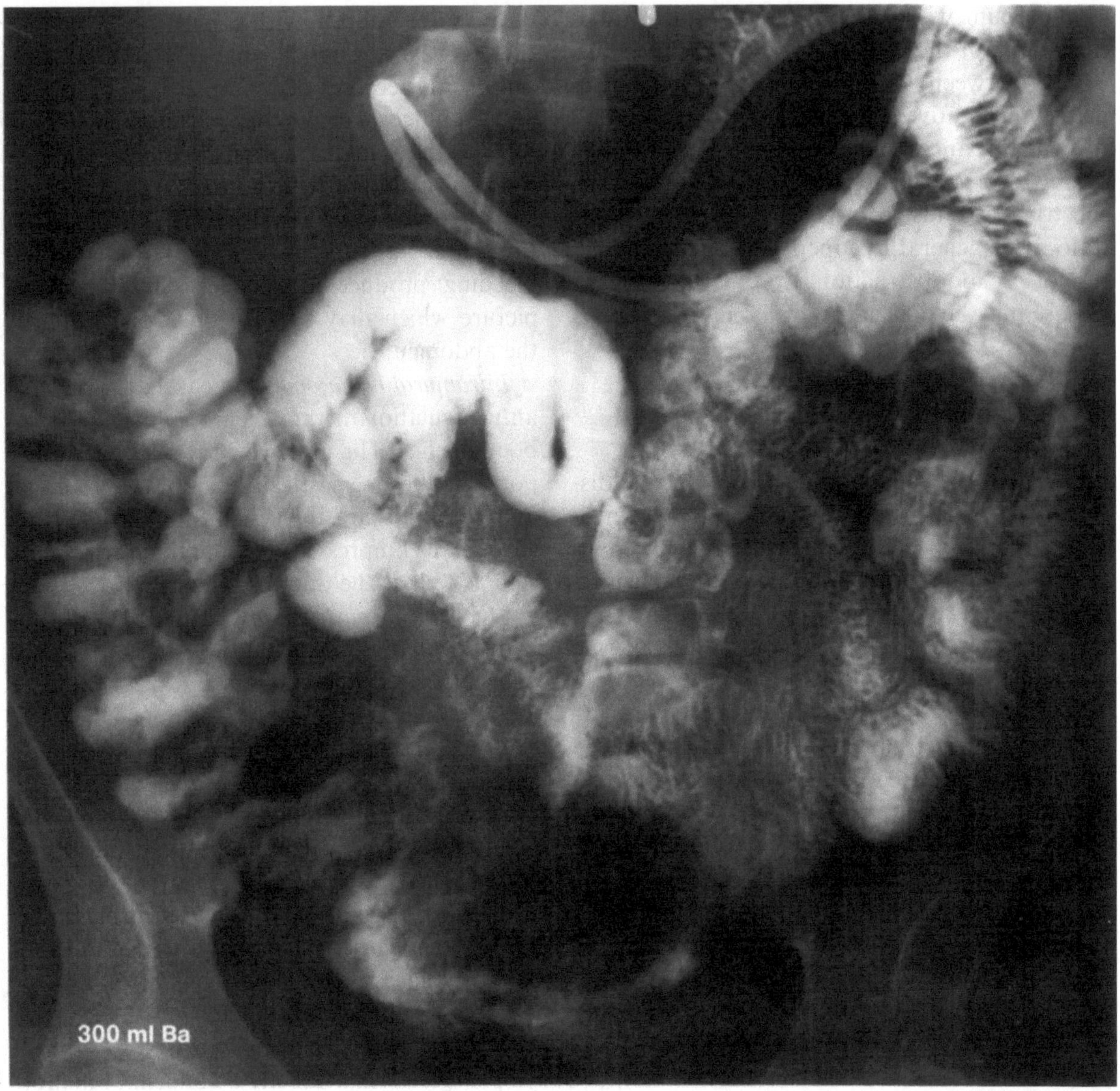

a

Fig. 5.4.-1 a and b. Hyperperistalsis, psychogenic, emotionally induced. Intestinal hurry in the barium phase (**a**), persistence of hyperperistalsis with adequate mucosal coating in the methylcellulose phase (**b**). Diminished diameter of bowel lumen. 36-year-old patient with uncharacteristic abdominal symptoms. Psychological problems

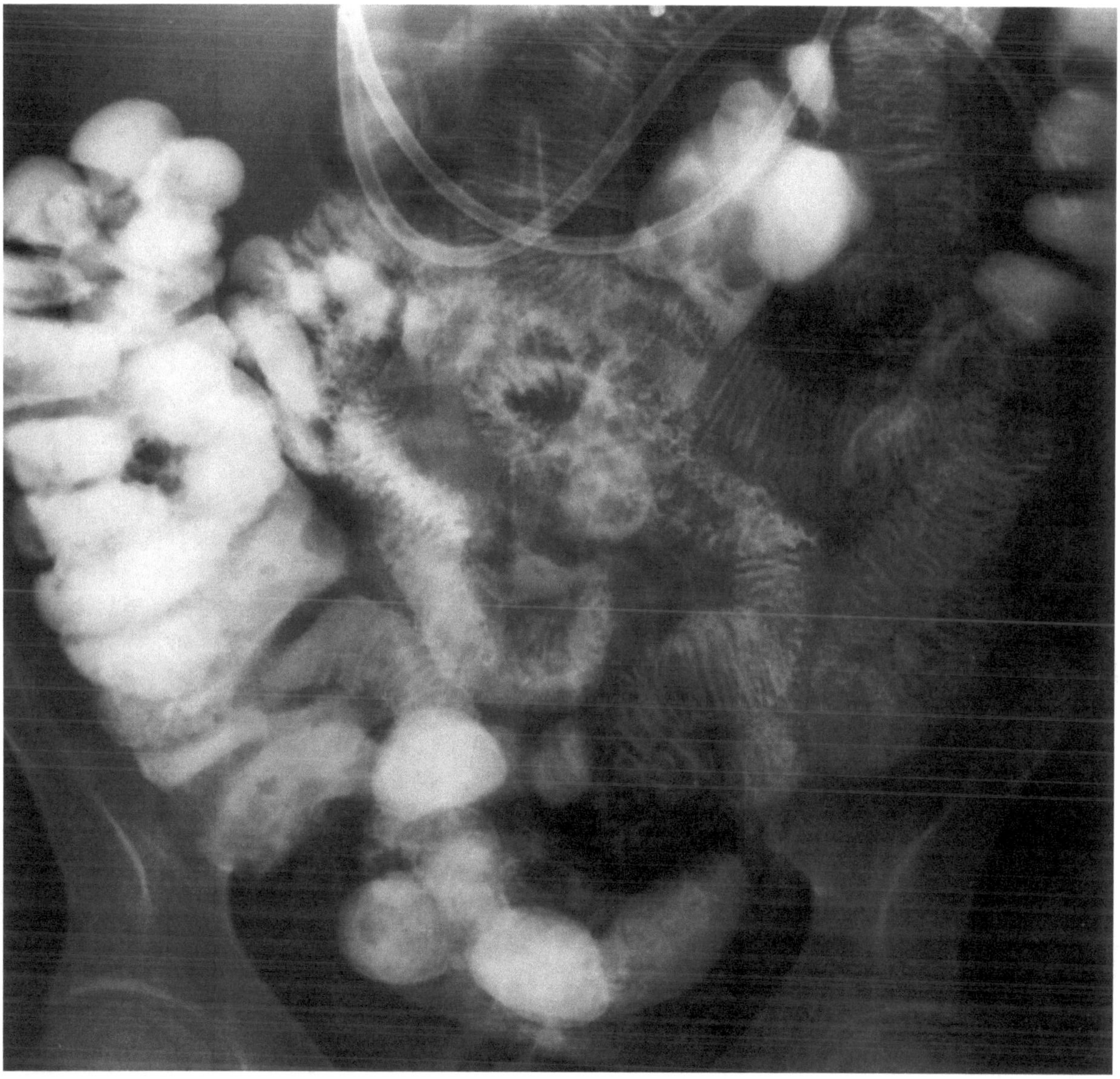

Fig. 5.4.-1 b

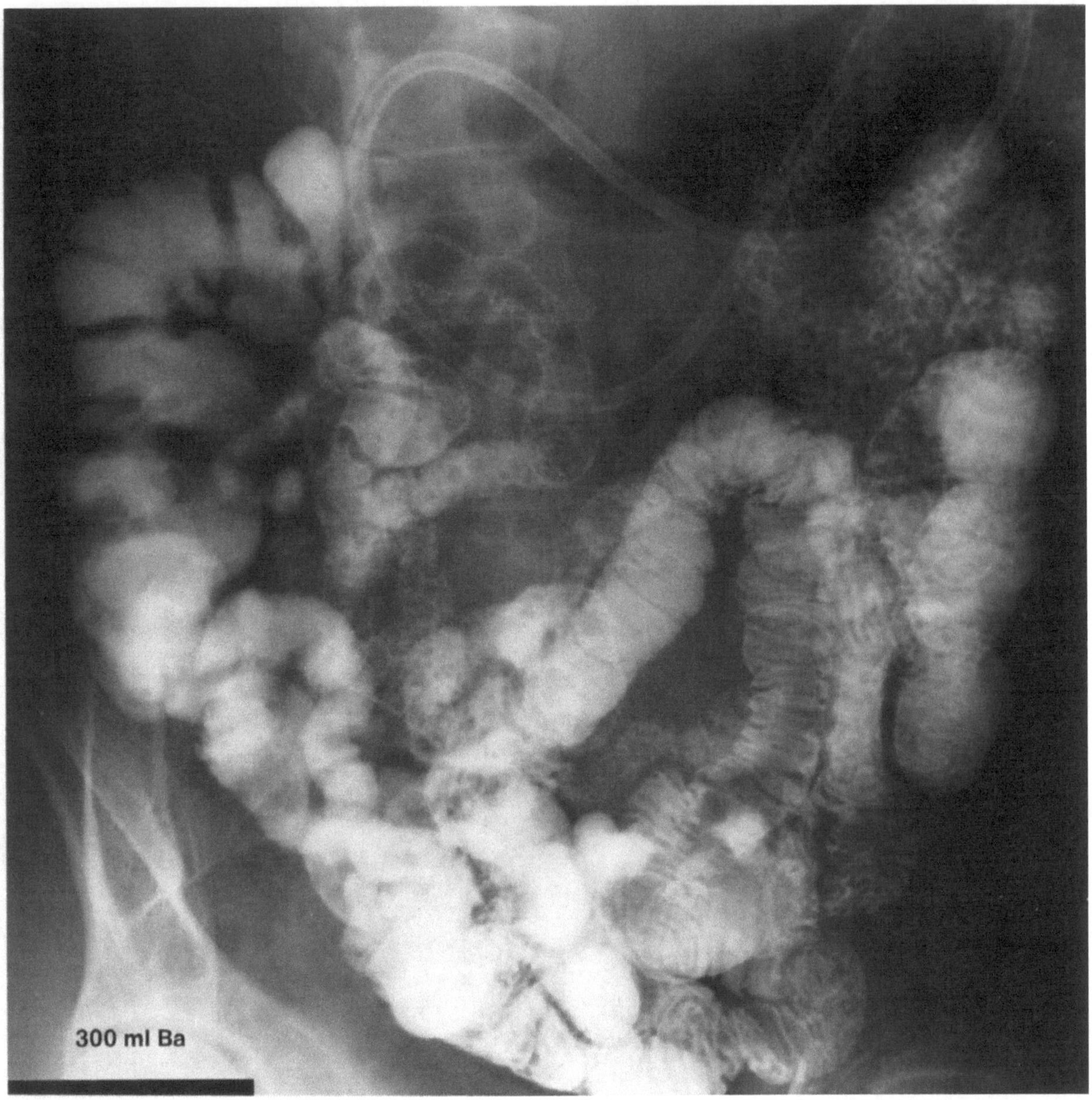

a

Fig. 5.4.-2 a and b. Hyperperistalsis, psychogenic, emotional. Intestinal hurry (**a**). Double contrast is already forming in the barium phase due to aerophagy. In the methylcellulose phase (**b**), the hyperperistalsis persists and the mucosal coating is maintained. Spastic colonic haustral pattern. No evidence of inflammatory changes. 52-year-old man with irritable bowel syndrome

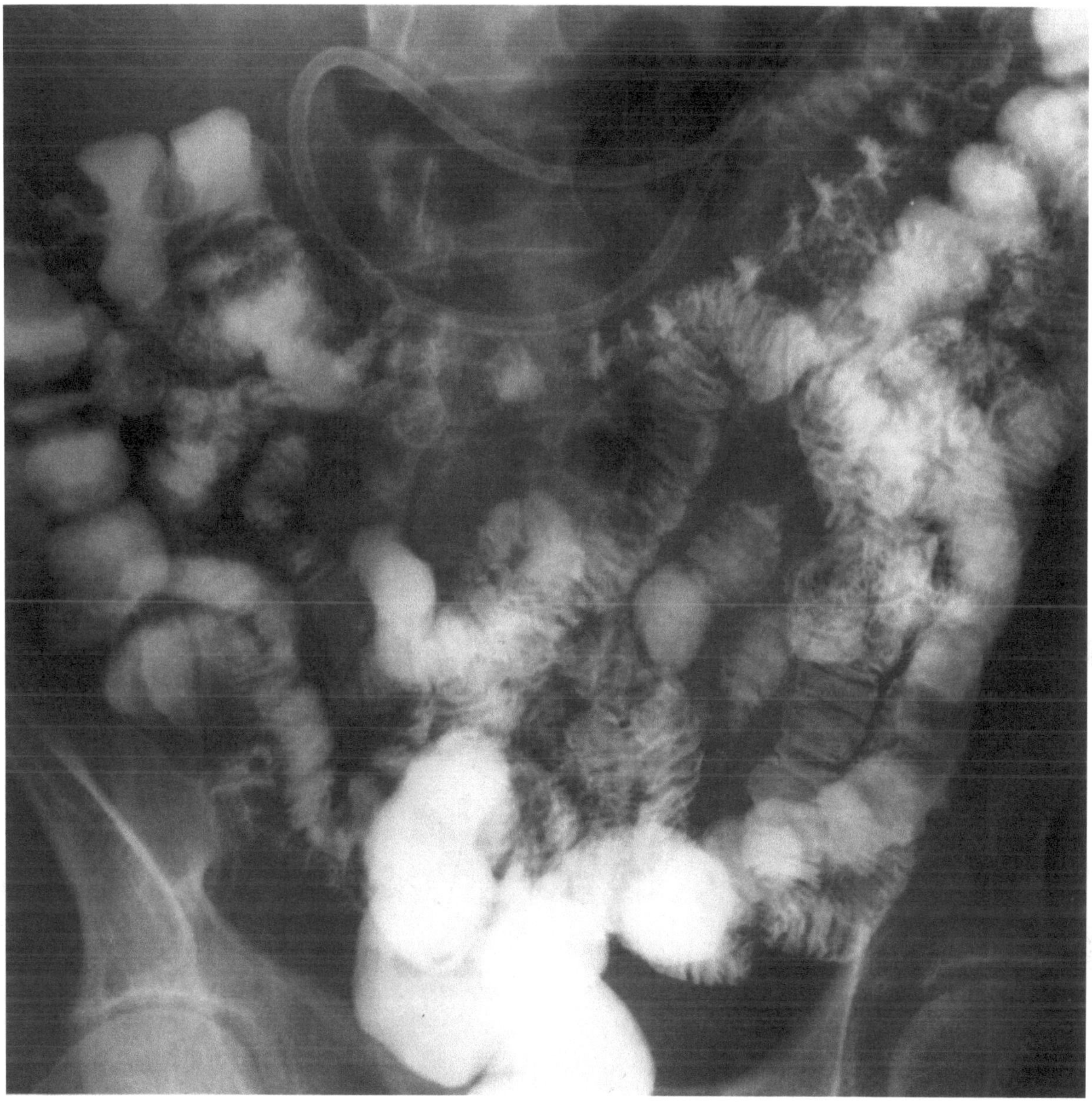

Fig. 5.4.-2b

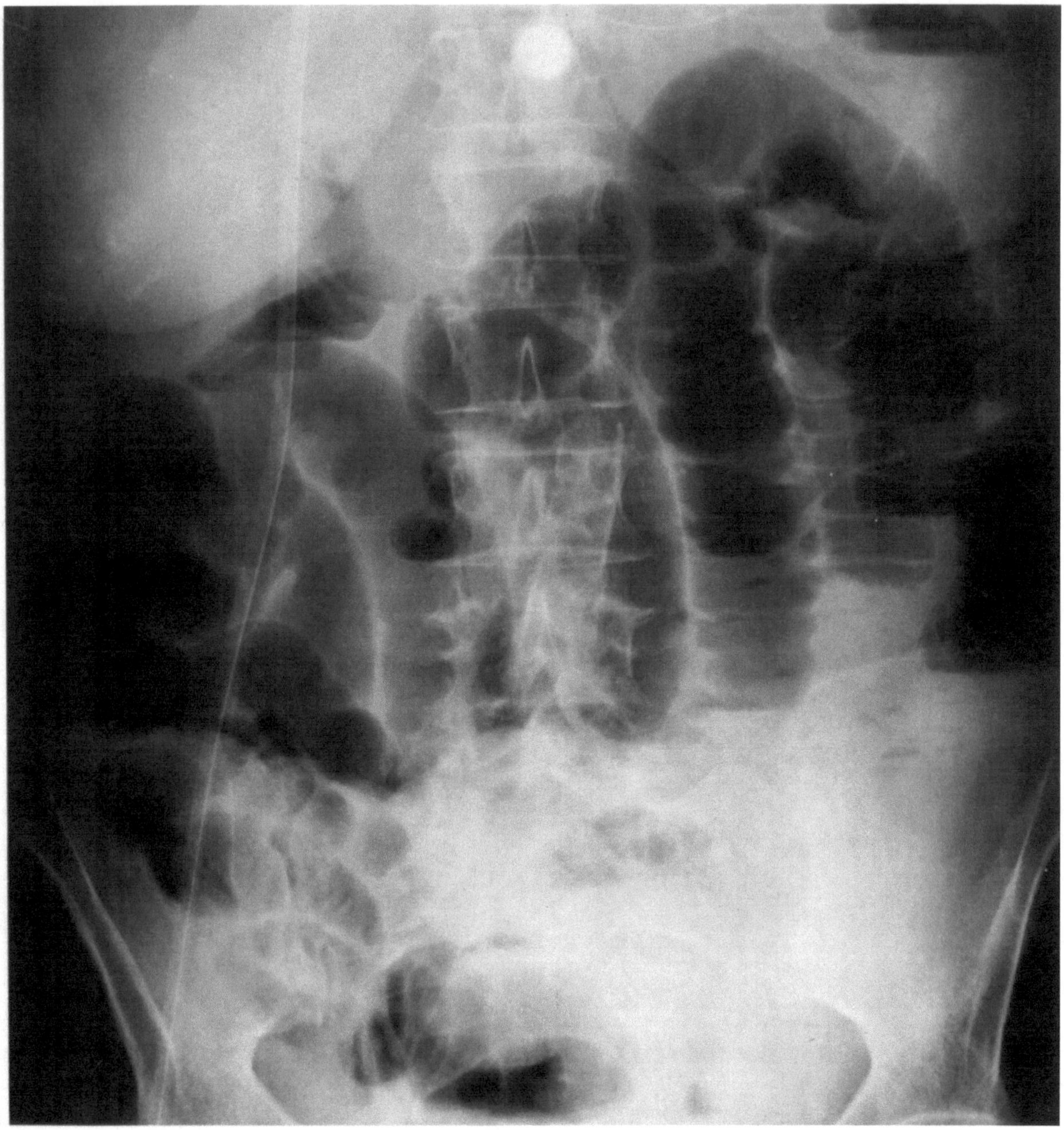

a

Fig. 5.4.-3 a to c. Hypoperistalsis, drug-induced. Female patient with ileus of unknown origin without peritonitis (**a**). Enteroclysis prior to an already planned operation shows all the signs of a marked general hypoperistalsis (**b**). Even after additional dosage of metoclopramide, there is no acceleration of passage (**c**). Normal mucosal coating, no inflammatory changes. After repeated questioning, the patient admitted to 30 years of laxative abuse. Additional findings: residual aqueous contrast medium after colon enema for the exclusion of stenosis, duodenal diverticulum and reflux into the common bile duct after papillotomy

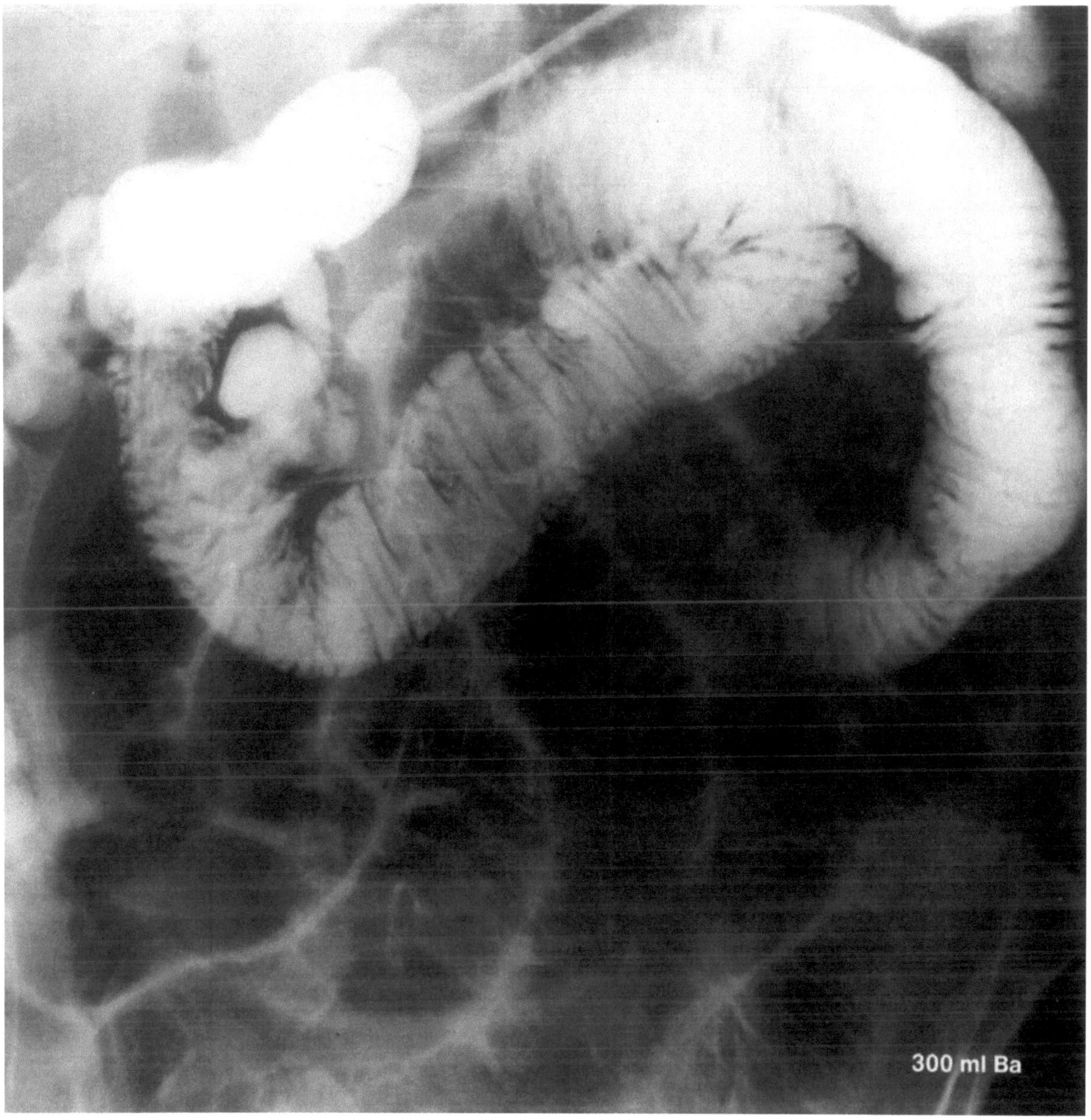

Fig. 5.4.-3b

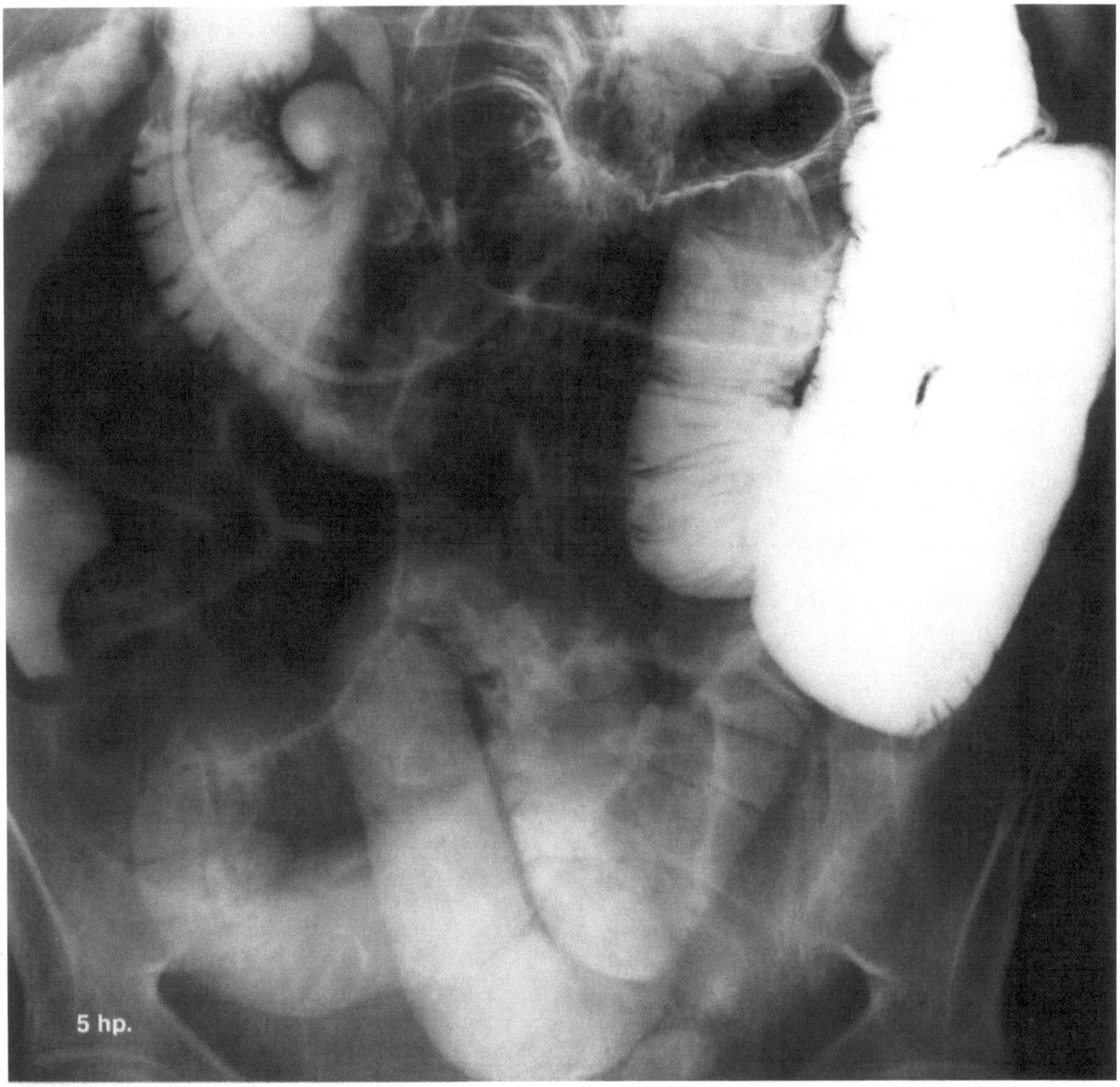

Fig. 5.4.-3c

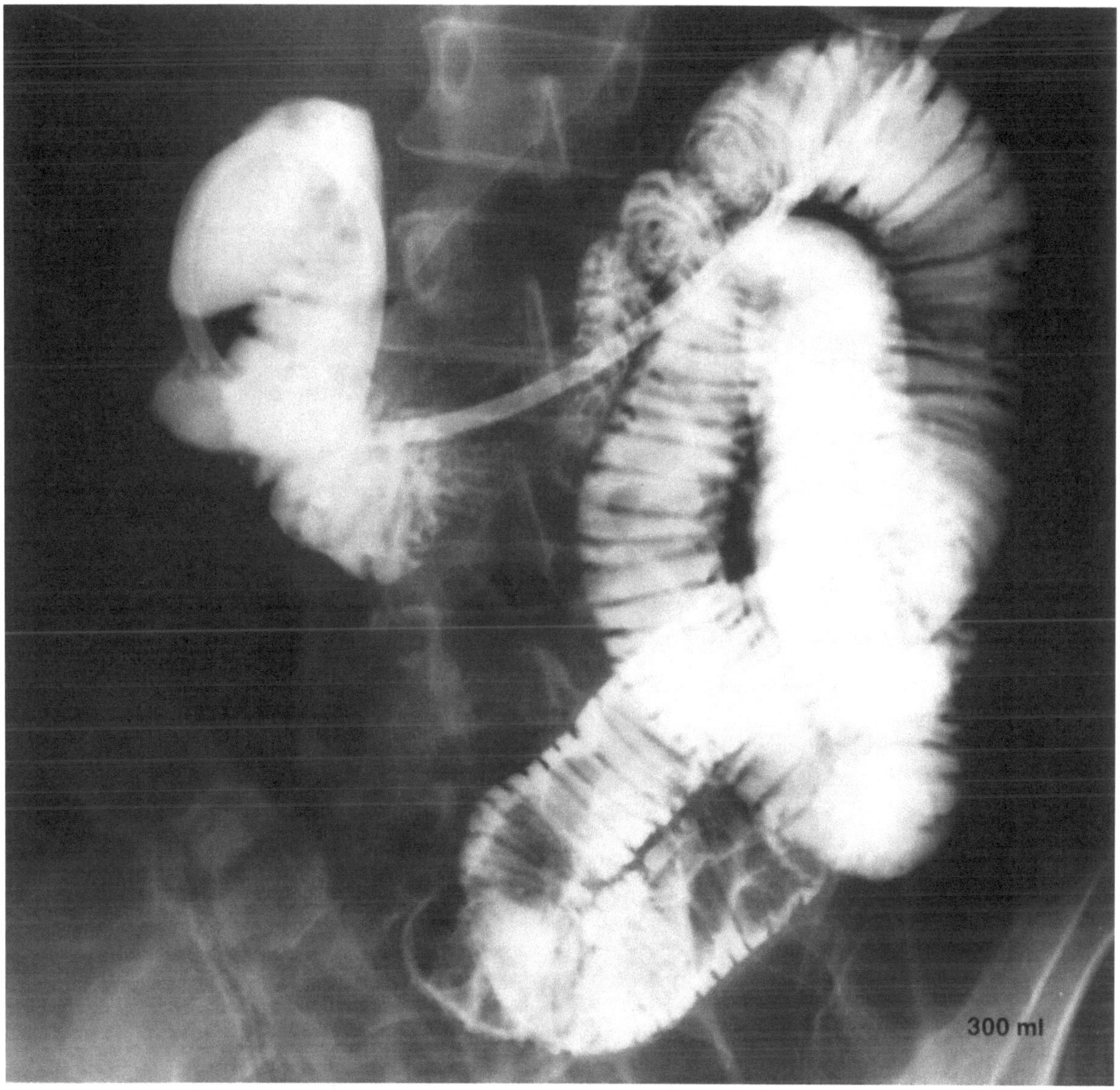

Fig. 5.4.-4. Hypoperistalsis, drug-induced. Distended hypomotile jejunum with residual food content. The patient who was underweight and suffering from diarrhea, was treated with loperamide. The loss of extraperitoneal fat resulted in a narrowing of the duodenum by the superior mesenteric artery (arteriomesenteric duodenal compression syndrome) which, together with the hypoperistalsis (loperamide-induced) prevented further advancement of the tube

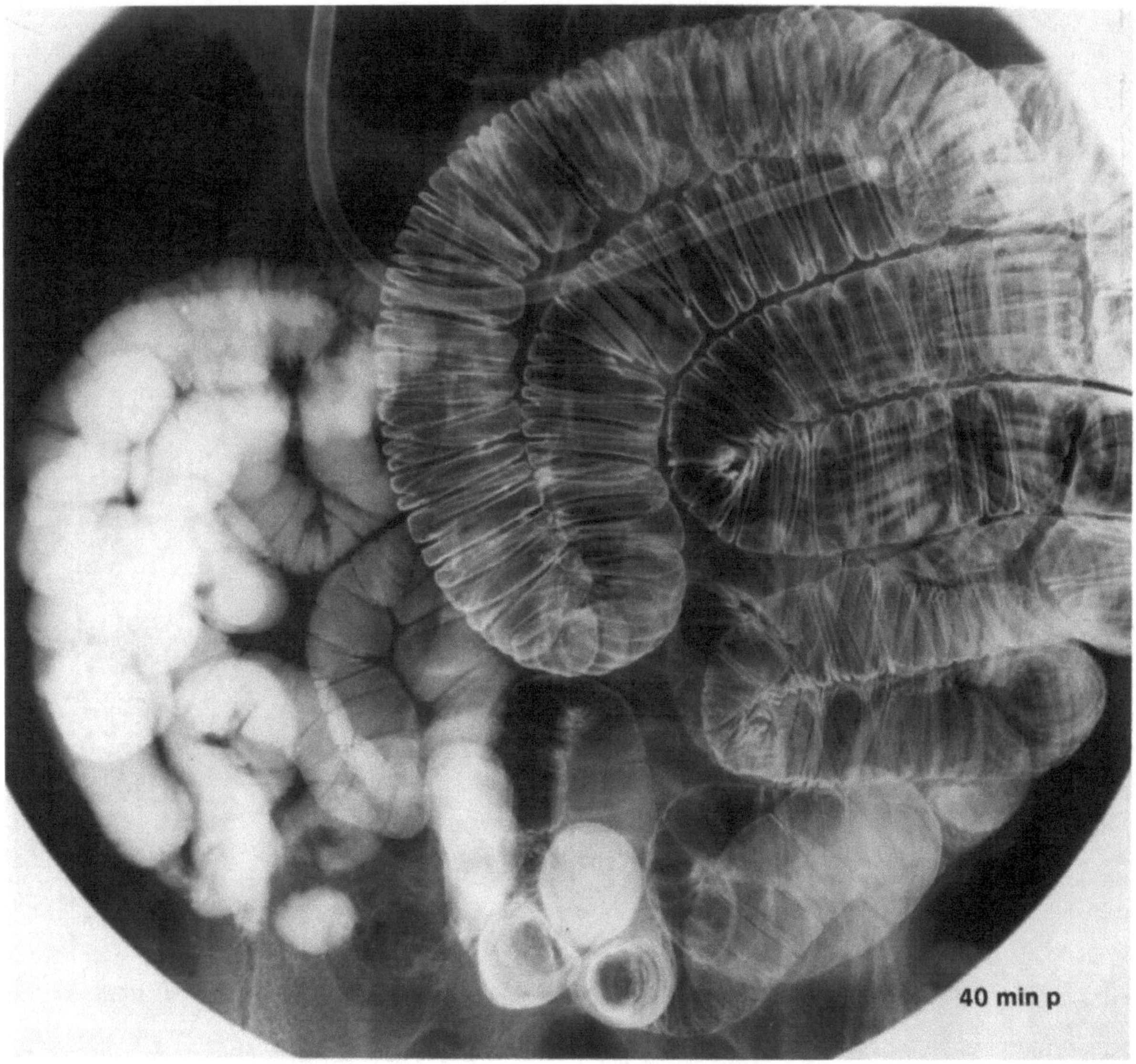

Fig. 5.4.-5. Hypoperistalsis, humoral-neurogenic induced. Dilatation and hypoperistalsis as far as the ileojejunal junction. Only after 40 min transit occurred into a nondistended ileum. 35-year-old patient with intermittent colicky abdominal pain and hypochondriac neurosis as well as considerable abuse of analgesics, spasmolytics and antipsychotic drugs. Status post vagotomy

a
b

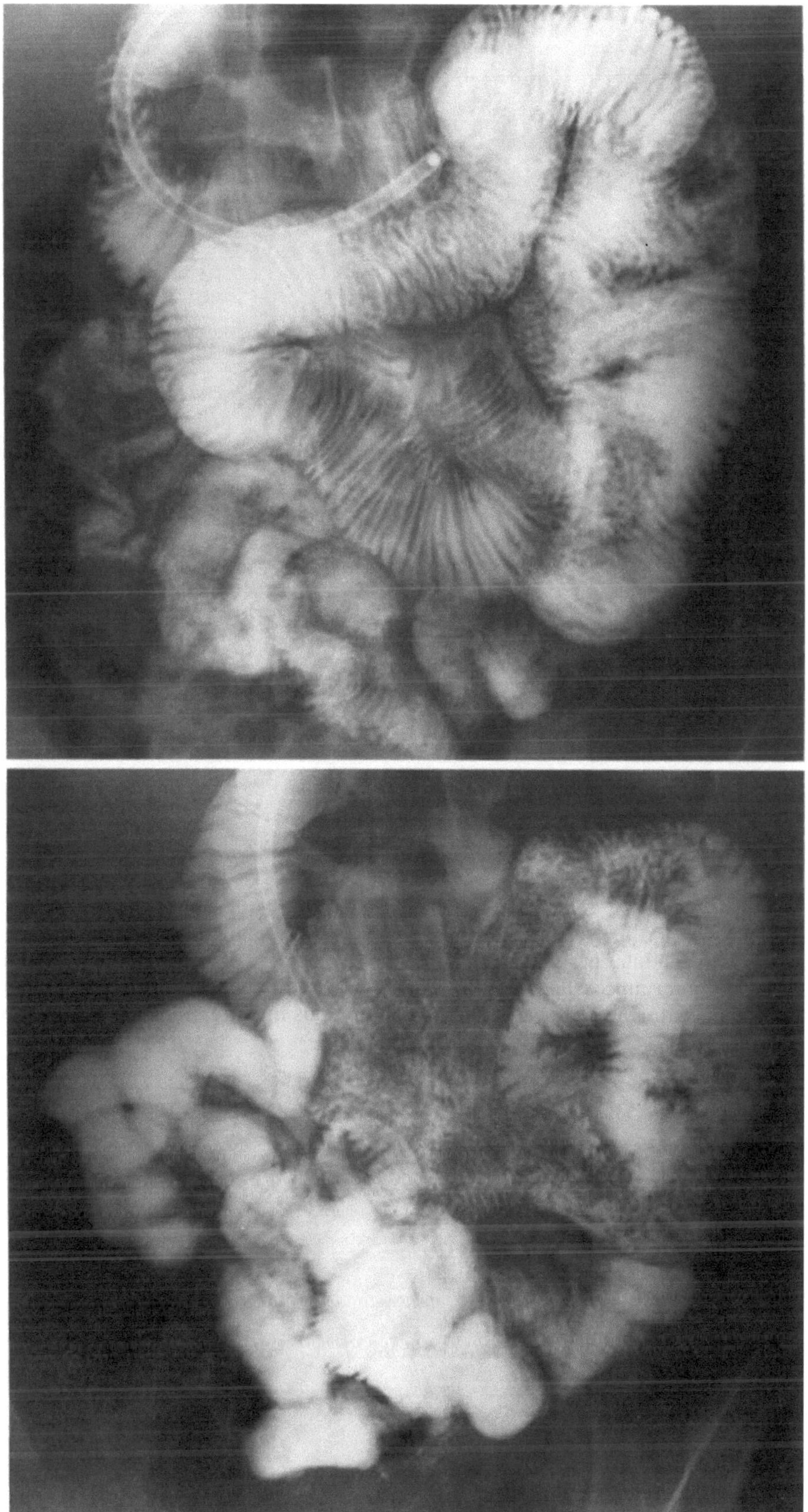

Fig. 5.4.-6a and b. Idiopathic pseudoobstruction. Considerable transit delay and hypoperistalsis with dilatation in the jejunum (**a**). After overcoming the ileojejunal junction, the peristalsis of the jejunum is normalized or even reactively increased due to rapid evacuation into the ileum (**b**). 21-year-old male with intermittent crampy periumbilical pain since childhood. A previous appendectomy because of this brought no improvement; all other investigations were unrevealing, too

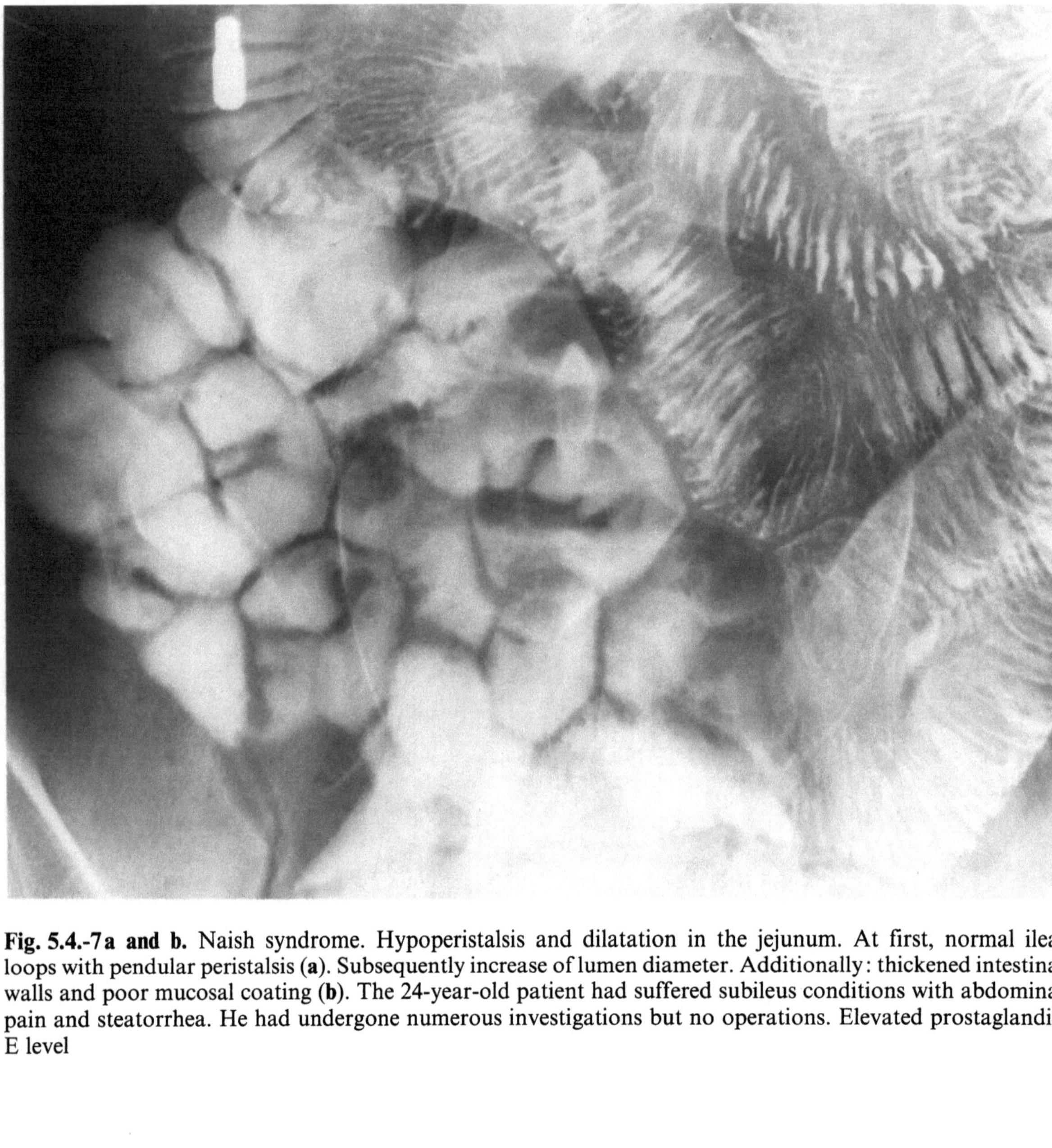

a

Fig. 5.4.-7a and b. Naish syndrome. Hypoperistalsis and dilatation in the jejunum. At first, normal ileal loops with pendular peristalsis (**a**). Subsequently increase of lumen diameter. Additionally: thickened intestinal walls and poor mucosal coating (**b**). The 24-year-old patient had suffered subileus conditions with abdominal pain and steatorrhea. He had undergone numerous investigations but no operations. Elevated prostaglandin E level

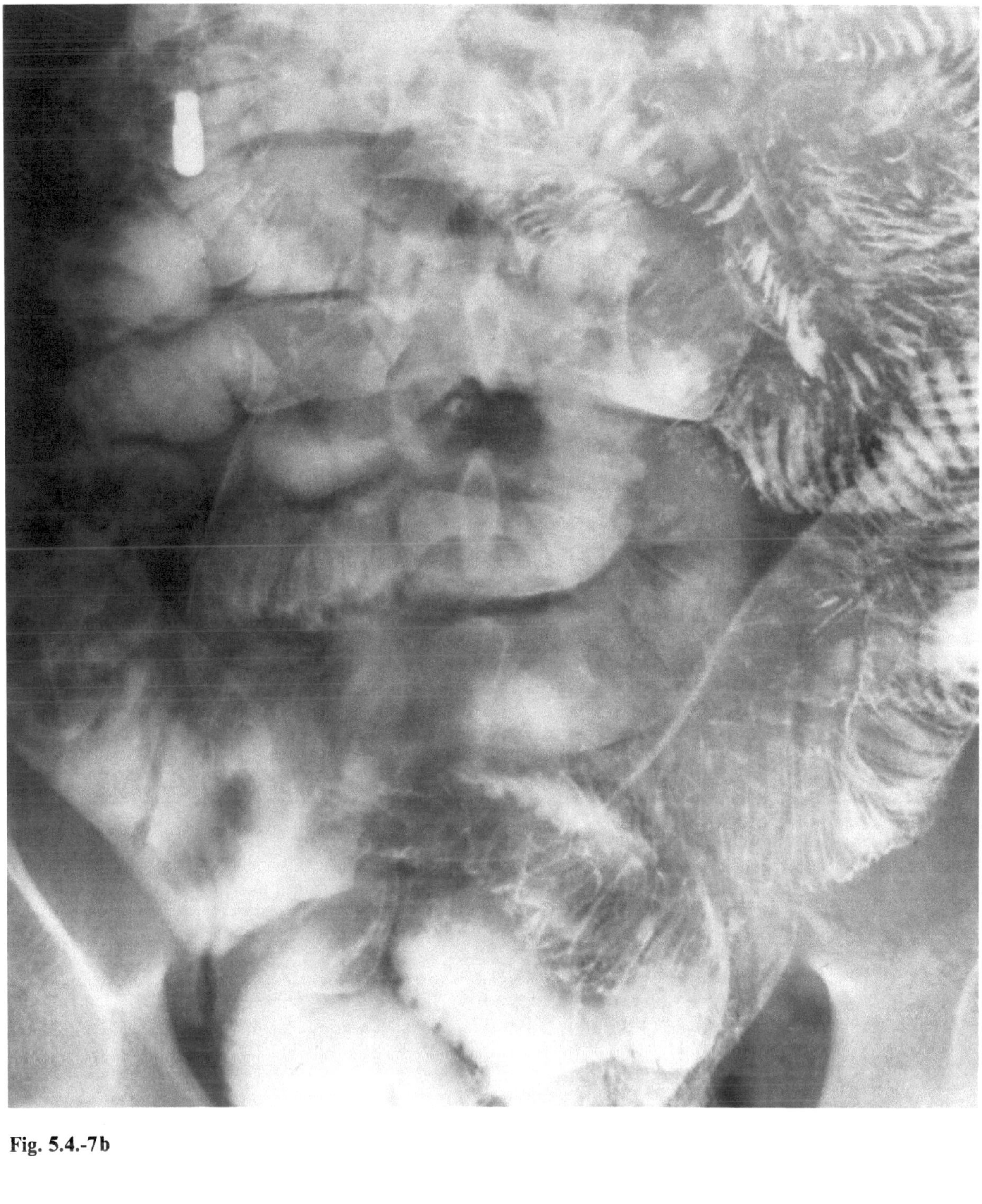

Fig. 5.4.-7b

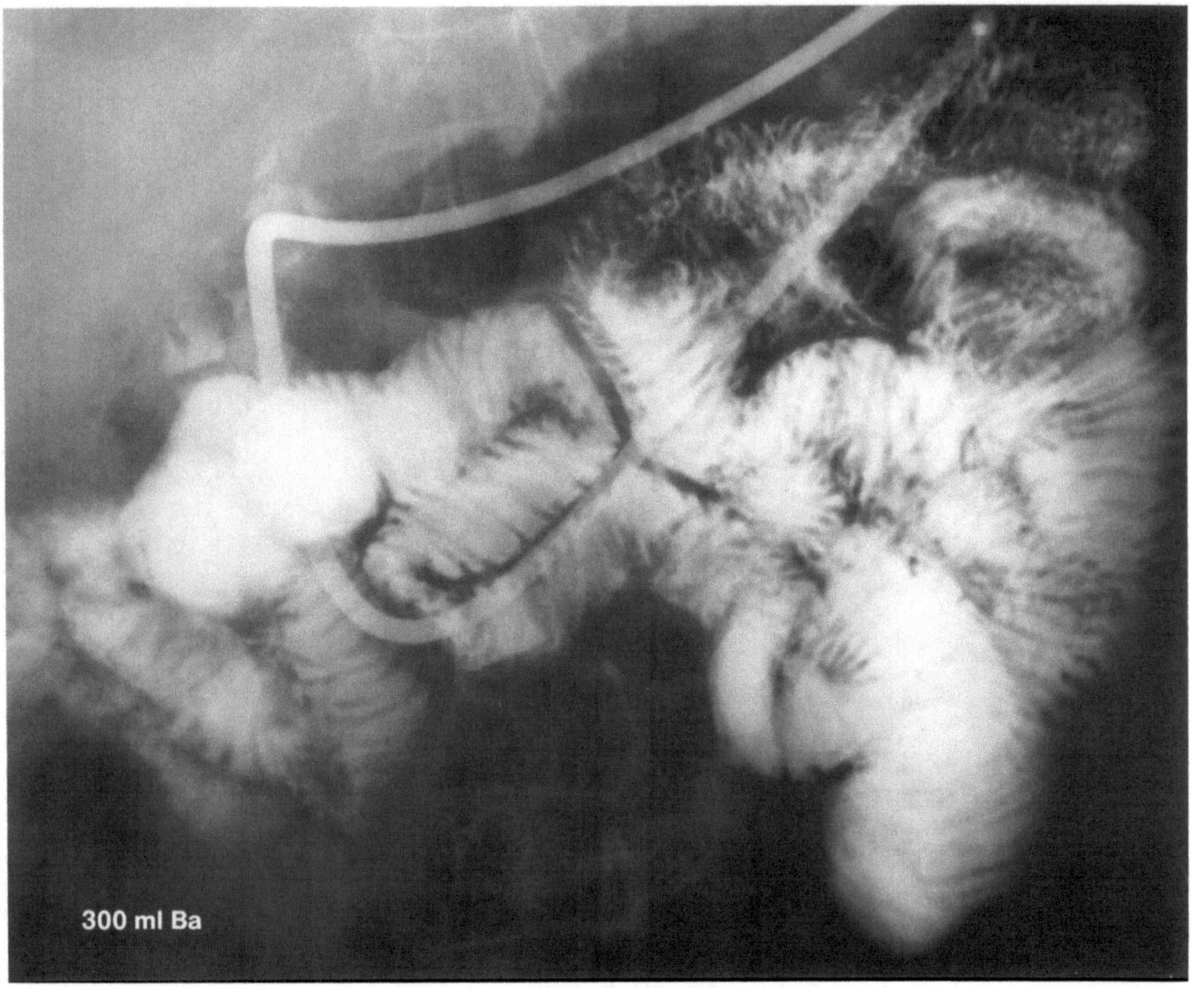

a

Fig. 5.4.-8 a and b. Malabsorption. Nonpropulsive hypermotility and premature flocculation. Thickened intestinal wall and folds (nonspecific enteritis and mucosal irritation). Patient with malabsorption in chronic pancreatic insufficiency, diabetic and alcohol-toxic polyneuropathy. **a** Barium phase. **b** Methylcellulose phase

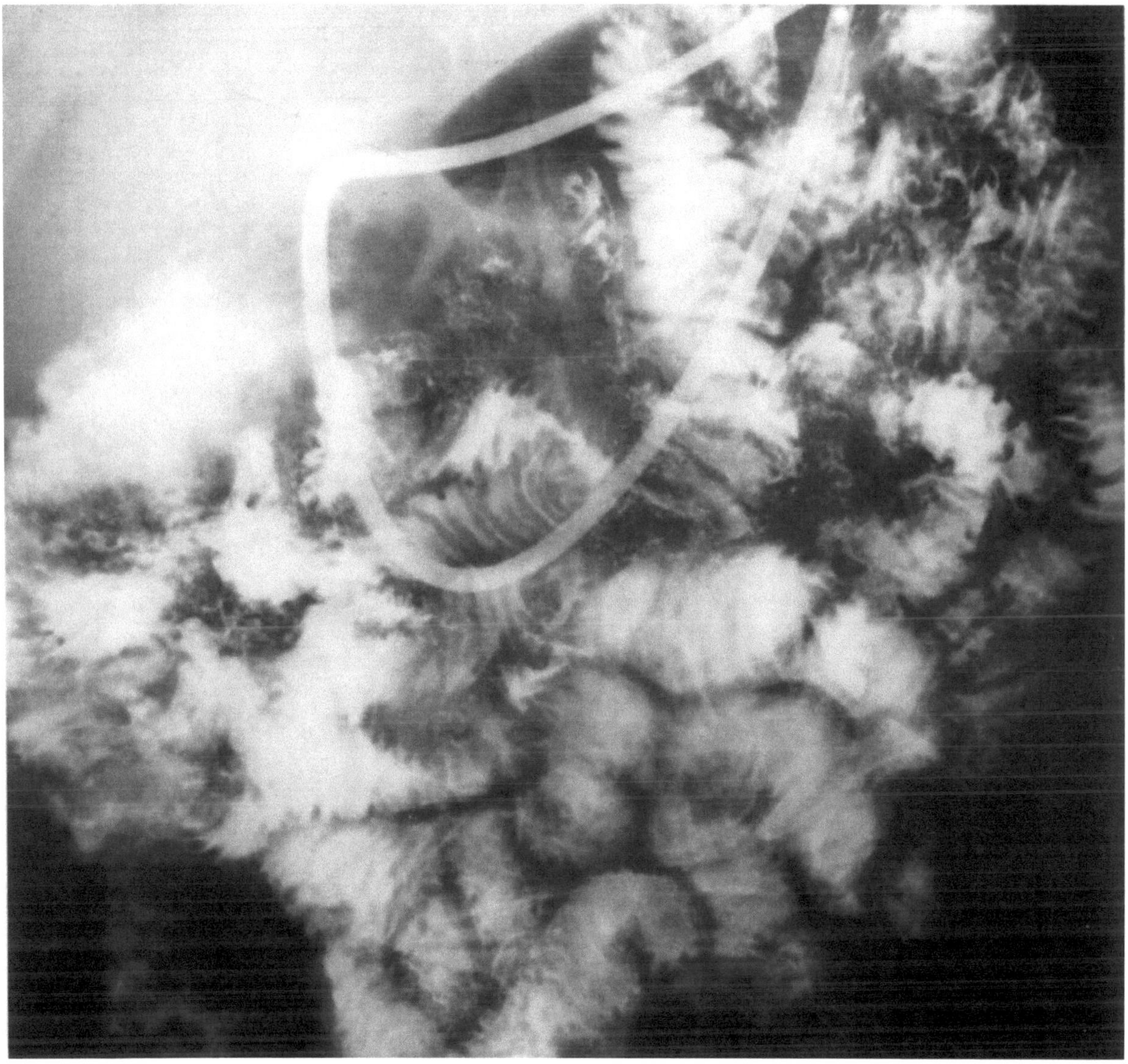

Fig. 5.4.-8 b

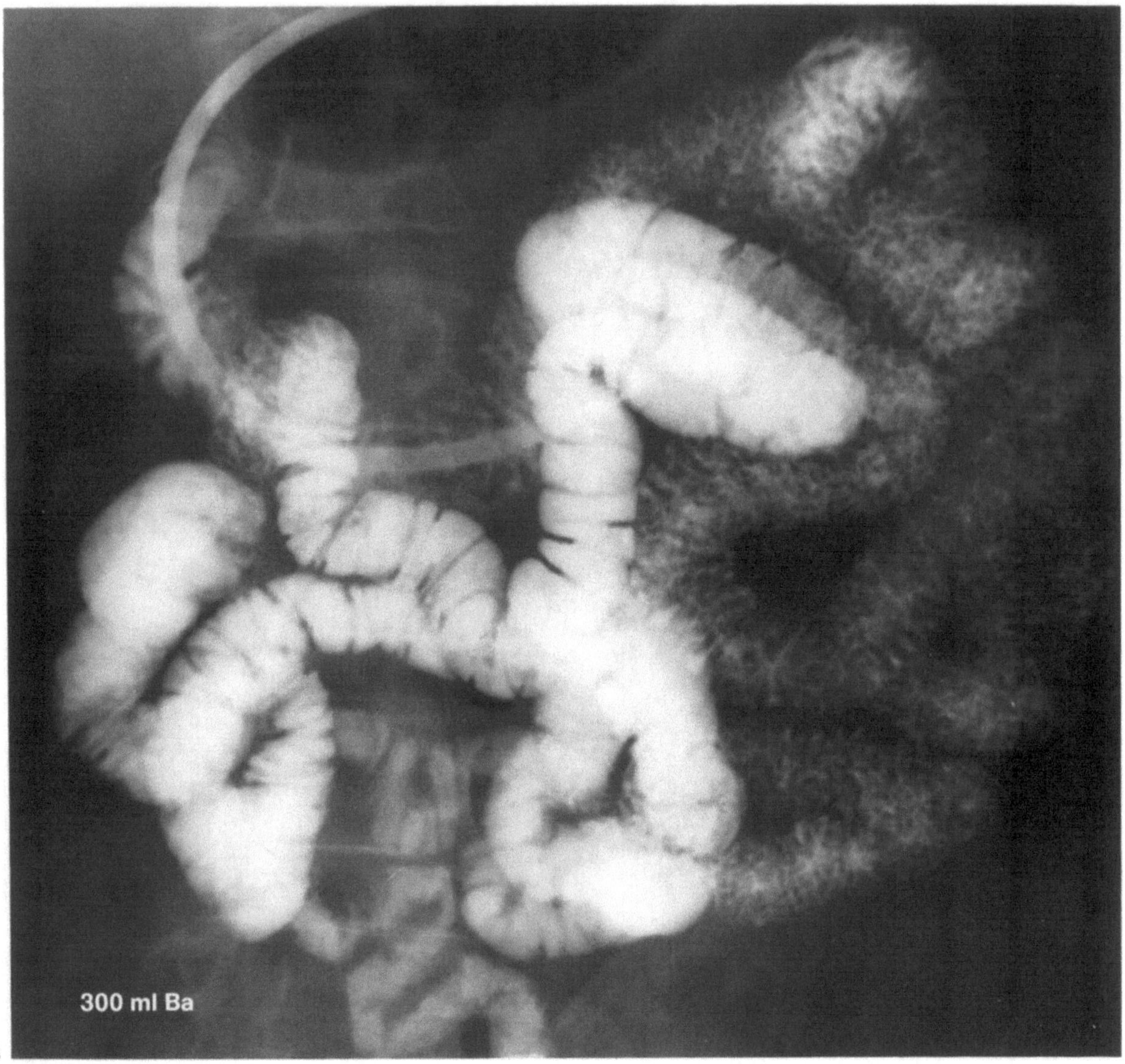

a

Fig. 5.4.-9 a and b. Lactose intolerance (disaccharidase deficiency). Hyperperistalsis, especially in the proximal jejunum (**a**). Poor mucosal coating and persistence of hyperperistalsis in the methylcellulose phase (**b**). 41-year-old male with diarrhea, also after beer consumption (maltase deficiency). Milk has been avoided since childhood. Proved deficiency of all disaccharidases

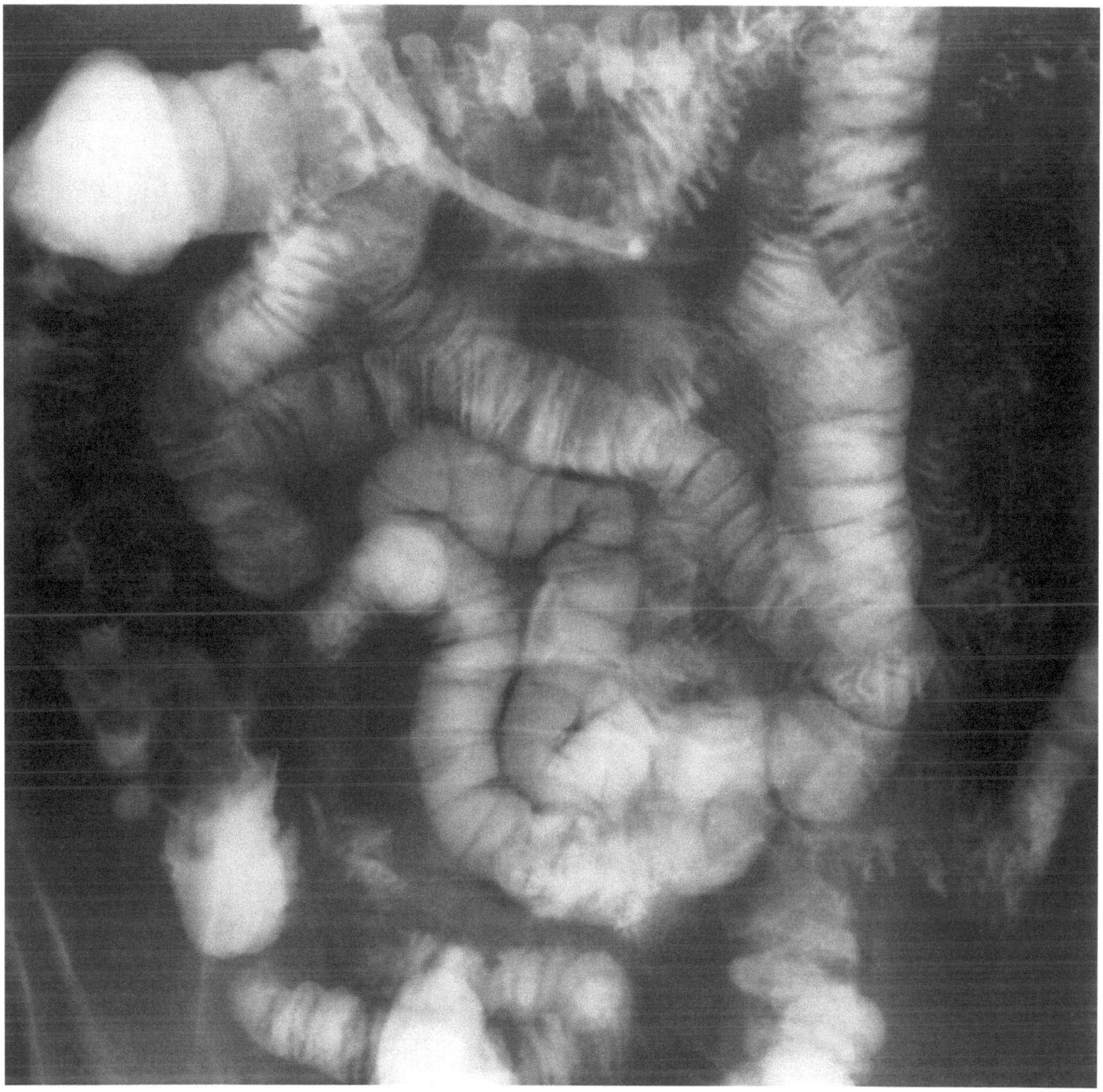

Fig. 5.4.-9b

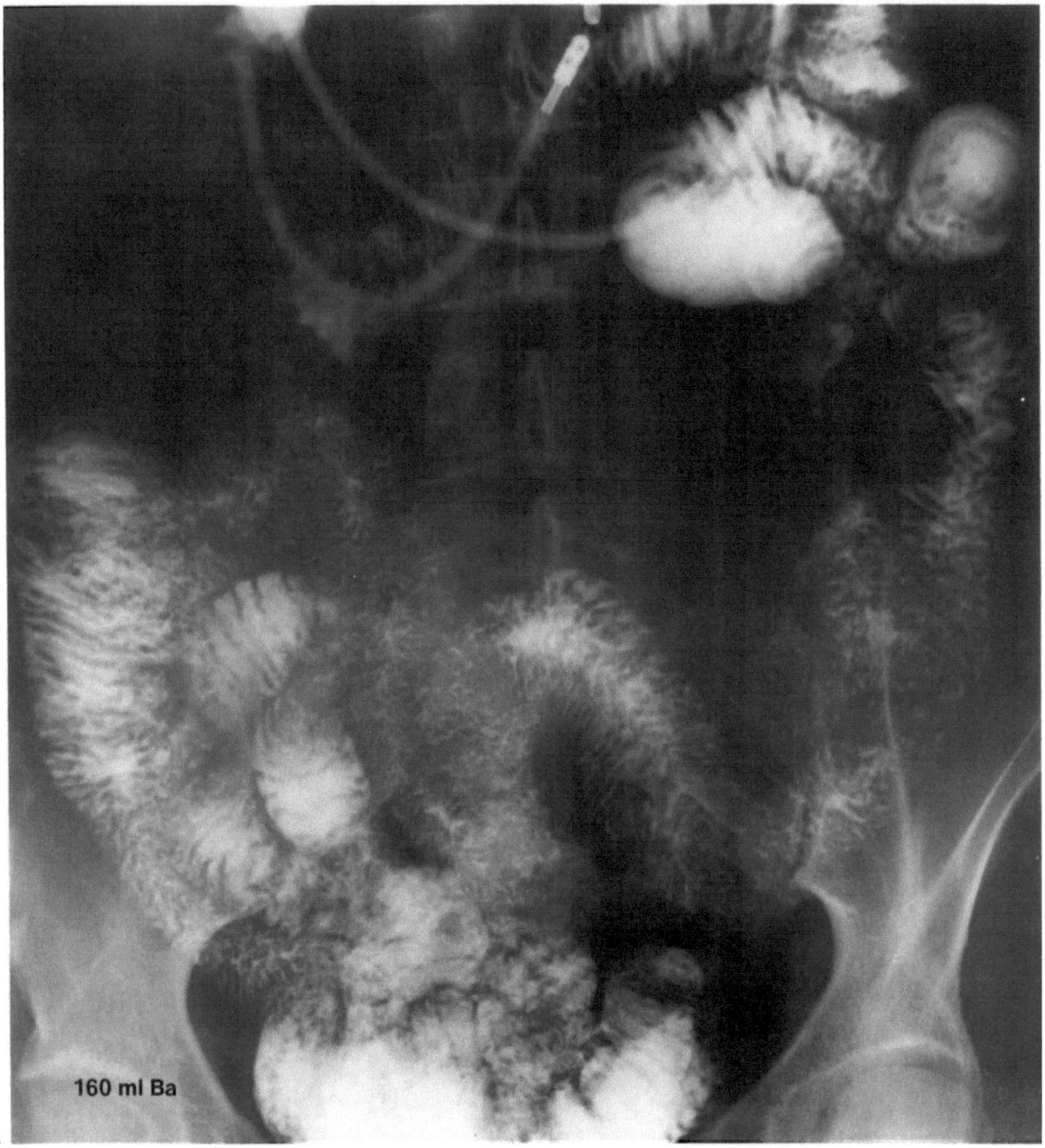

a

Fig. 5.4.-10 a and b. Celiac disease. General hyperperistalsis, incipient colonization in the duodenum and proximal jejunum. Jejunization of the ileum, reduced mucosal coating. 40-year-old patient with chronic diarrhea, meteorism, anorexia, weight loss and fatigue. Biopsy: subtotal villous atrophy and marked chronic inflammation. Improvement with gluten-free diet. **a** Barium phase. **b** Methylcellulose phase

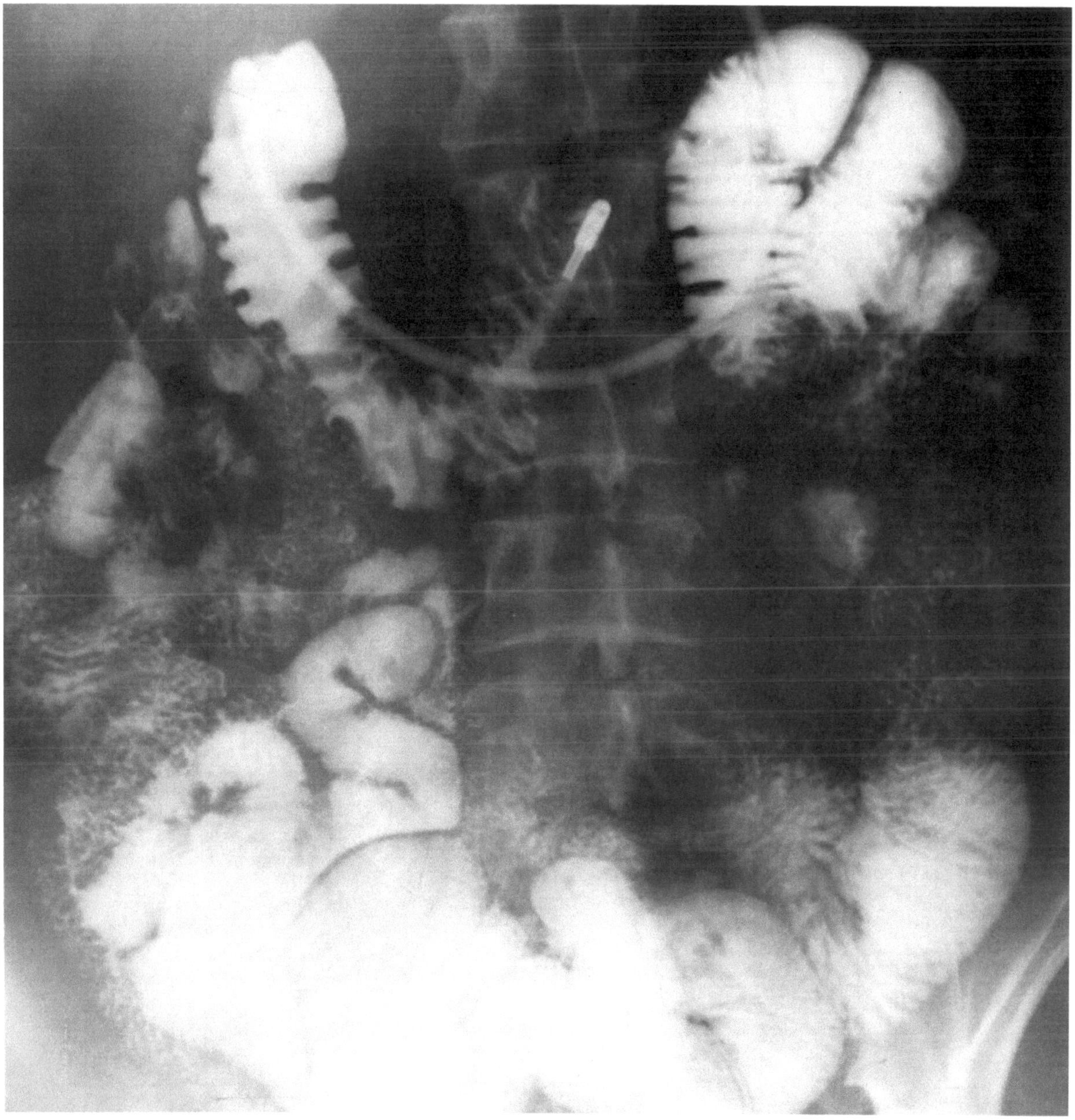

Fig. 5.4.-10b

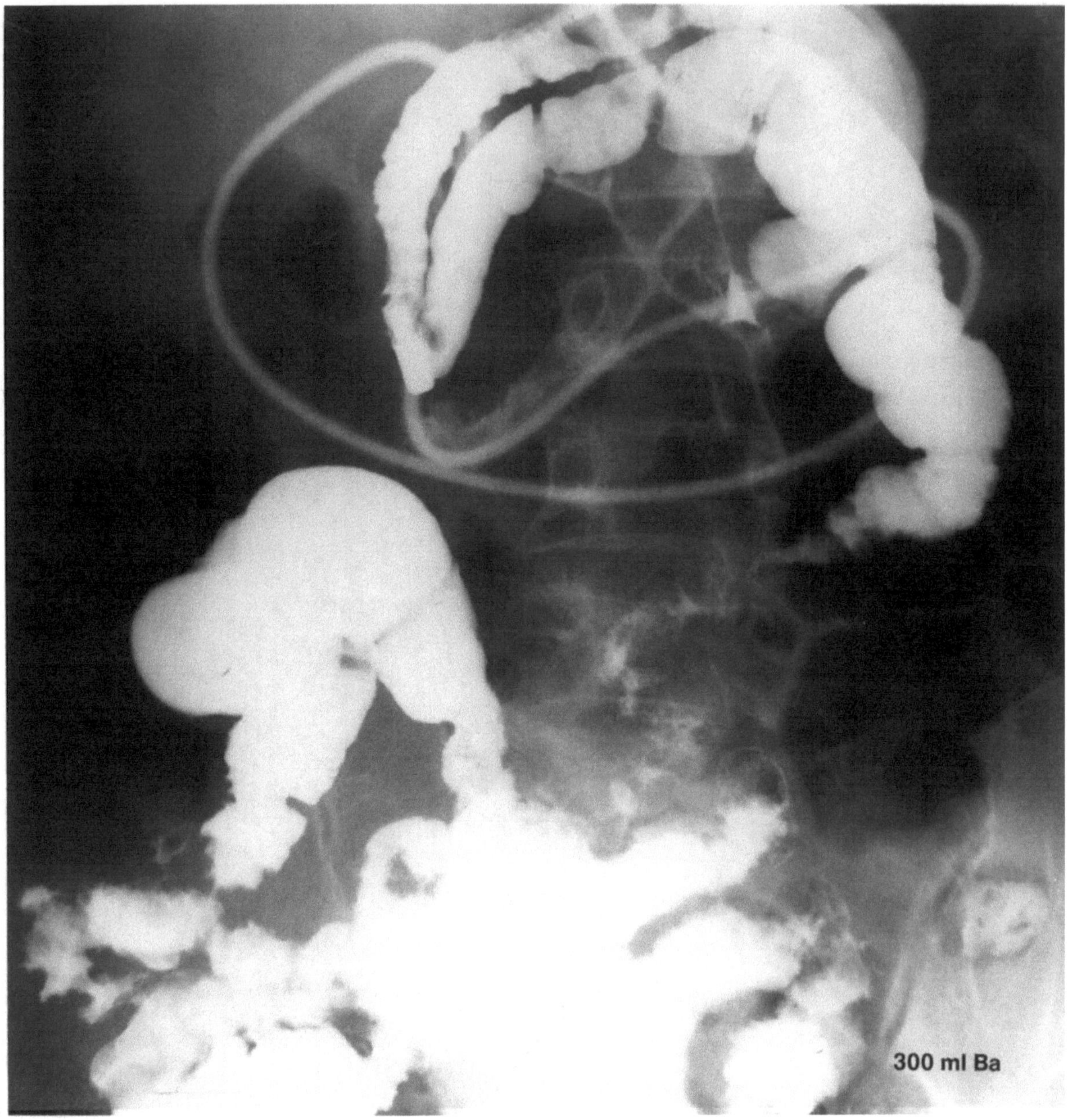

a

Fig. 5.4.-11a to c. Celiac disease. Colonization of the jejunum and distension of the ileum with loss of folds (**a**). Marked atrophy of the mucosa with pseudopolypoid mucosal remnants or regenerations (**c**). Poor mucosal coating due to inflammation (**b**). 54-year-old female with chronic diarrhea

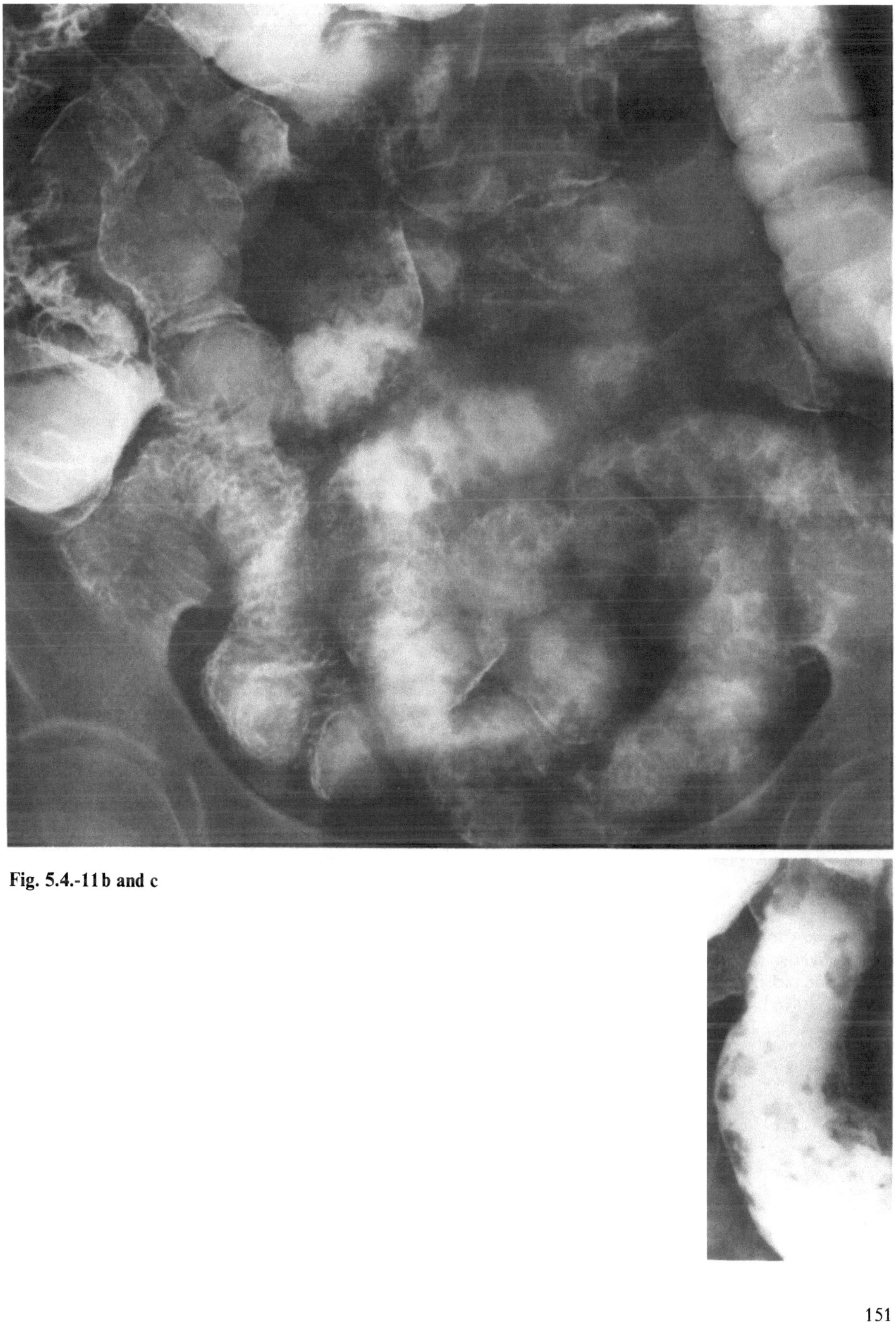

b

Fig. 5.4.-11 b and c

c

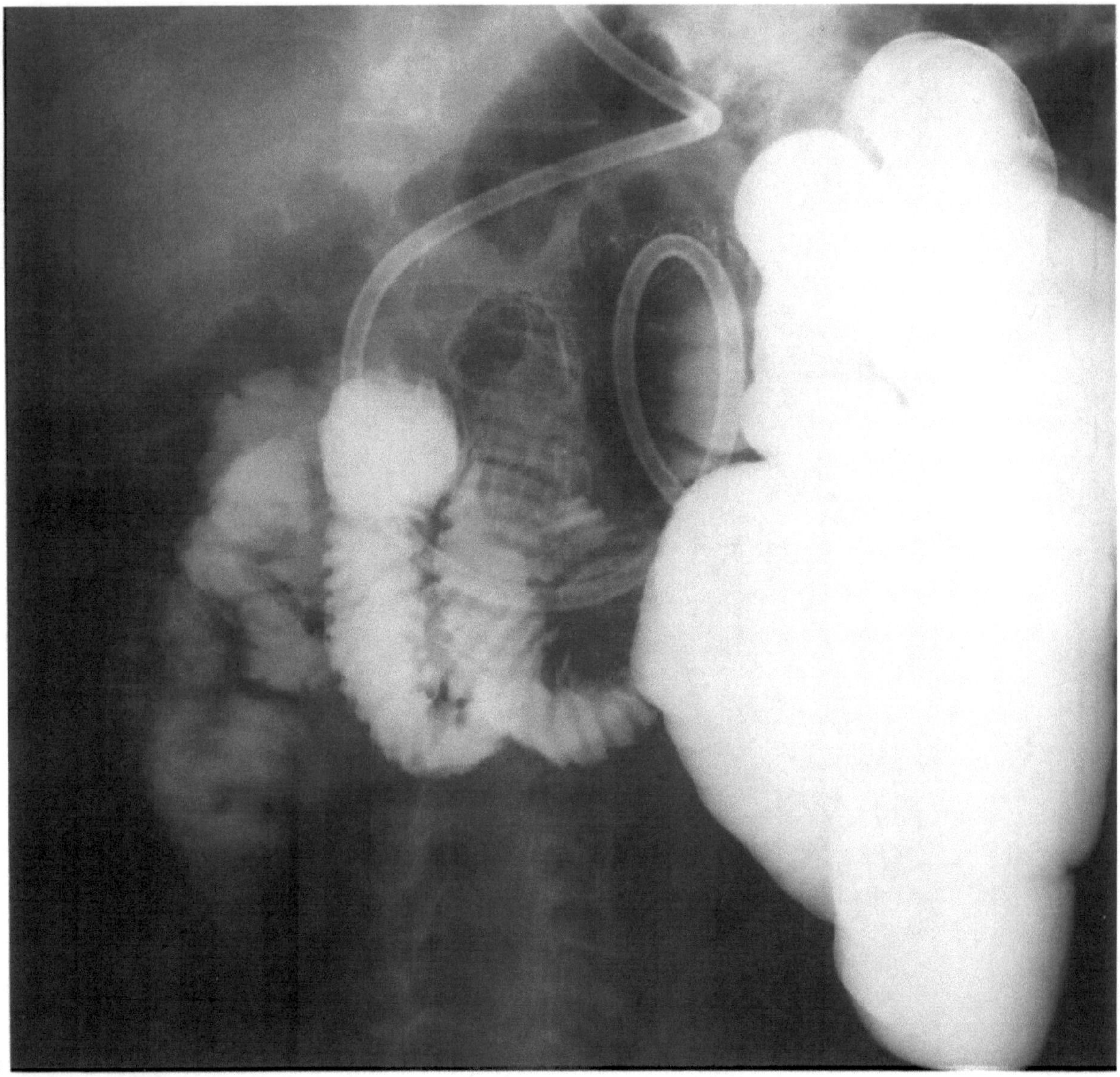

a

Fig. 5.4.-12 a and b. Sprue syndrome. Marked colonization of the jejunum and atrophy of the ileal folds. Transit delay due to hypoperistalsis in the jejunum and nonpropulsive peristalsis in the ileum. Wall and fold edema. Clouding of transparency due to increased intestinal fluid. 57-year-old male with long-standing chronic diarrhea and severe malabsorption syndrome. In spite of thorough investigations, a definitive diagnosis was not possible. With antibiotic therapy for a secondary bacterial overgrowth, the malabsorption syndrome improved. **a** Barium phase. **b** Methylcellulose phase

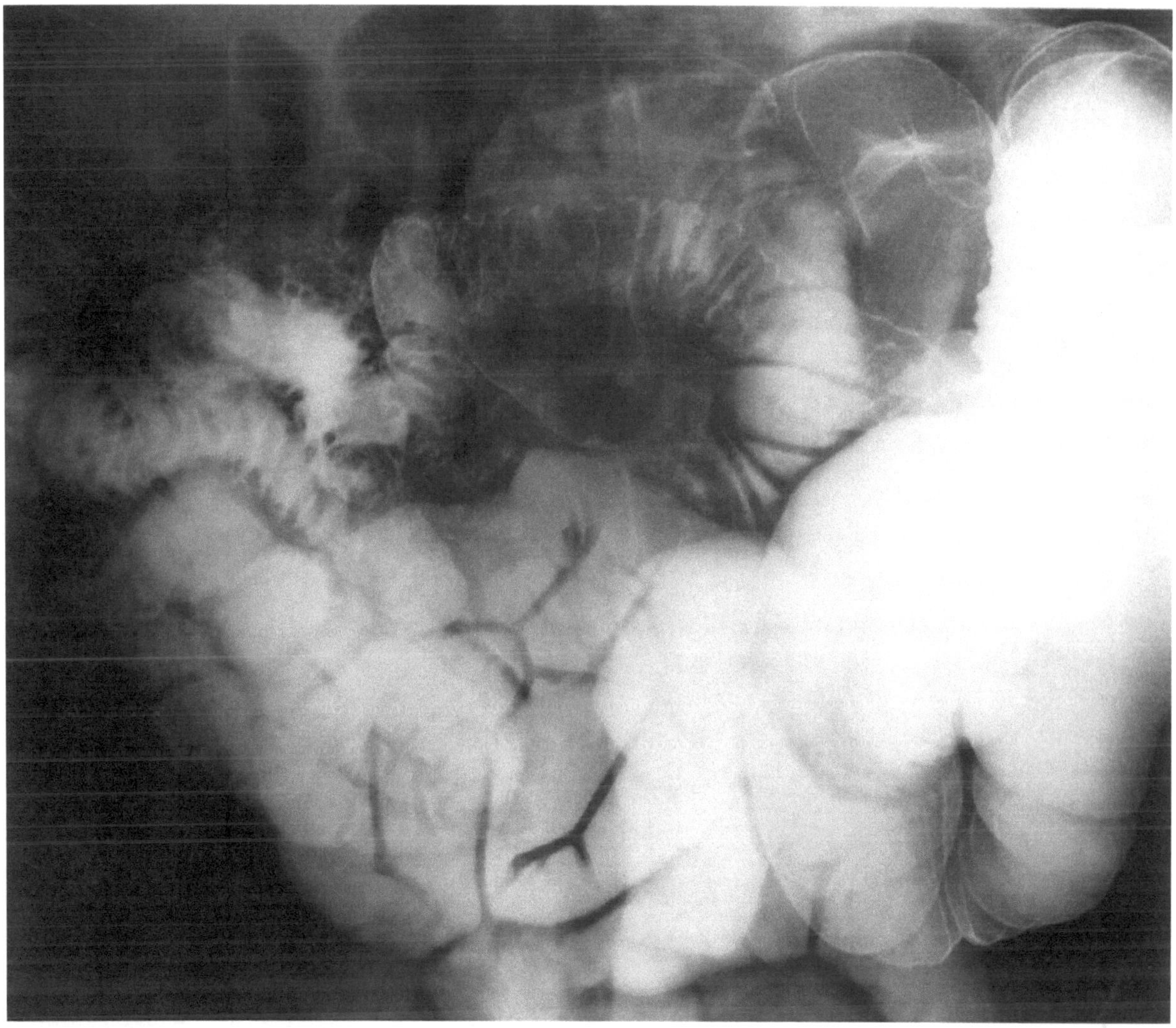

Fig. 5.4.-12 b

a

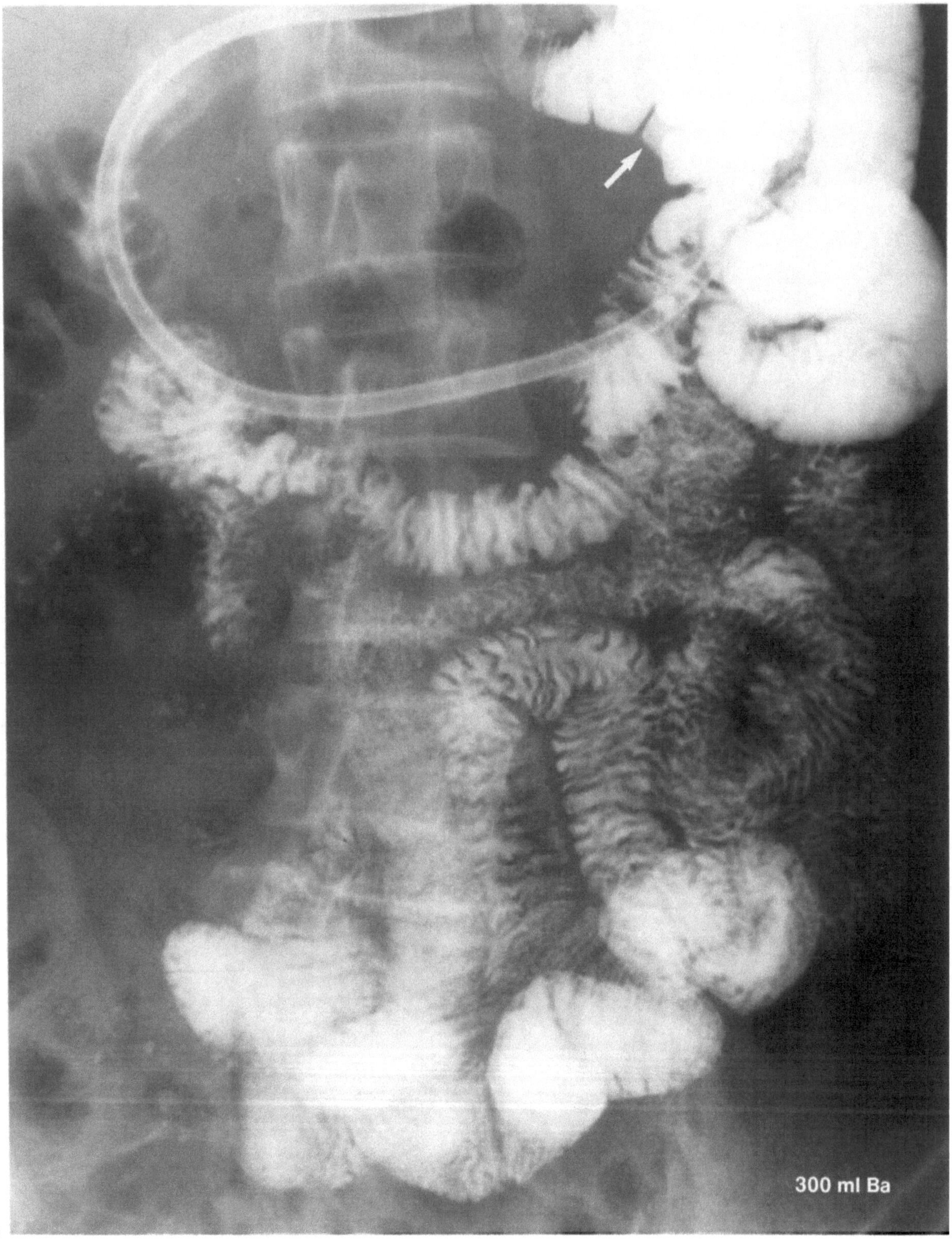

Fig. 5.4.-13 a and b. Celiac disease. Colonization (→) with local hypoperistalsis and jejunization with hyperperistalsis. Normal mucosal coating. 37-year-old asymptomatic female with known glutenenteropathy in remissior on diet. Control investigation for exclusion of tumor. **a** Barium phase. **b** Methylcellulose phase. Identical findings 2 years later

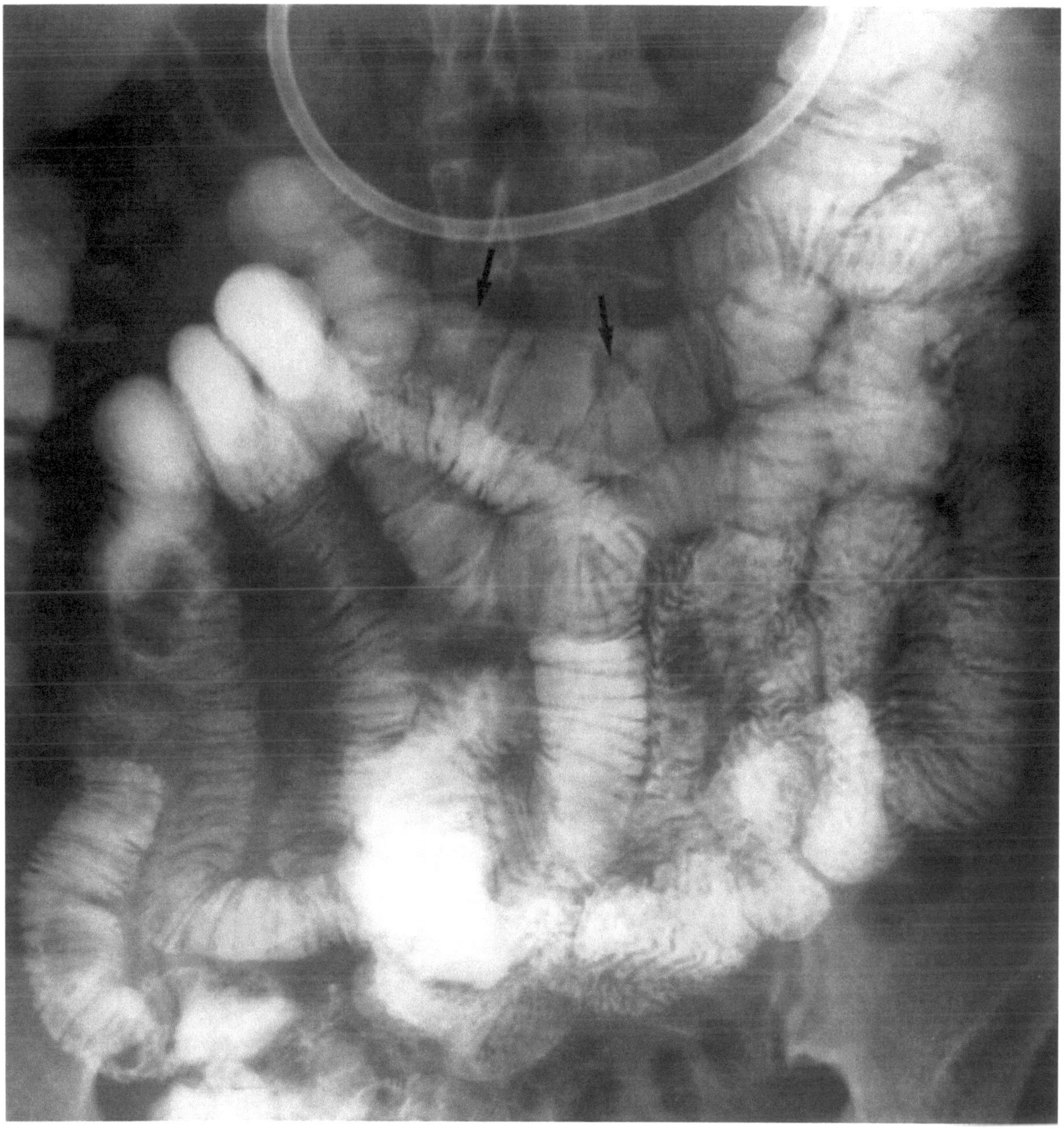

Fig. 5.4.-13b

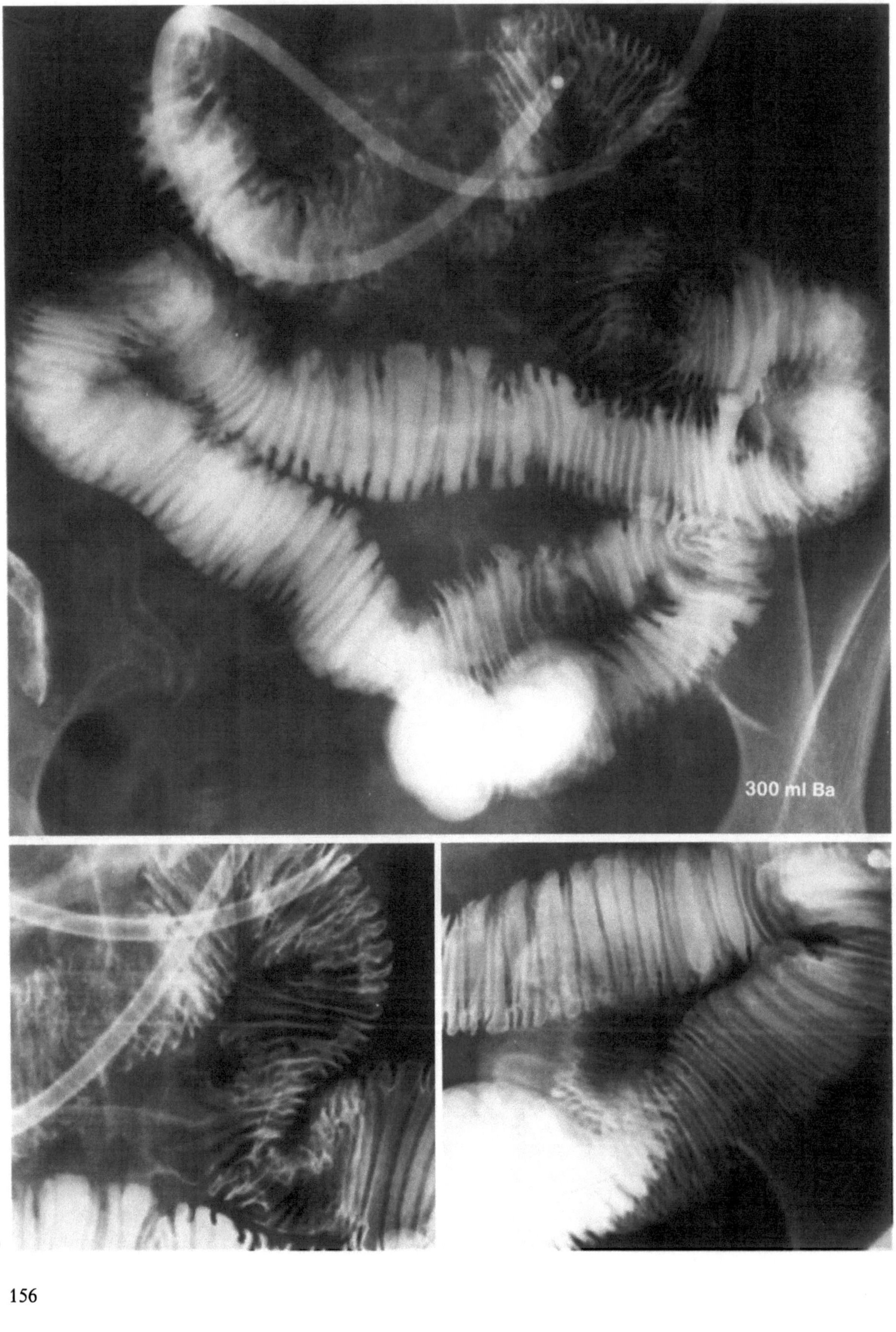

a

b

c

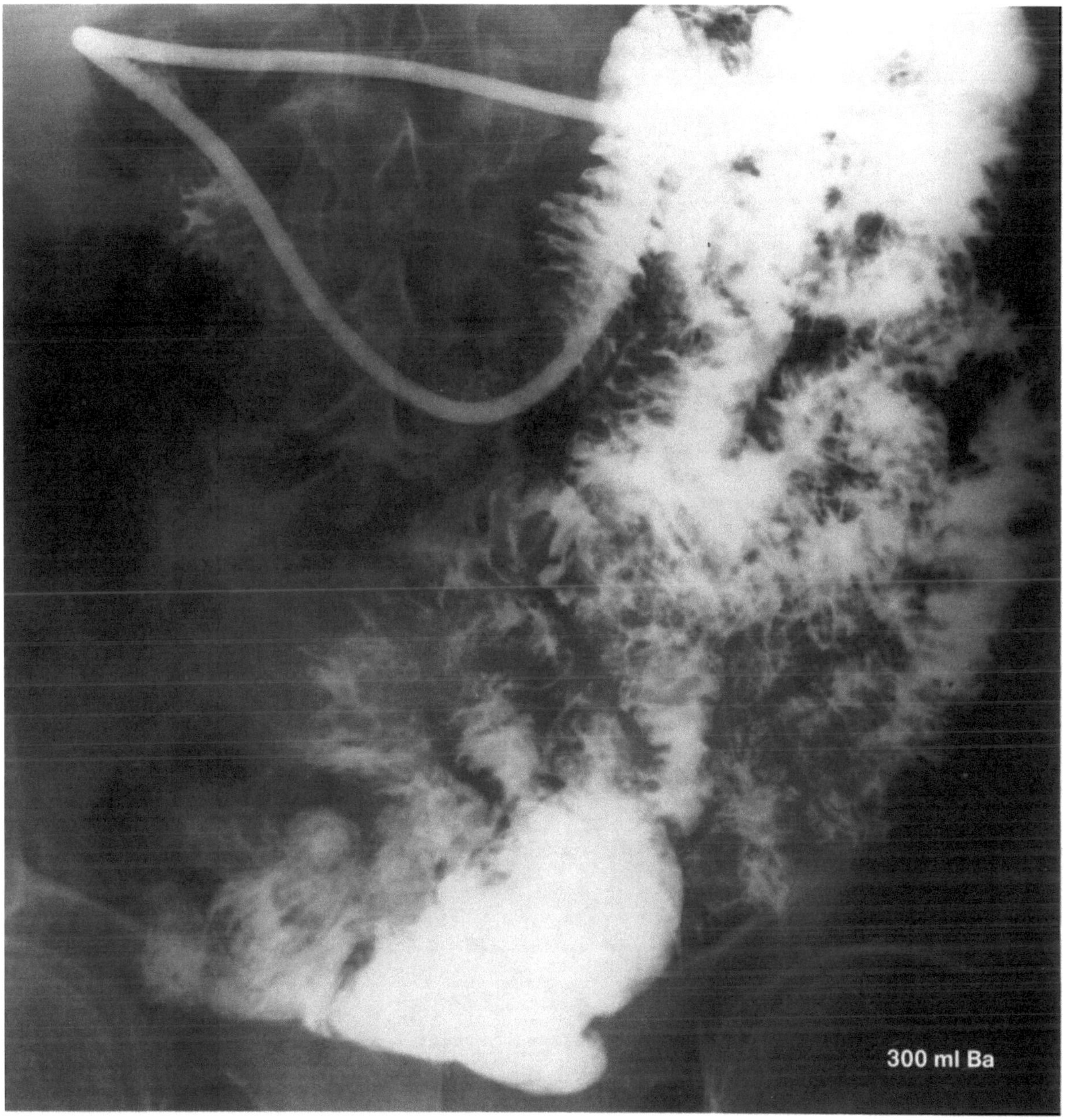

a

Fig. 5.4.-15a to c. Amyloidosis, primary. Hyperperistalsis, thickened, deformed folds (**a**), adequate coating (**b**). The intestinal wall thickening is easily recognized by ultrasound (**c**). Patient with anemia due to chronic gastrointestinal blood loss. No abdominal symptoms

Fig. 5.4.-14a to c. Scleroderma. Hypoperistalsis, segmental dilatation, hide-bound sign (**a** and **c**) and broad-based diverticula (**b**). Patient with severe esophageal involvement but mild abdominal complaints

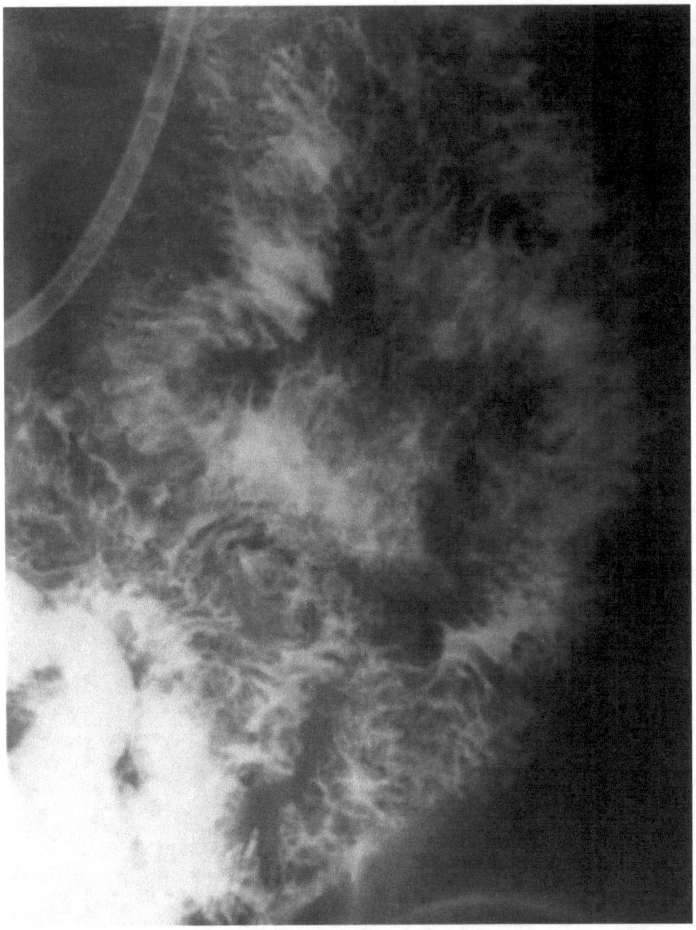

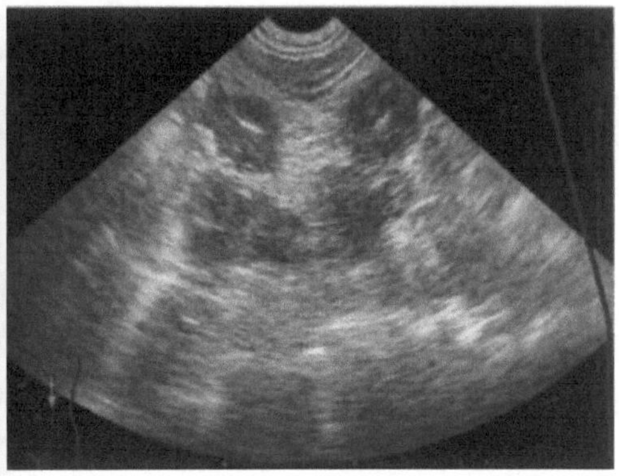

Fig. 5.4.-15c

Fig. 5.4.-15b

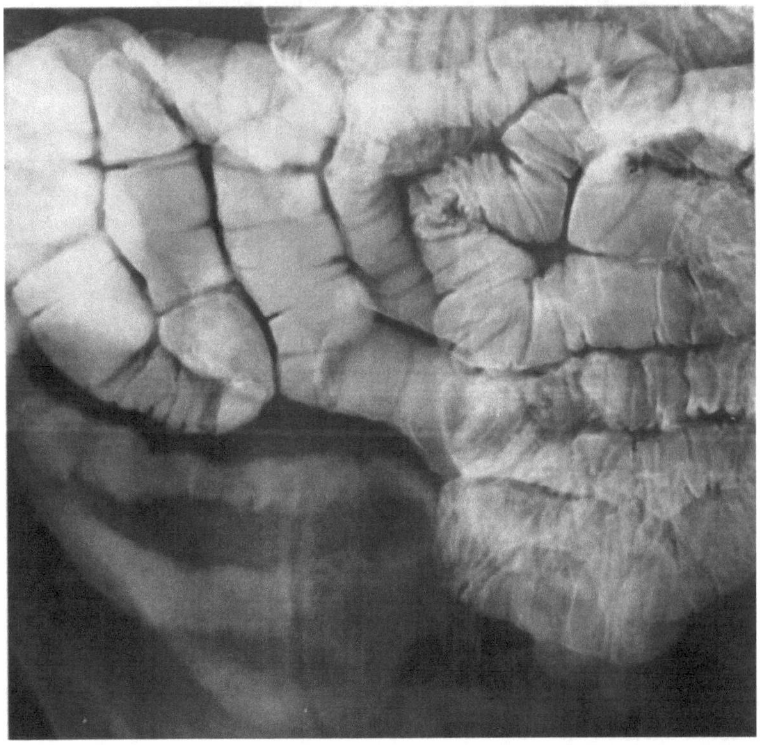

Fig. 5.4.-16. Amyloidosis, primary. Hypoperistaltic rigid ileum with thickened wall. Nodular infiltration, ulcerations, loss of folds. Patient with diarrhea and crampy abdominal pain. Involvement of other organs, especially the colon

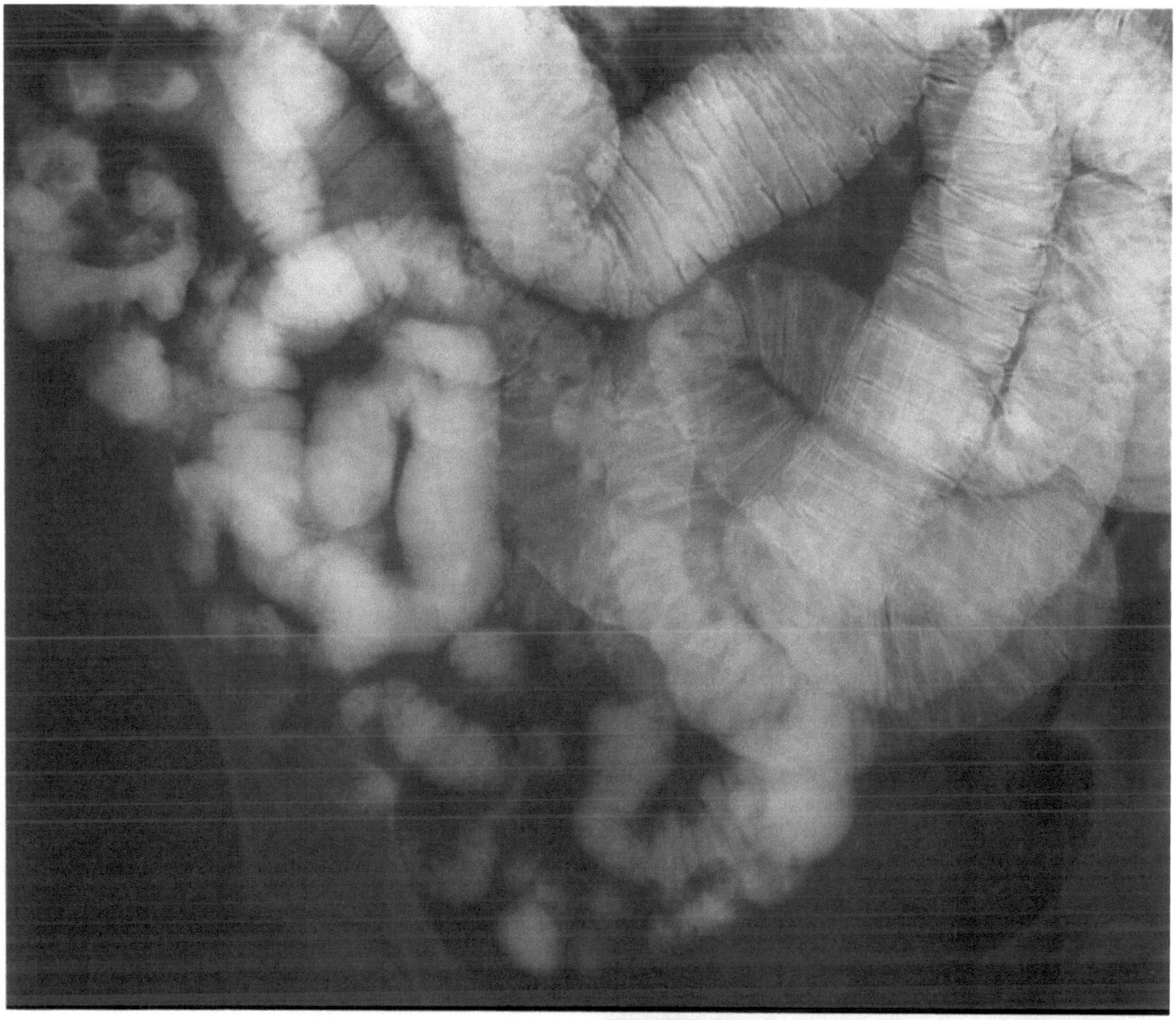

a

b

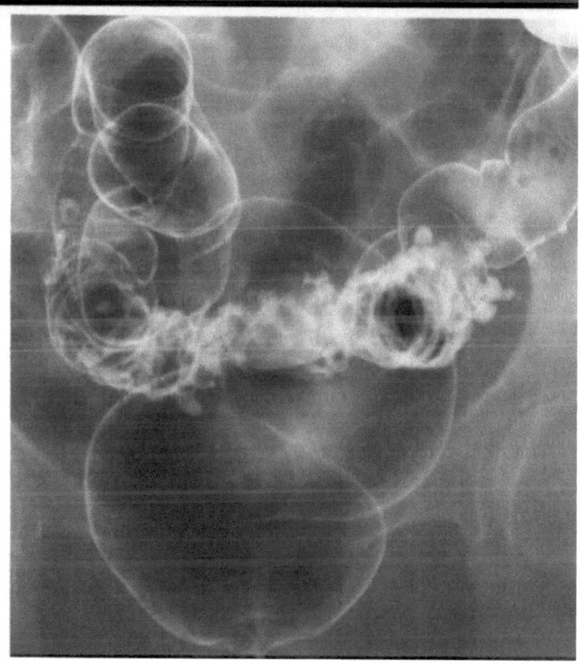

Fig. 5.4.-17 a and b. Adjacent inflammation. Transitory local hyperperistalsis and passage delay with dilatation (**a**) as a reaction to a severe diverticular disease (**b**). Regression of this functional disturbance in the later course of the examination. Patient with intermittent lower abdominal pain and transitory subileus due to diverticulitis

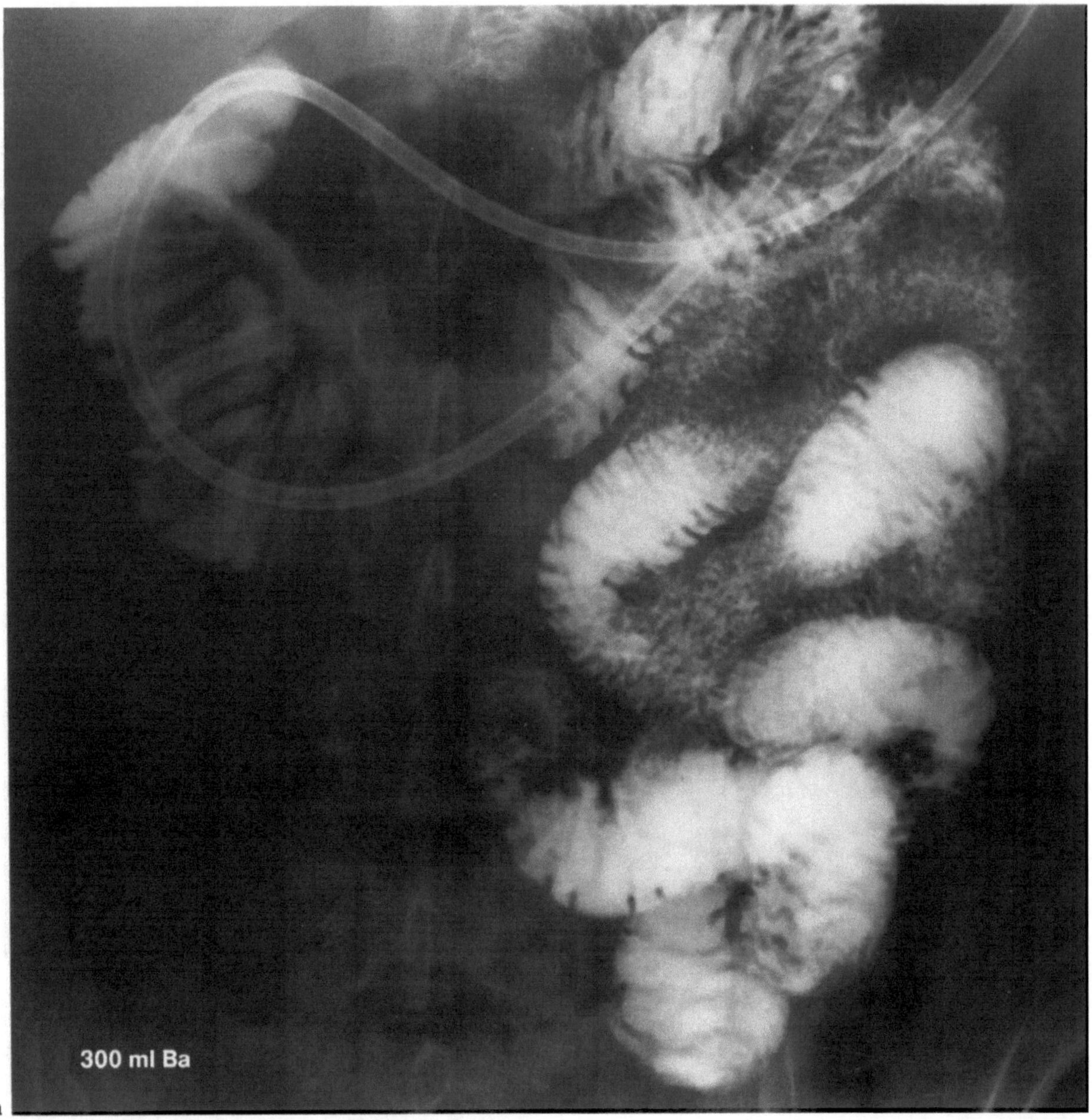

a

Fig. 5.4.-18 a and b. Diabetic angiopathy. Nonpropulsive hyperperistalsis (**a**). Distension of the duodenum. In the MC phase poor mucosal coating, normal folds (**b**). 23-year-old female with crampy left-sided upper abdominal pain. Juvenile diabetes, gangrenous large toe, renal insufficiency, retinopathy, slight exocrine pancreatic insufficiency

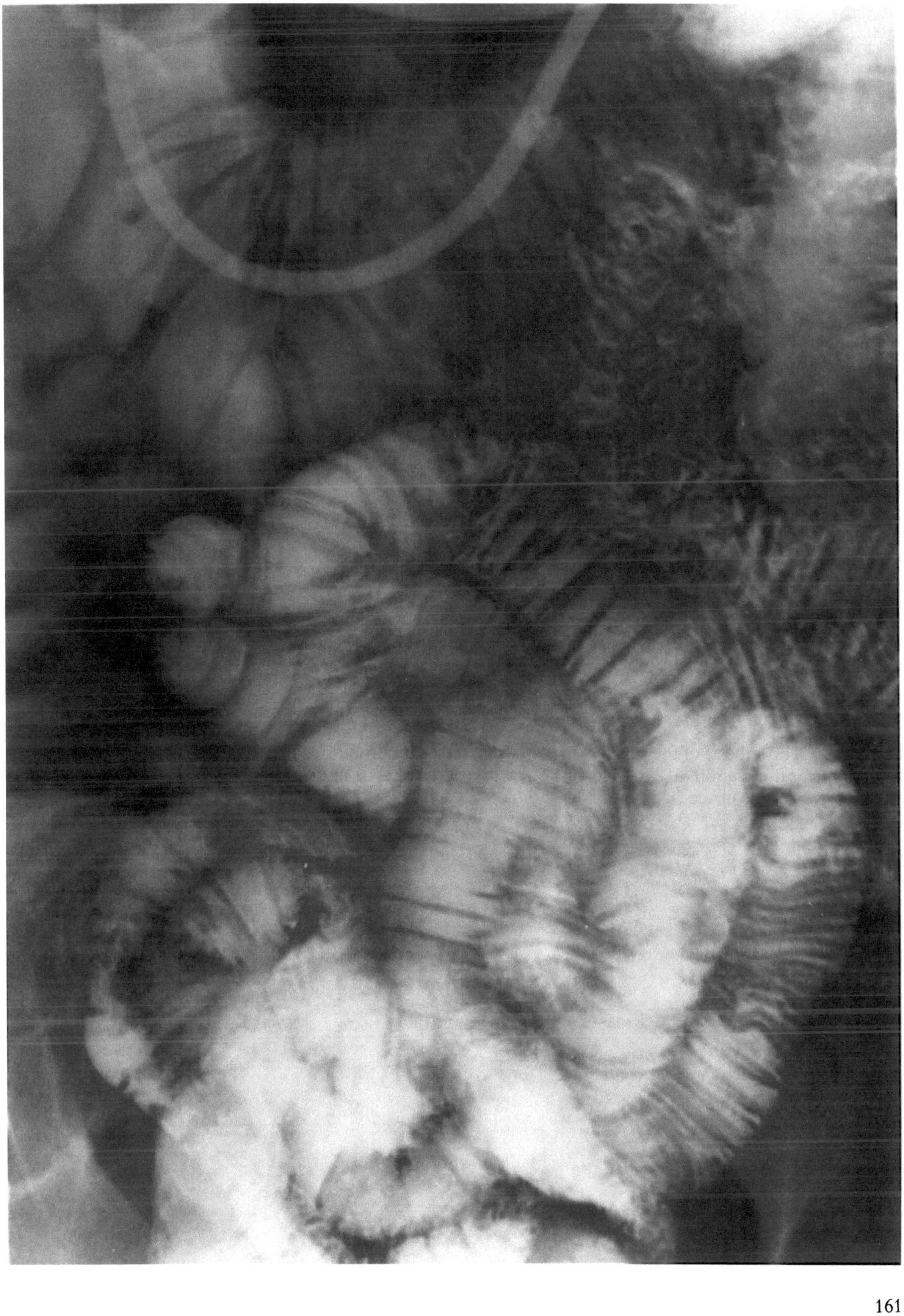

b

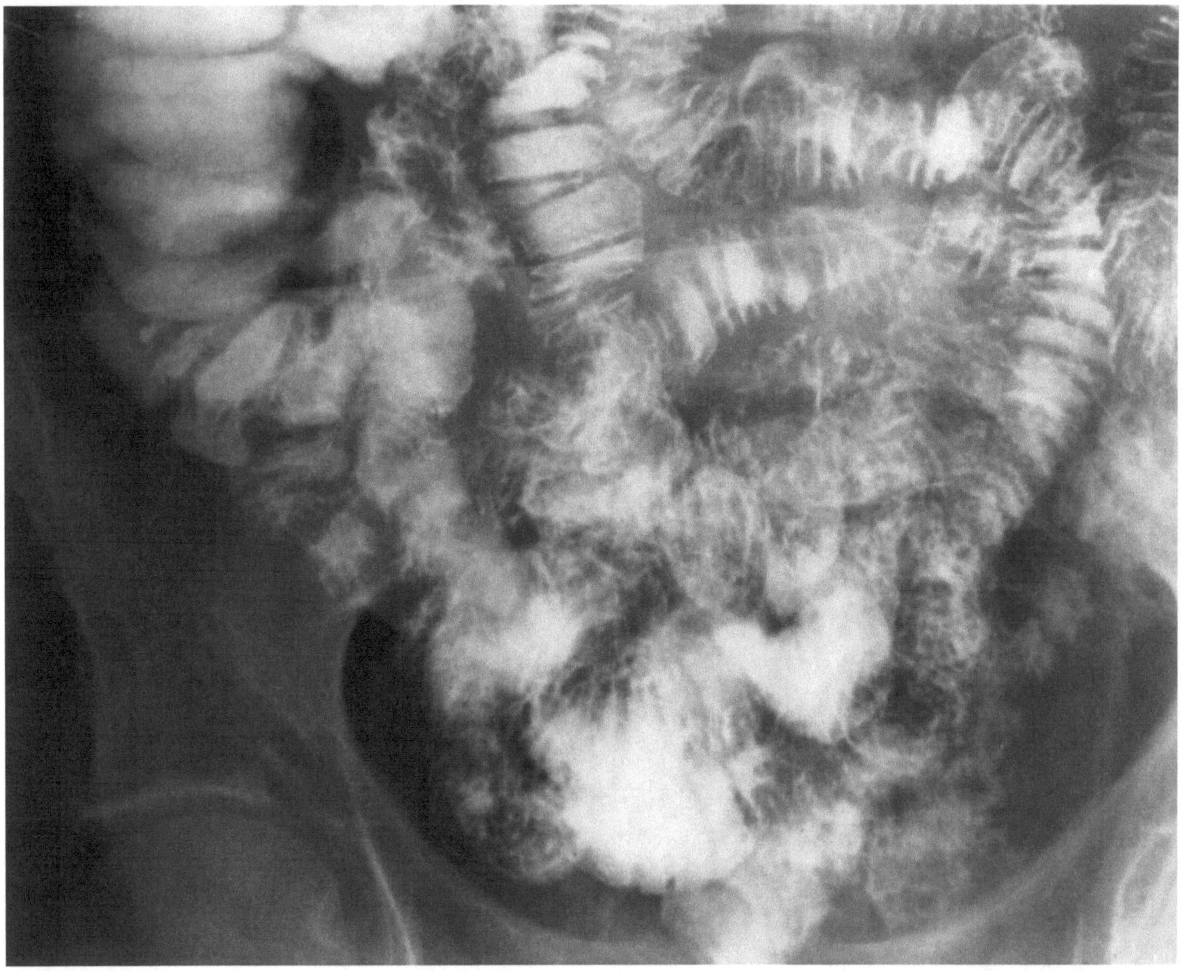

Fig. 5.4.-19. Thrombosis of the superior mesenteric artery. Nonpropulsive hyperperistalsis, nonspecific enteritis and mucosal irritation. 51-year-old smoker with arterial occlusion disease, abdominal pain and diarrhea. At surgery, necrosis of the small bowel was found

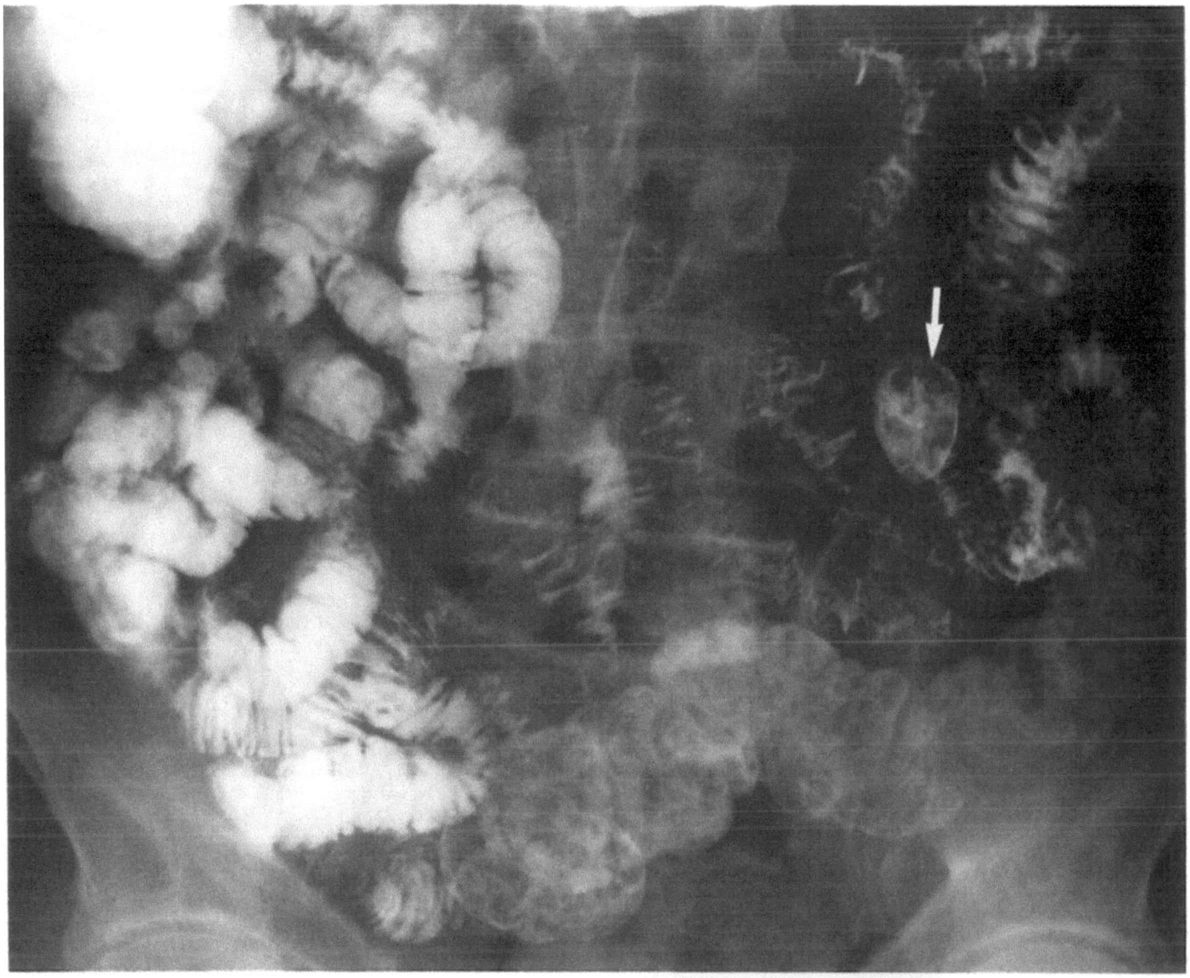

a

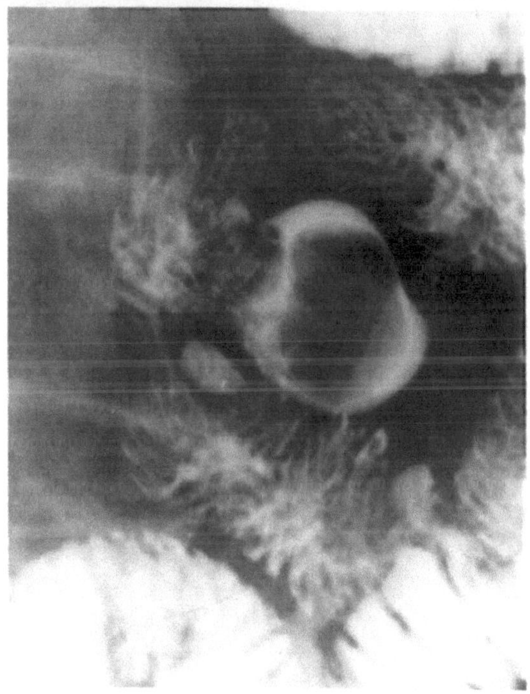

b

Fig. 5.4.-20 a and b. Intestinal hemorrhage. Hyperperistalsis and poor mucosal coating due to intestinal blood emanating from a bleeding jejunal diverticulum (→)

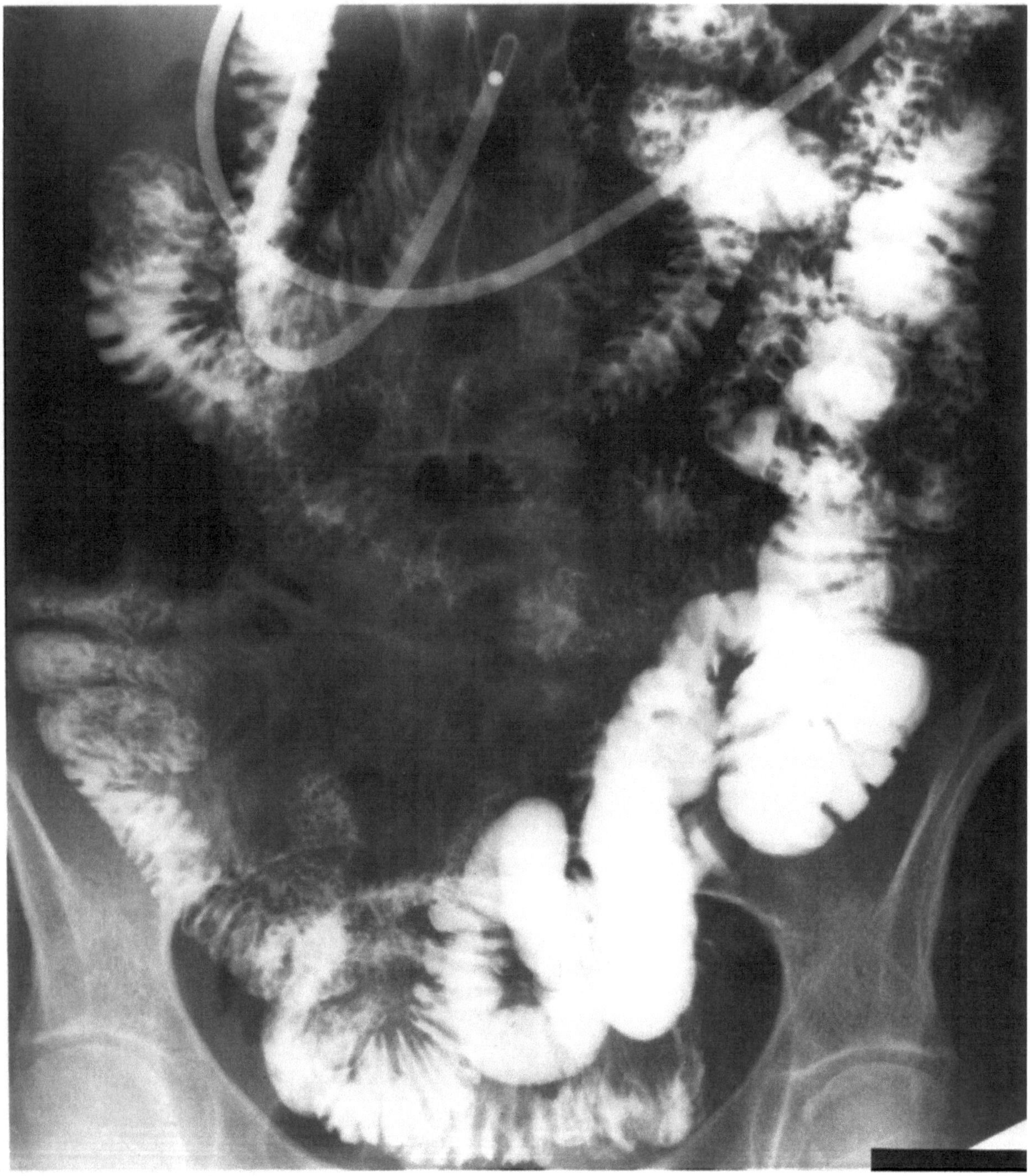
a

Fig. 5.4.-21 a and b. Intestinal lymphangiectasia. Hyperperistalsis, thickening of folds and nodular infiltrations, premature flocculation. 37-year-old female with hypoproteinemia and edema. Barium phase (**a**), methylcellulose phase (**b**)

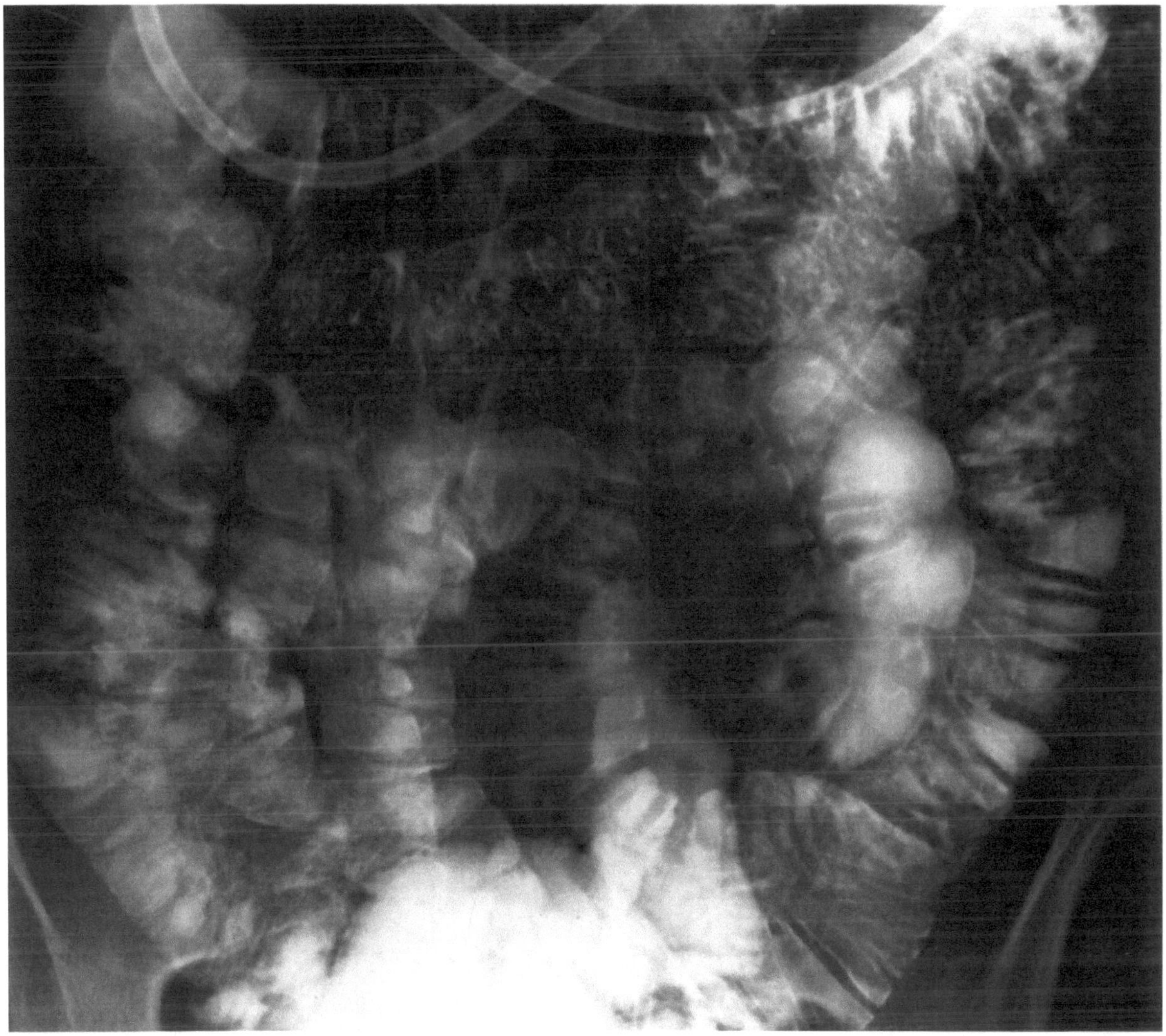

Fig. 5.4.-21 b

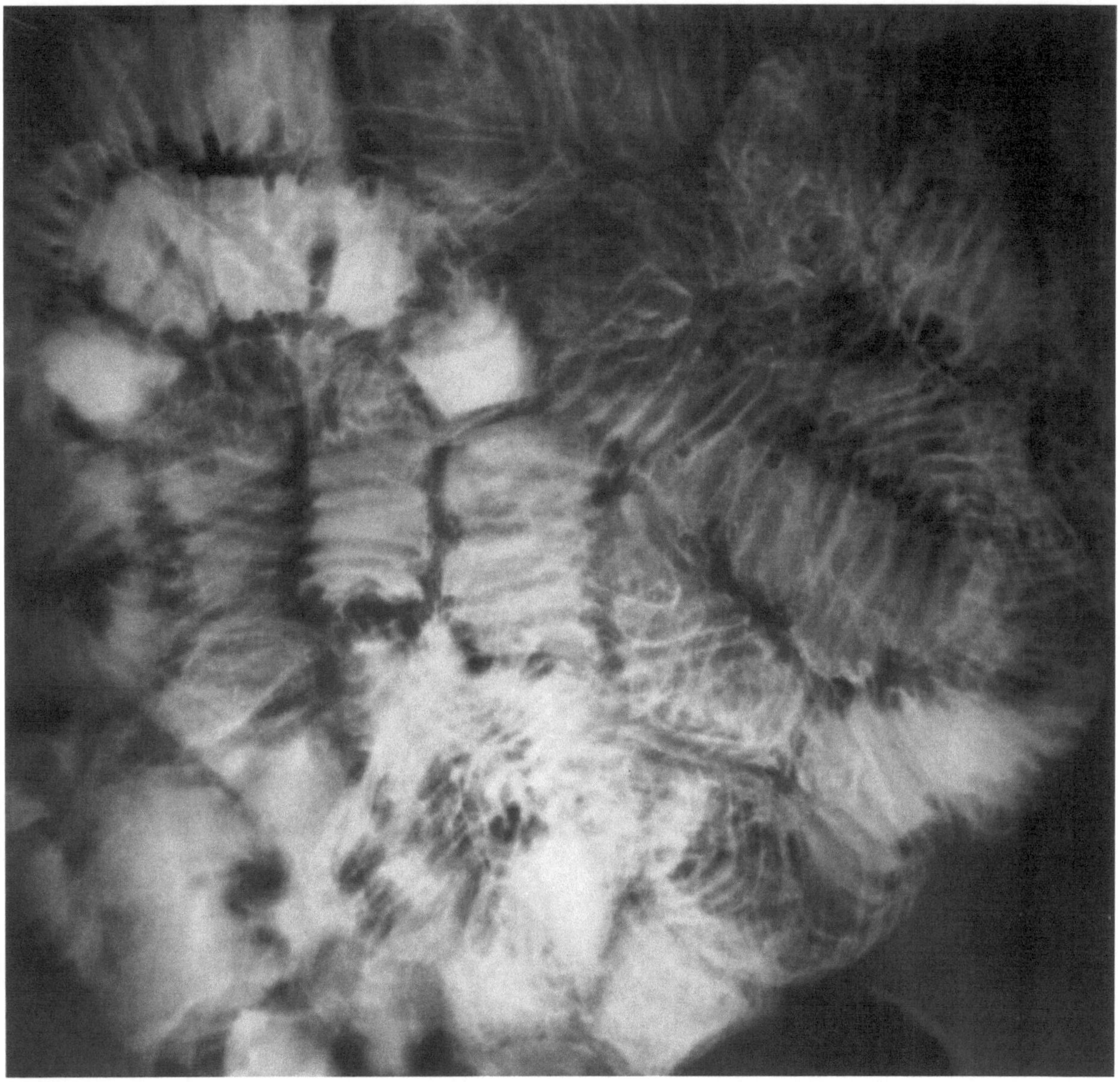

Fig. 5.4.-22. Intestinal lymphangiectasia. Nonpropulsive hyperperistalsis, edematous, thickened folds and intestinal walls, poor mucosal coating. 23-year-old female with severe hypoproteinemia and malabsorption syndrome

5.5 Obstructions

Every sixth patient admitted to hospital with acute abdominal complaints is reported to suffer from small bowel obstruction (Caroline et al. 1984). The plain upright abdominal film is the first radiological examination for these patients, but often fails to yield exact information regarding location, extent and cause of the obstruction (Fig. 5.5.-1). If the diagnosis remains unclear, enteroclysis – which is superior to all other contrast medium investigations – is indicated (Ott et al. 1985; Maglinte and Miller 1984; Maglinte, Peterson et al. 1984).

In the search for stenoses, the enteroclysis technique has to be adjusted for each individual case. This is particularly important concerning the flow rate and the frequently large amounts of barium and methylcellulose. Fundamentally, the barium bolus should be monitored carefully, so that short stenoses are not overlooked (see Fig. 2.8.-3, p. 19). Palpation and compression of the bowel with spot filming yields information about the mobility of the intestinal loops and the elasticity of the intestinal wall.

Advanced stenoses may be more difficult to demonstrate than partial obstructions, since dilated, fluid-filled and therefore inadequately contrasted proximal intestinal loops may superimpose the stenosis. However, delayed filming (up to 24 h) can show up the stenosis also in these cases (Fig. 2.8.-4c, p. 22). In any case, sufficient information about the localization can be provided for the surgeon.

The fear shared by many surgeons of worsening of the ileus condition by the barium during enteroclysis is unfounded: There is no condensation of the contrast medium in the small bowel. The only contraindications for enteroclysis, therefore, are perforation and large bowel obstructions.

In suspected perforation, enteroclysis with a water-soluble contrast medium in single contrast is indicated. An ionic water-soluble contrast medium (Gastrografin®) can also be used to treat a subileus condition. This positive "therapeutic" effect on the peristaltic stimulation has to be weighed up against possible side effects on the circulation and electrolyte metabolism.

The typical picture of obstruction (see e.g. Fig. 5.5.-5) shows dilated prestenotic loops and hyperperistalsis in the proximal jejunum. At the stenosis, there is an abrupt change in lumen caliber which is dependent on the degree of obstruction, and there is local hyperperistalsis. The hyperperistalsis along the proximal intestinal loops is a remarkable differential diagnostic sign against the so-called pseudoobstruction e.g. in drug-induced (see chapter 4.5 and Fig. 5.4.-3, pp. 136–138) or paralytic ileus. This abnormal motility behavior should be recognized at the beginning of the investigation, since it may subside with increased filling of the intestinal loops.

In the newborn, meconium ileus in cystic fibrosis is more common than intussusception which occurs mainly in infants. The main cause of small bowel obstructions in adults are in ca. 75% of cases postoperative *adhesions and fibrous bands* (Figs. 5.5.-1 to 6). They have to be differentiated from metastases and tumors. In both adhesions and metastases, which have not yet infiltrated the mucosa, an intact surface persists in spite of distortion of folds. Absolute distinction between benign and malignant causes of an obstruction is seldom possible on radiographs alone.

As a rule, solitary fibrous bands lead to more severe stenoses than multiple adhesions (Caroline et al. 1984). In very extended adhesions, *retractile mesenteritis* should not be overlooked concerning differential diagnosis.

Ileus due to *small bowel intussusception* is rare in adults. In older individuals the causes of intussusception are increasingly malignant tumors (Fig. 5.5.-7), benign tumors (Figs. 5.5.-8 and 9) and Meckel's diverticulum, as well as lymphatic hyperplasia mainly at the ileocecal valve. Foreign bodies (e.g. undigested fruits, bezoars), worm ileus and intussusception of an intestinal anastomosis (Fig. 5.5.-10) are also found. In children these obstructions are mostly localized in the ileocecal region. Tumors or large polyps are to be mentioned in the radiological differential diagnosis. A configuration, whereby the valvulae conniventes converge concentrically at the stenosis ("coiled spring sign"), may also appear in intussusception and volvulus of the small bowel (Fig. 5.5.-7b).

$^{2}/_{3}$ of *volvulus* cases involve the small bowel. Causes for volvulus are anomalies of rotation and fixation of the mesentery and adhesions, around which the small bowel can twist. Necrosis of the intestine often ensues.

The *inguinal hernia* is sometimes observed as coincidental finding and rarely presents an indication for enteroclysis. The radiological diagnosis of *internal hernias* (Fig. 5.5.-11) and *abdominal wall hernias* is, however, important. Fluoroscopic investigation in lateral position with coughing maneuver is of special significance here (Maglinte, Miller and Lappas 1984).

Other causes for small bowel obstructions are a gallstone ileus (Fig. 5.5.-12), radiation enteritis (Fig. 5.5.-13), fatty tissue necrosis (Fig. 5.5.-14), foreign body reactions (Figs. 5.5.-15 and 16), endometriosis (Fig. 5.5.-17).

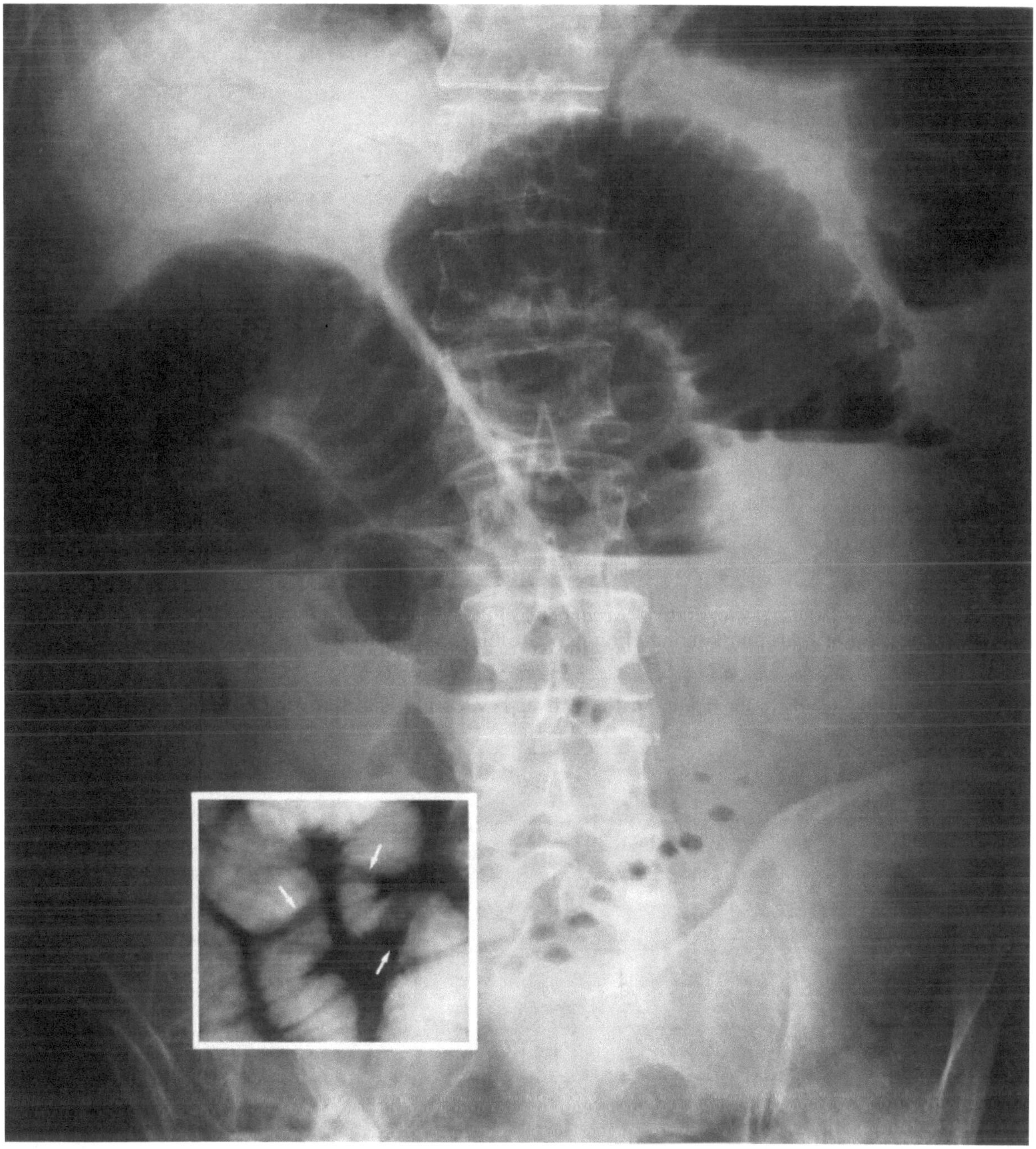

Fig. 5.5.-1. Small bowel ileus due to multiple fibrous bands in the ileum. Distinct air-fluid levels in rigid jejunal loops on the erect abdominal film. The detail of enteroclysis is inserted at the actual site of the obstruction. It shows multiple fibrous bands (→) with luminar narrowing. **Please observe:** 1. In case of "proximal small bowel ileus", the strictures mostly lie considerably more distal than assumed (the immediate prestenotic loops are already filled up with intestinal fluid). 2. There is no certain correlation between the severity and quantity of strictures and the clinical and radiological extent of the ileus. 3. Frequently in contrast medium investigation, even in severe clinical signs of obstruction, there is no marked prestenotic dilatation or transit delay visible (e.g. in intermittent partial obstructions). 4. One band seldom comes alone!

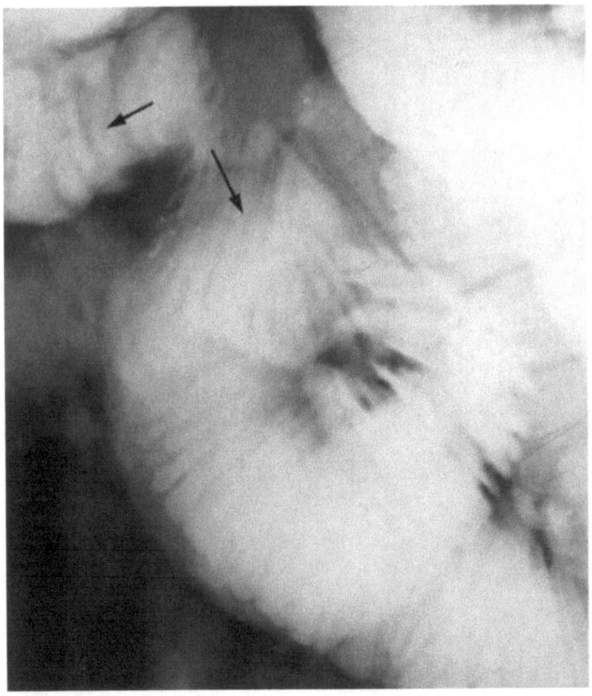

Fig. 5.5.-2. Multiple bands, postoperative. Accordion-like distortion of folds and kinking of an entire loop (→)

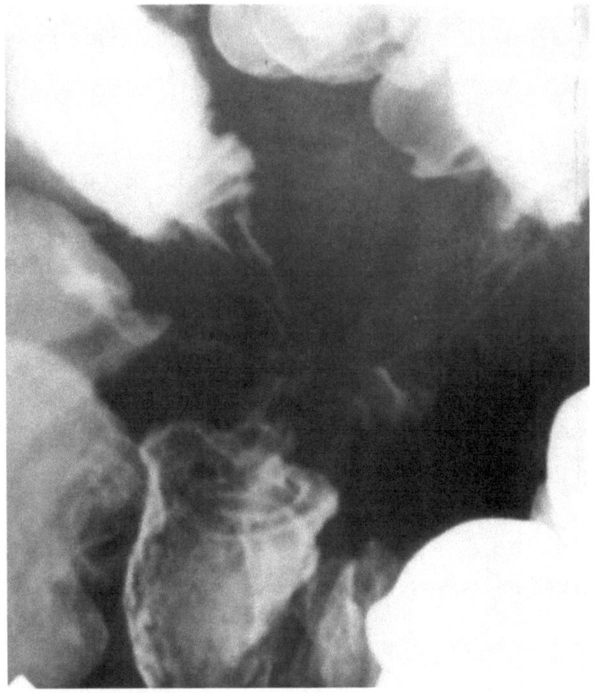

Fig. 5.5.-4. Crossed bands, postoperative. The bowel lumen is constricted due to considerable inflammatory thickening

Fig. 5.5.-3. Multiple bands in the ileum, postoperative. Two easily visible crossing bands (→) and in addition a marked stenosis (⇒)

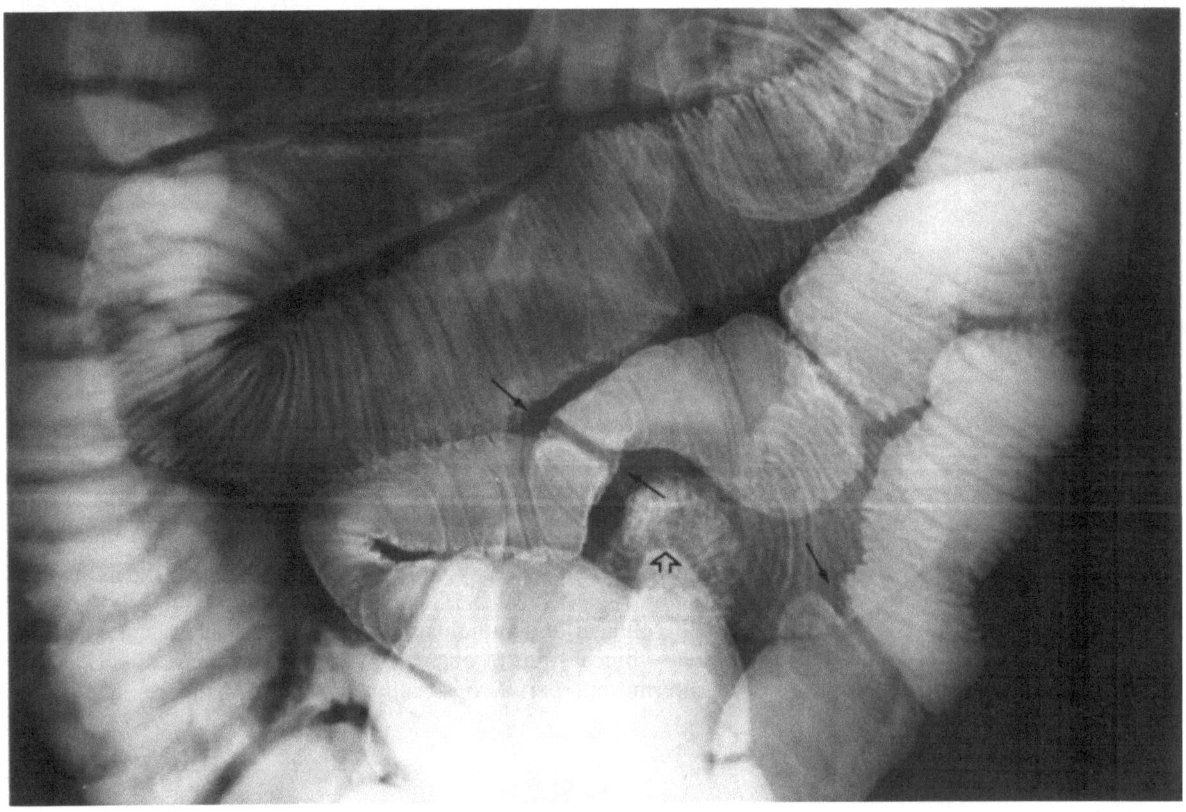

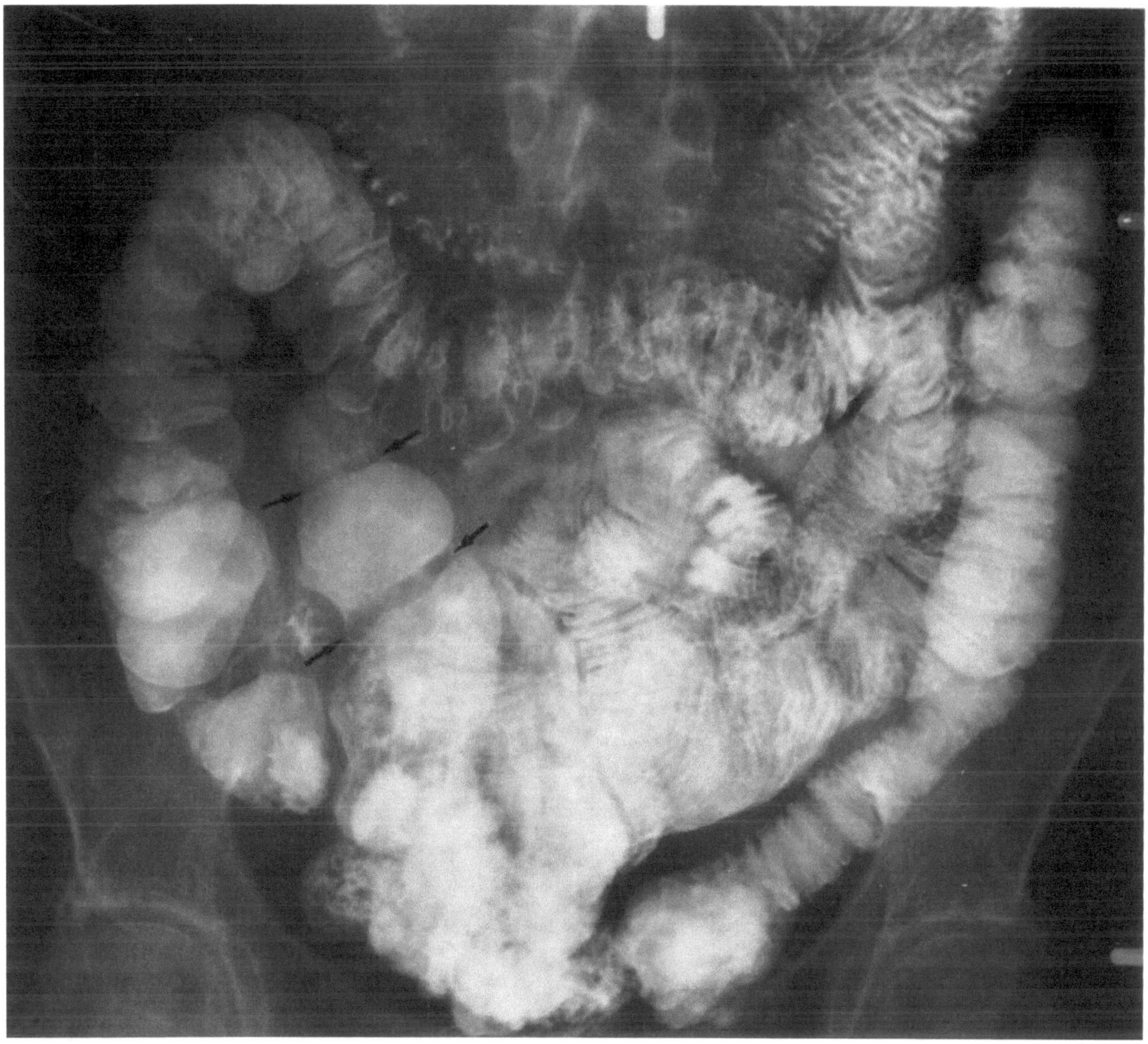

Fig. 5.5.-5. Multiple bands, postoperative. Typical image of obstruction due to bands (→) with prestenotically distended loops

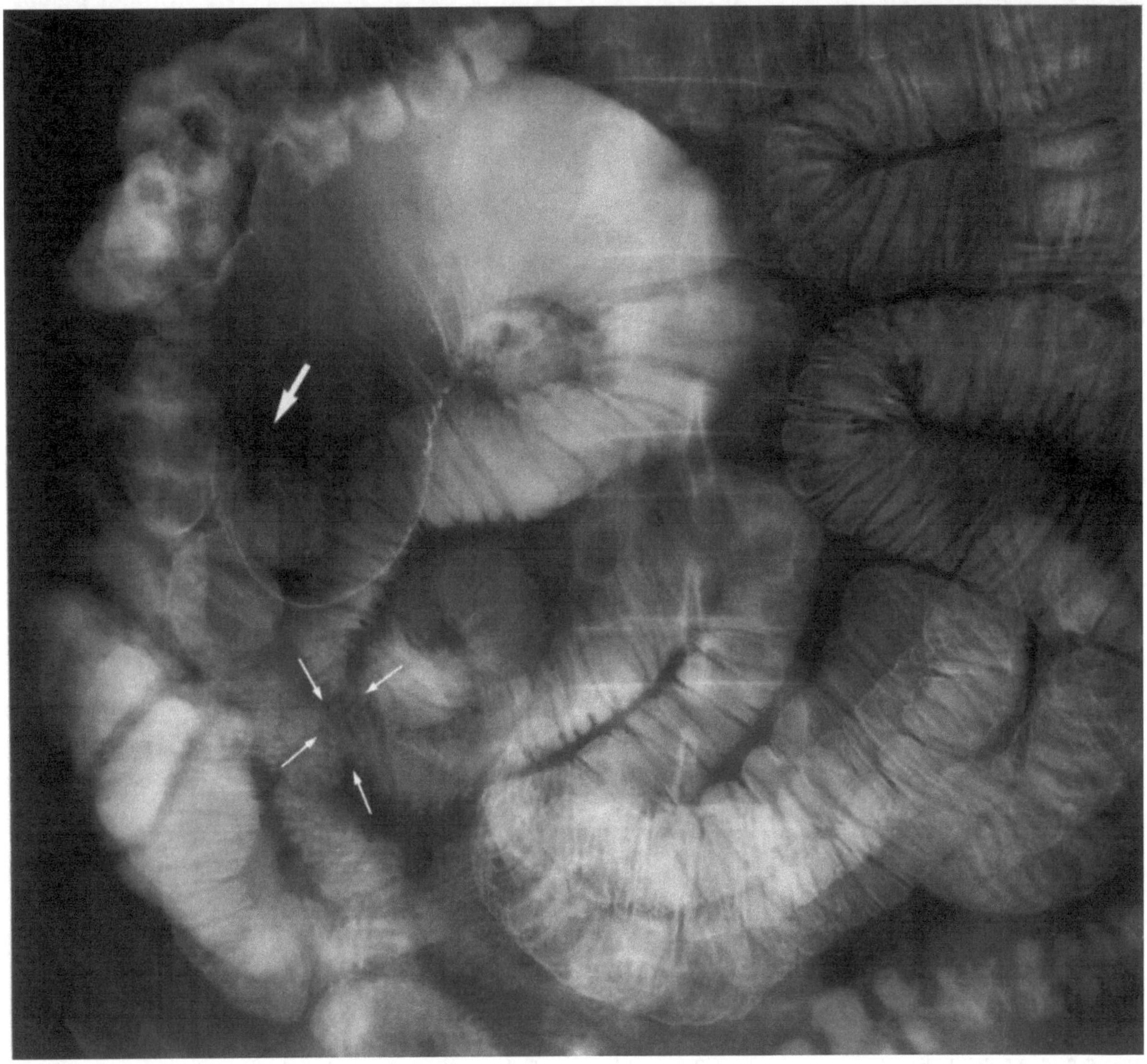

Fig. 5.5.-6. Bands and adhesions, postoperative. Star-like configuration in the ileum (→) caused by adhesion of three intestinal loops. Additional advanced stenosis with prestenotic dilatation and abrupt change in luminal caliber due to a fibrous band (➡)

a 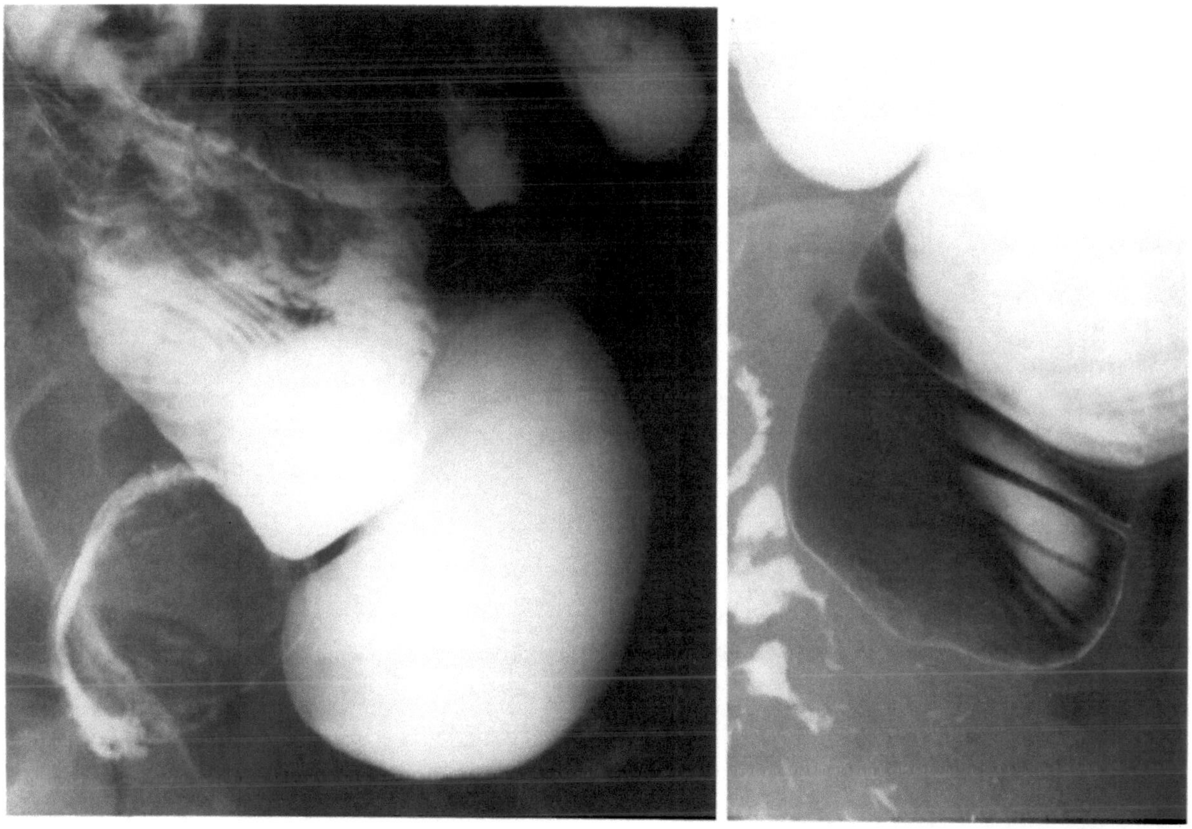 b

Fig. 5.5.-7 a and b. Intussusception by a leiomyosarcoma. **a** The intussuscipiens together with the tumor subtotally occludes the intestinal lumen, leading to a massive prestenotic dilatation. The contrast medium flows around the intussuscipiens. **b** The prestenotically dilated intestinal loop shows concentrically convergent folds ("coiled spring sign")

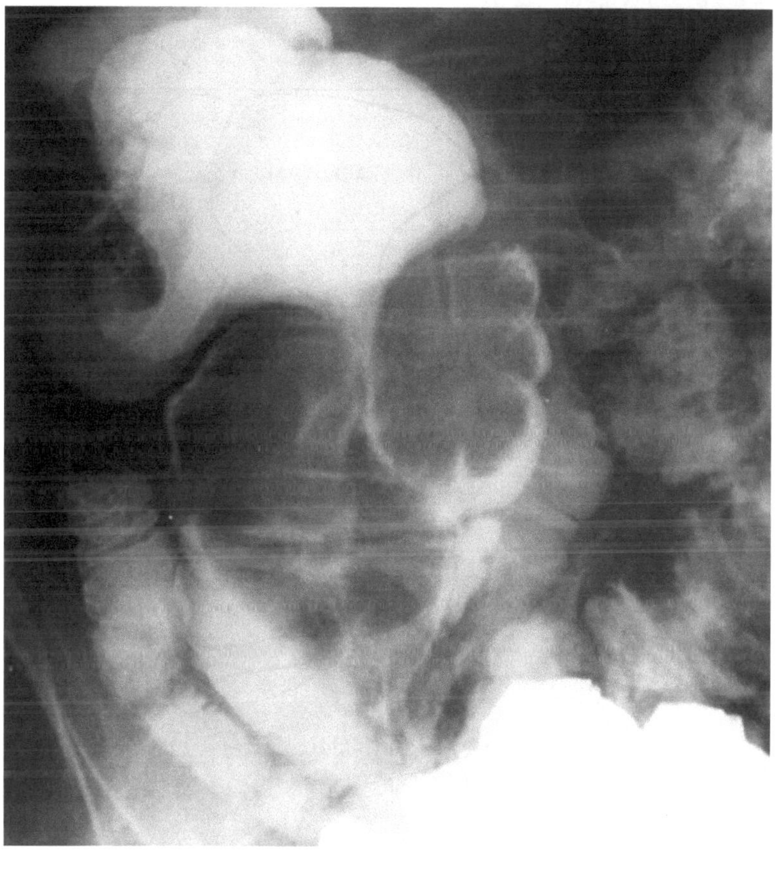

Fig. 5.5.-8. Intussusception of an ileocecal lipoma. The intussuscipiens in the cecum consists of the lipoma and a part of the ascending colon

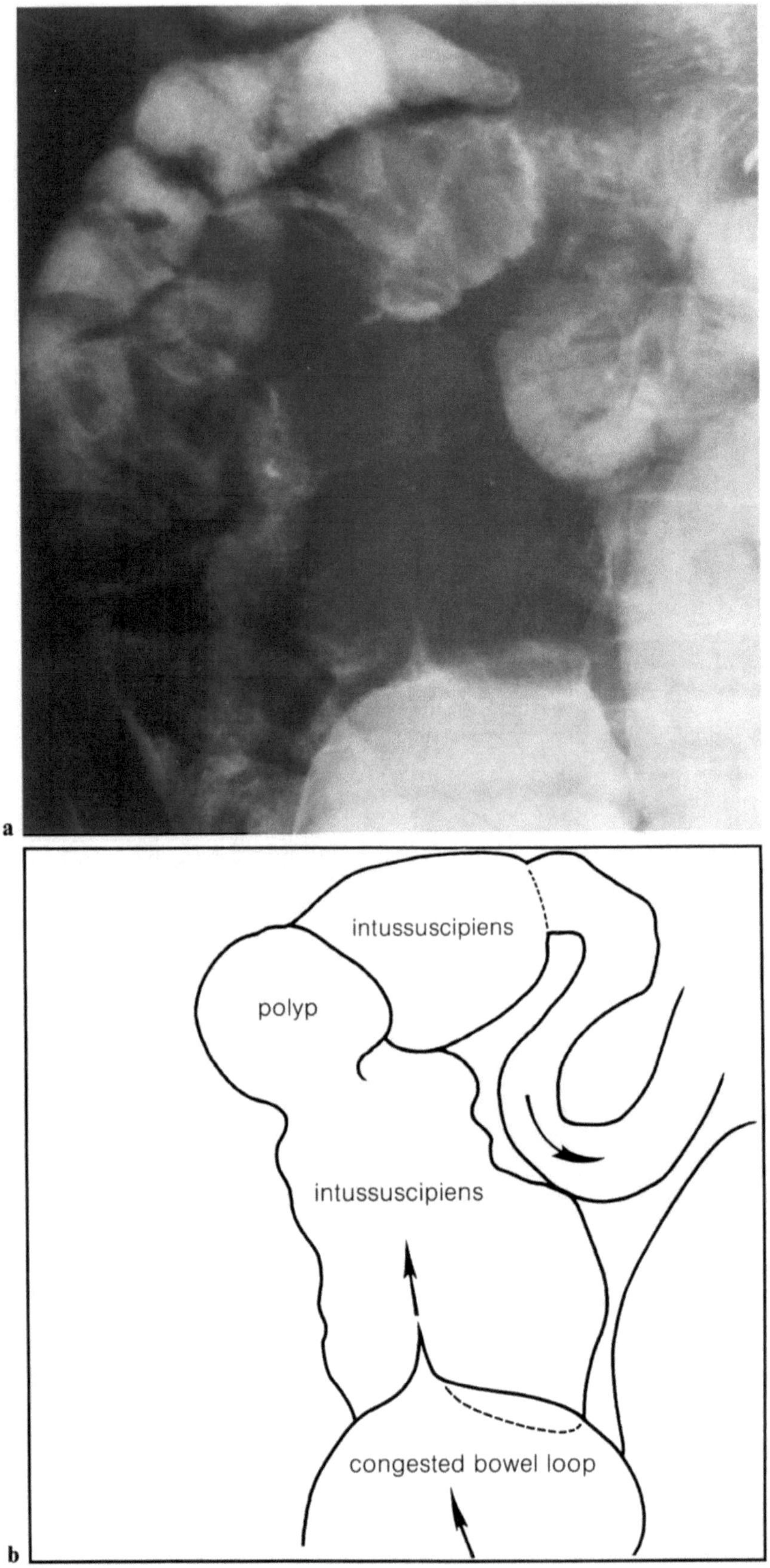

Fig. 5.5.-9 a and b. Intussusception by a polyp. Inflammatory fibroid polyp (histologically) is visible in the distal $^1/_3$ of the intussuscipiens

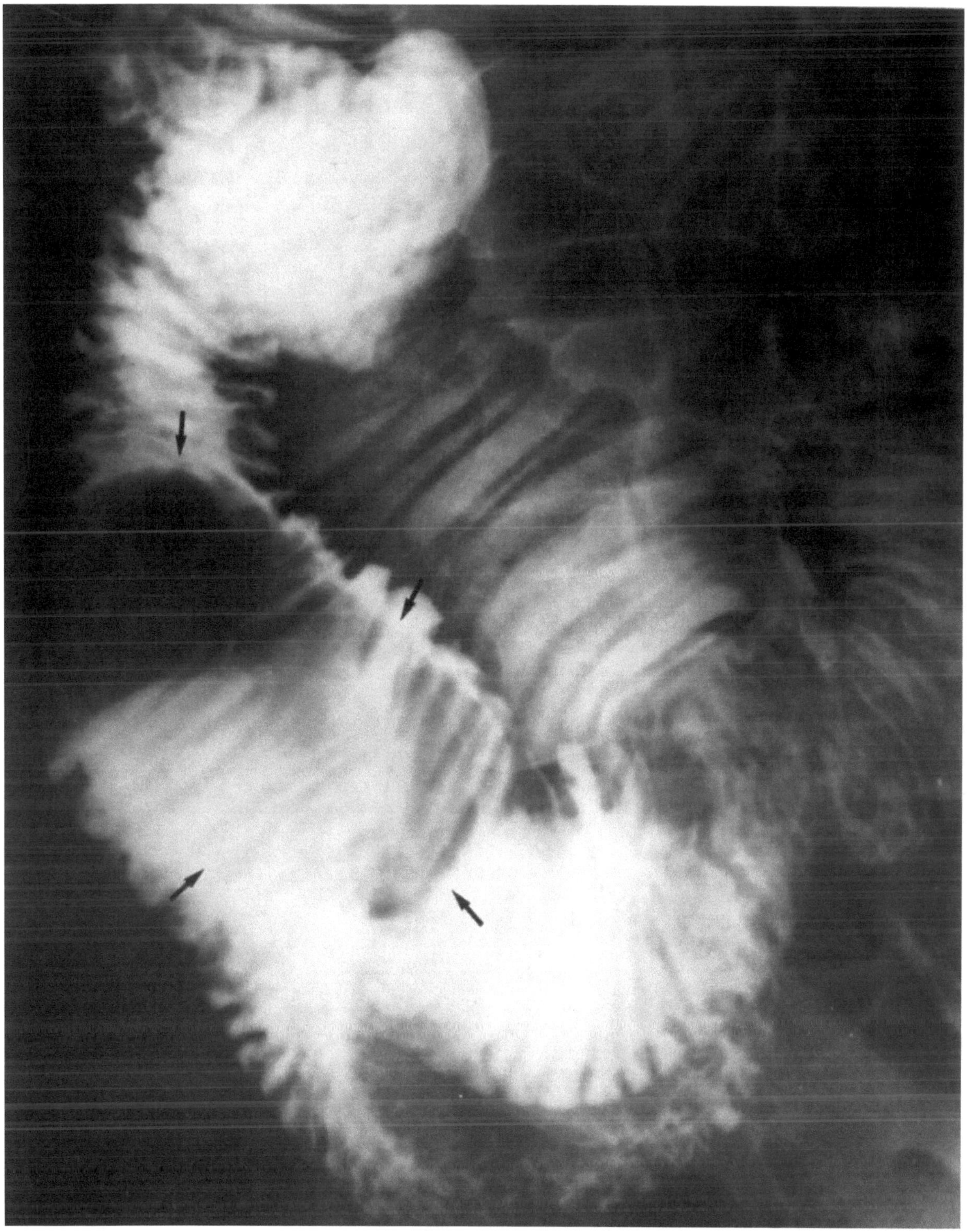

Fig. 5.5.-10. Intussusception of intestinal anastomosis. The intussuscipiens (→) in the efferent loop simulates a tumor. This is a very rare complication after gastrectomy. Intussusception after gastrointestinal anastomosis is more frequent

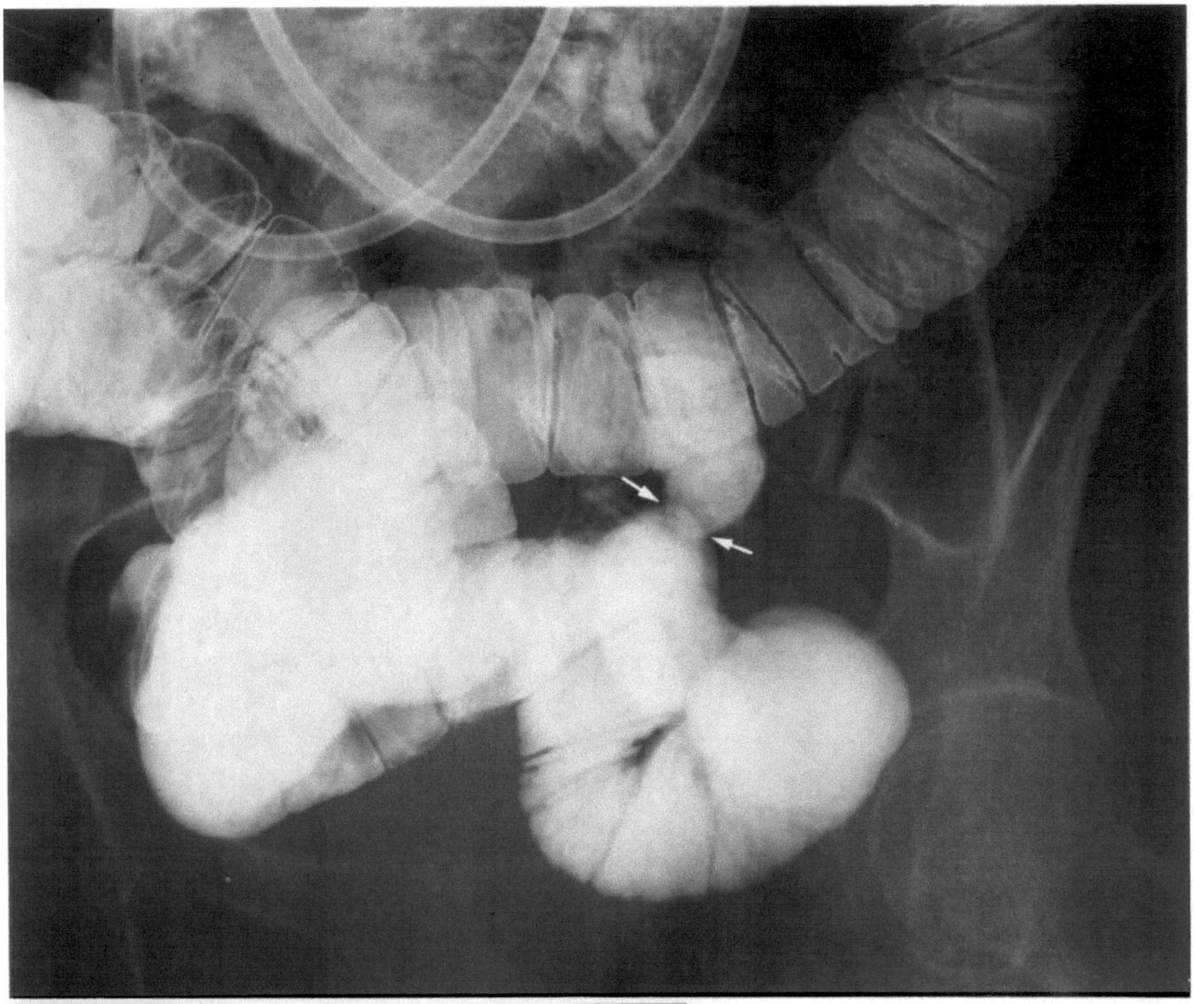

a

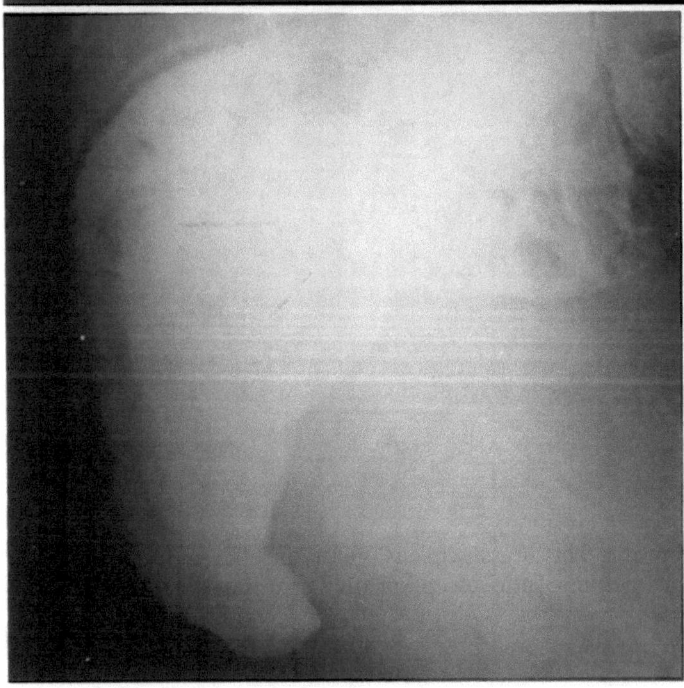

b

Fig. 5.5.-11 a and b. Internal hernia. The jejunum proximal to the hernial opening (→) is prestenotically dilated (**a**). The ileum is displaced into the presacral cavity and descends farther down with coughing maneuver (**b**). Female with intermittent subileus condition for years

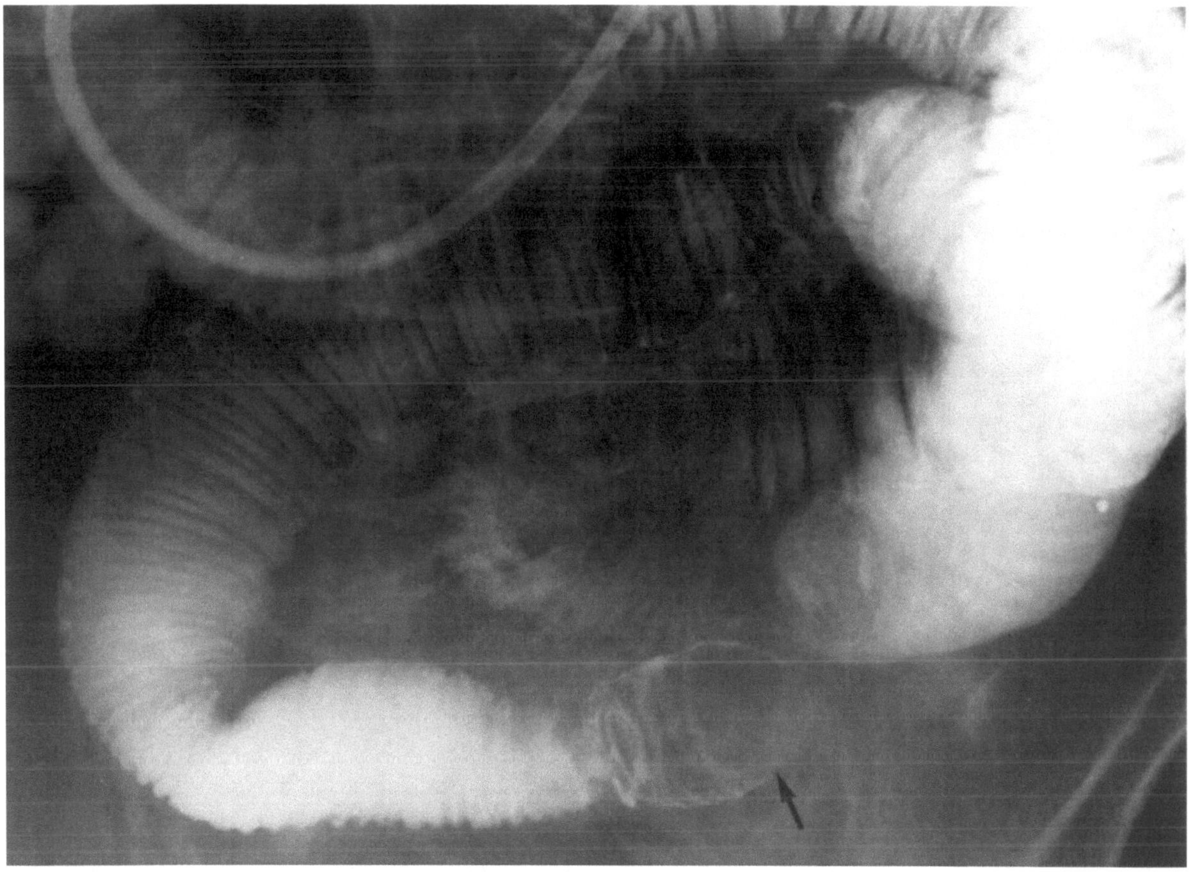

Fig. 5.5.-12. Intestinal occlusion by a gallstone. The concrement (→) obstructs the intestinal lumen. Status after gallstone perforation and subsequent bile duct surgery a week previously. Thereafter progressive ileus condition. Surgery after enteroclysis revealed a penetration of the stone into the mesentery

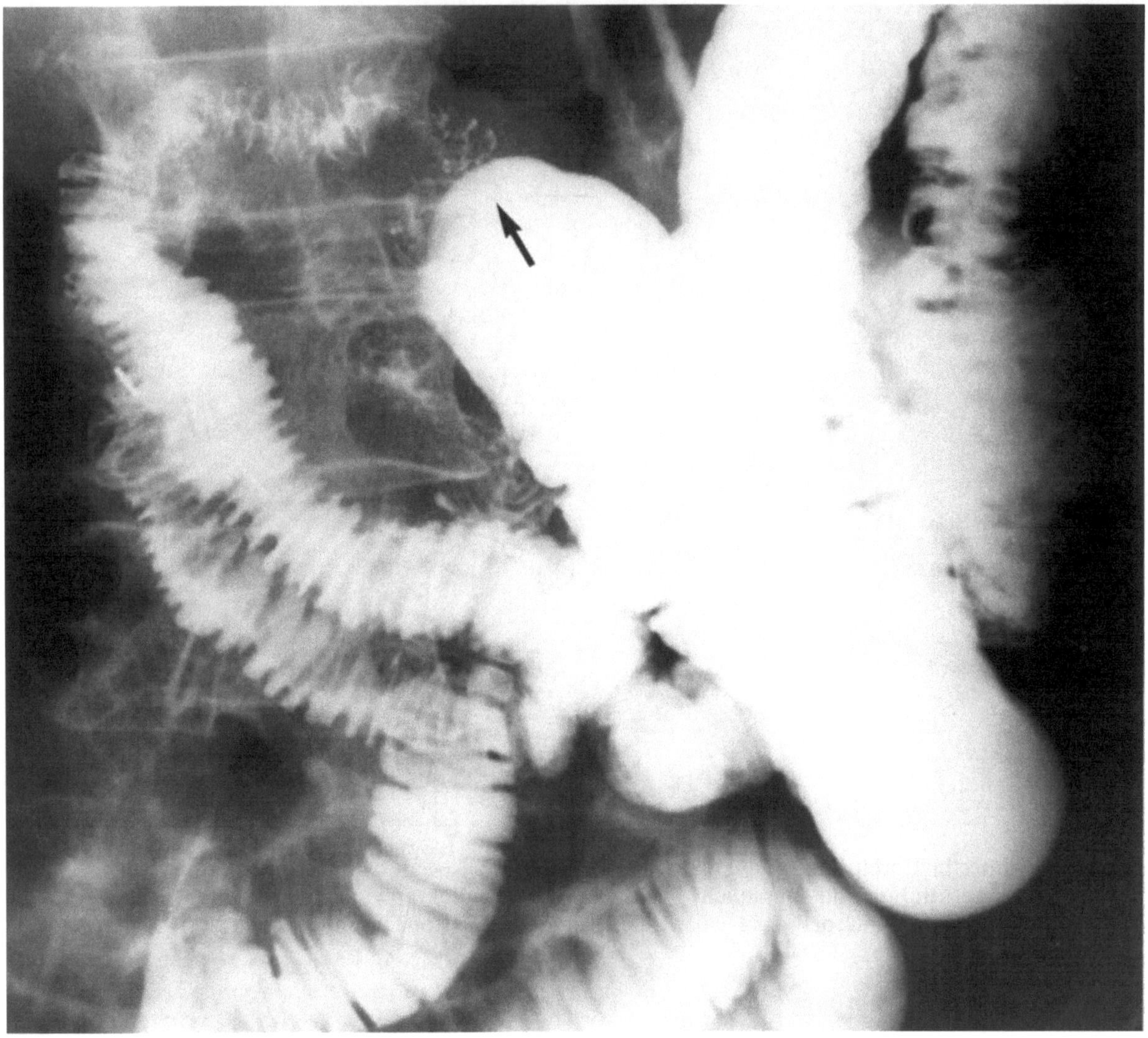

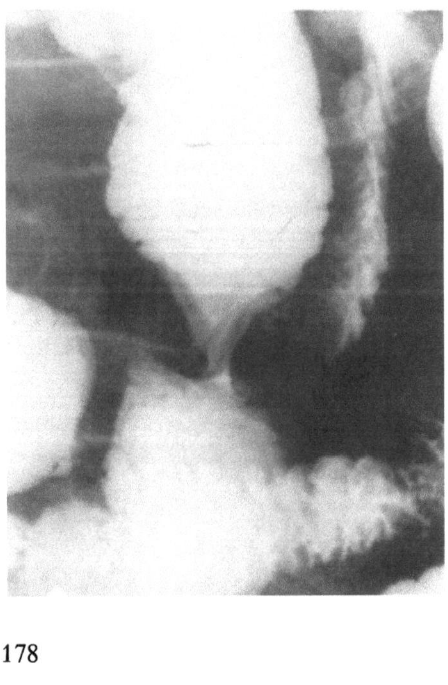

Fig. 5.5.-13. Irradiation stenosis. Short advanced stricture (→). Prestenotic dilatation. Two of the loops reveal changes of radiation enteritis (barium phase)

Fig. 5.5.-14. Stenosis by mesenteric fatty tissue necrosis. The stenosal contours are smooth, the mucosa is intact as evidence of an external process. Surgery detected postoperative fatty tissue necroses with scarry constriction of the intestinal wall

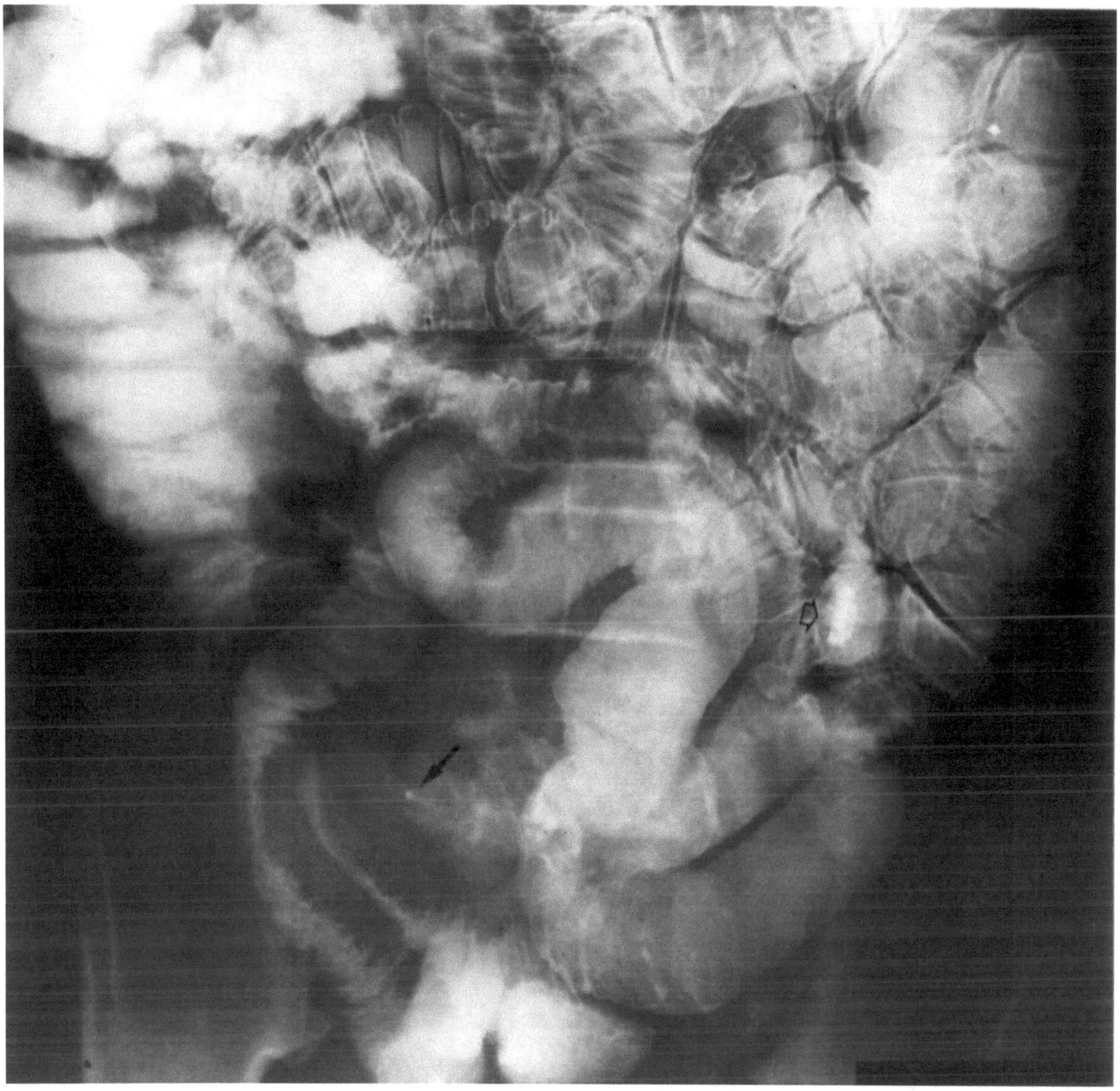

Fig. 5.5.-15. Stenoses due to foreign body reaction. Thickened intestinal loops and irregular mucosal folds with prestenotic dilatation at the tip of a ventriculoperitoneal shunt (→). After removal of the shunt, complete healing of the obstructing inflammation ensued. Measuring device (⇒)

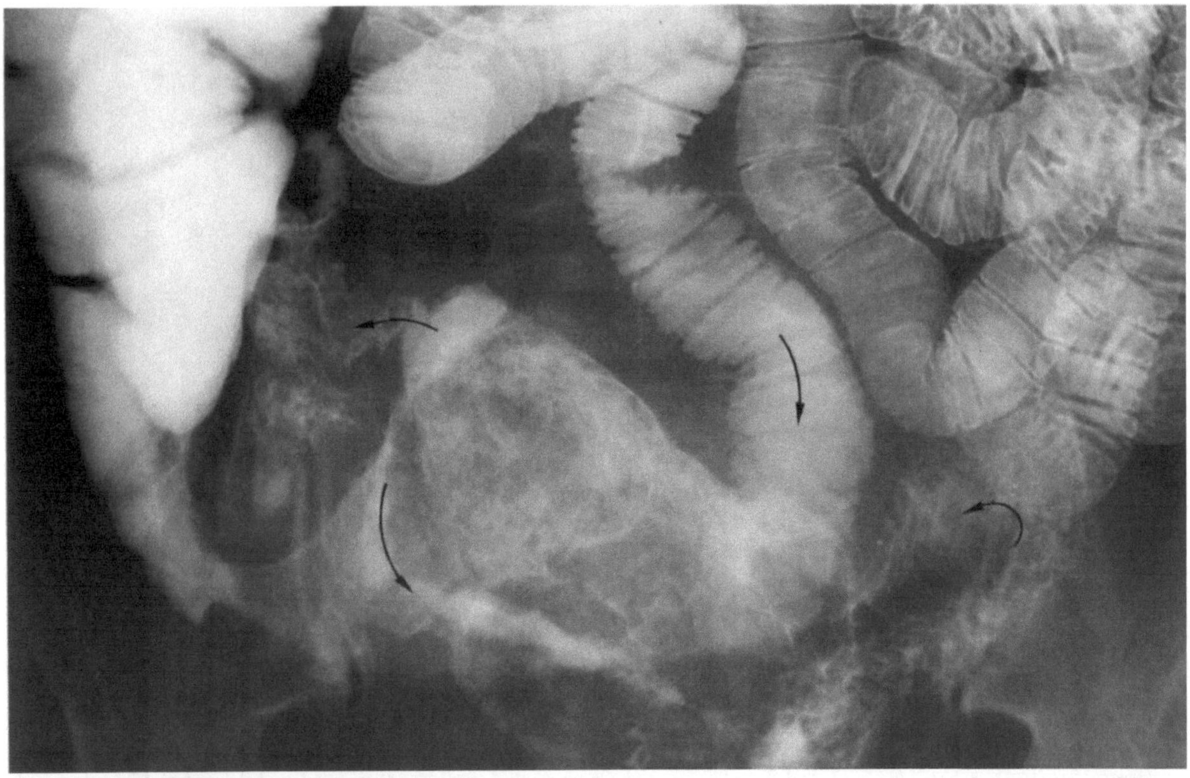

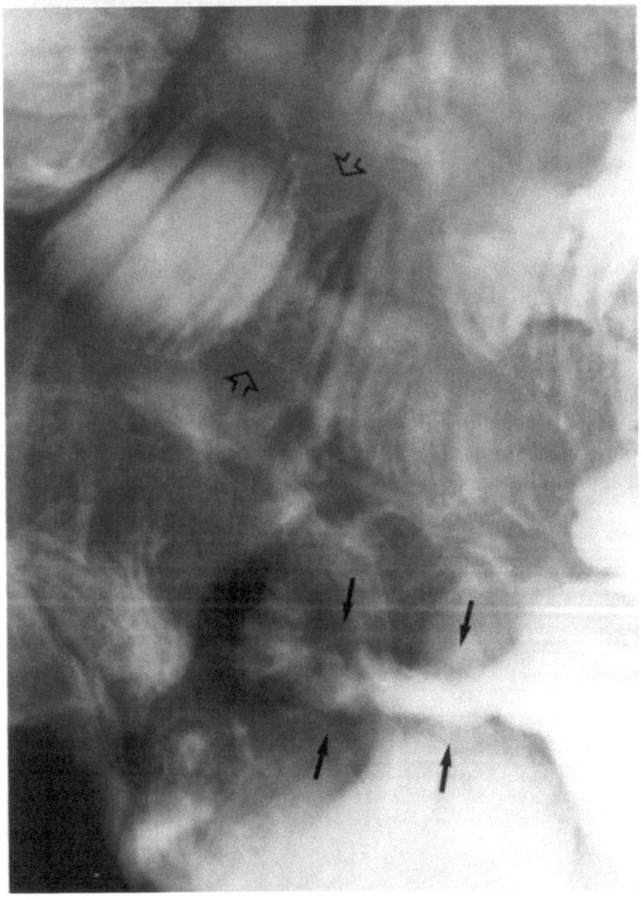

Fig. 5.5.-16. Obstruction due to foreign body abscess. Chronic abscess around an operation towel left in the peritoneal cavity. Infiltration in several ileal loops. Blockage of afferent intestinal loop, hyperperistalsis of the efferent loops due to inadequate filling

Fig. 5.5.-17. Obstruction in endometriosis. Luminar narrowing of varying degree due to mucosal infiltration

5.6 Malformations

Abnormalities are mostly detected by coincidence and bear no pathologic significance. In some cases, they may cause considerable trouble, however.

5.6.1 Disturbed Rotation and Fixation

Rotation disturbances of the gastroduodenal loop and those of the umbilical loop have to be differentiated; but both may present together.

The most frequent malformation is the *mobile duodenum* whereby a free mobile mesoduodenum is maintained (Sandera 1931). This can lead to intubation difficulties. If these are overcome, the tube may show a curly course (Fig. 5.6.-1). A barium test injection is helpful for orientation. If the tube cannot be brought over the inferior duodenal flexure, it should be left there (see chapter 2.4).

The radiologist should be aware of malformations and should not be surprised if the tube advances to the right rather than to the left.

In order to place the rapidly growing gut into the fetal abdomen, a rotation of the umbilical loop around the vitelline duct ensues. The amount of rotation is demonstrated by the 270–300° anticlockwise migration of the cecal pole. This process may arrest at various places or the fixation which takes place after rotation of a certain bowel segment either occurs prematurely at the posterior abdominal wall or not at all (Ferner 1964).

The most varied position anomalies of the small and large bowels result from these rotatory and fixatory disturbances (staging see Grob 1953).

Radiographs alone will not always clarify the type of rotation/fixation anomaly. Evaluation of these anomalies is especially important for the surgeon, who will thus avoid confrontation with an unexpected situation (Figs. 5.6.-2 and 3). The patient should therefore be informed about the abnormal position of his gut. Malrotation, however, can cause complaints, especially if the jejunum is twisted in the presence of a long movable mesentery, possibly resulting in temporary ischemia (Fig. 5.6.-4a and b; Aldrich et al. 1955; Gardner and Hart 1934).

The jejunum is usually situated in the left upper quadrant and the ileum in the right lower quadrant.

Nonrotation

The umbilical loop rotation comes to a standstill after the first normal turn of 90° (Figs. 5.6.-2 and 3). The whole of the small bowel lies in the right half of the abdominal cavity, whereby the descending duodenum passes directly into the jejunum. The ileum opens into the cecum from the right and the entire colon lies in the left half of the abdomen (Altschul 1924).

Malrotation I

The umbilical loop rotation comes to a standstill at 180°. The duodenojejunal junction lies farther to the right than usual (Fig. 5.6.-4a). The jejunum is more orientated medially but also extends partially towards the left abdomen (Fig. 5.6.-4b).

Malrotation II

The rotation ensues in alternating directions (90° in normal and 90° in alternating direction). The duodenum and the small bowel have a similar position as in "nonrotation" in the right abdomen, or are medially located. The proximal colon comes to rest behind the small bowel.

5.6.2 Internal Hernias

If there is a disturbance of fixation after umbilical loop rotation, openings may develop, into which bowel loops can herniate. Such locations are found at the ileocecal junction (retrocecal hernia), at the duodenojejunal junction (right and left paraduodenal hernia, hernia of Treitz), in the region of the epiploic foramen and finally as a defect in the mesentery or transverse mesocolon (Parsons 1953).

Internal hernias are clinically difficult to diagnose. In enteroclysis it is important to pursue the contrast medium bolus carefully. In the hernial region, local motility disturbances may be observed, which result from the obstruction. In most cases, there is a local hyperperistalsis and the patient complains of pain in the hernial region. Lateral viewing is important as in a.p. view the hernial opening may be overlooked (Fig. 5.5.-11, p. 176).

5.6.3 Duplications

Duplication abnormalities can occur along the whole length of the gastrointestinal tract. The small bowel is most frequently affected, mainly the distal ileum (Gross et al. 1952). The duplication lies at the mesenteric border of the bowel and has the same wall structures as the gut itself. The mucosal lining may but does not have to correspond with the adjacent bowel segment. In most cases, there is no bowel connection so that a direct demonstration of the malformation is not possible (Moore and Battersby 1952; Smith 1960). Demonstration may be brought indirectly by impression on the neighbouring intestinal loops or better still by means of ultrasound or CT.

5.6.4 Diverticula

Acquired ("false") diverticula arise in relation to sites of penetration of the bowel wall by the vasa recta, which enter on the mesenteric border, therefore lying on the concave side of the small bowel in the mesenteric attachment region.

Diverticula are most frequently found in the duodenum (5.2–23%; Rösch 1978). They are mostly situated in the papilla area. In the remainder of the small bowel diverticula are found in 0.2–0.5% (Prévôt 1968; Sellink 1976) and diminish in quantity and size from the jejunum to the ileum. Diverticula in the terminal ileum are rare (Fig. 5.6.-8). Diverticula are mostly found incidentally and have no pathological significance (Fig. 5.6.-5). However, sometimes they lead to retention of food matter (Fig. 5.6.-6) or hemorrhage (Figs. 5.6.-7 and 5.4.-20, p. 163), torsion with necrosis and perforation or volvulus. The retention of bowel contents in diverticula can lead to bacterial overgrowth in the small bowel and chronic diarrhea.

Congenital diverticula are found at the antimesenteric border. As "true" diverticula, they have the same characteristics as the intestinal wall and are therefore contractile. Differentiation between congenital and acquired diverticula is not always possible and in practice, not necessary (see chapter 4.3).

5.6.5 Meckel's Diverticulum

Meckel's diverticulum occurs when the omphalomesenteric duct does not obliterate completely. Autopsies discover ca. 1–4% (Christie 1931; Ladd 1942). It is always found at the antimesenteric side, between 20–100 cm proximal to the ileocecal valve – usually at 80 cm. The size can vary considerably, between 1–30 cm in diameter.

Arey (1947) discriminates three different types of Meckel's diverticula, corresponding to the obliteration of the omphalomesenteric duct. Type A, the most frequent type, is a mobile blind sack (Figs. 5.6.-9 and 11). Type B, less frequent, is fixed to the umbilicus by a fibrotic strand, therefore projecting always at the same place (Figs. 5.6.-10 and 12). Type C is very rare and consists of an open connection to the outside, which can be demonstrated by a fistulogram.

Usually, the blind sack is lined with ileal mucosa (70%). It can, however, possess ectopic gastric, duodenal or colonic mucosa (15–20%) or even pancreatic tissue (4%), thus precipitating bleeding or ulcers (Prévôt 1968).

The radiological demonstration by follow-through examination was disappointing (Berne 1959; Stein et al. 1958). Enteroclysis has brought considerable improvement (Maglinte et al. 1980); failures, however, are not excluded. For example we missed a Meckel's diverticulum in a baby with intestinal bleeding and classical medical history, but were successful by radioisotope study with technetiumpertechnetate (Ber-

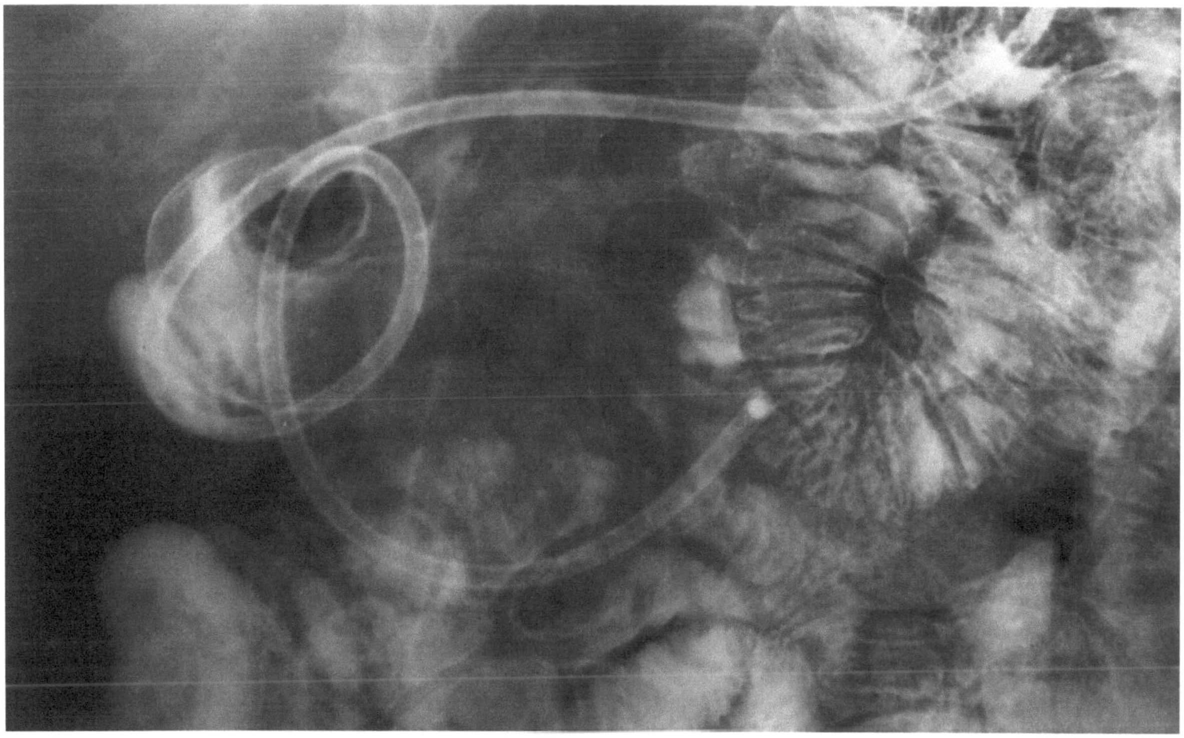

Fig. 5.6.-1. Mobile duodenum. Curly course of the duodenal tube. Rather difficult, but nevertheless successful intubation

quist et al. 1973; Duszynski et al. 1971; Rosenthal et al. 1972) (Fig. 5.6.-13).

During examination it is necessary to pursue the contrast medium bolus carefully and to pay attention to triangular array of folds which may lead to the diverticulum. After the methylcellulose has been administered, the barium-filled diverticulum shows up more intensely and is therefore more easily recognizable (Fig. 5.6.-9).

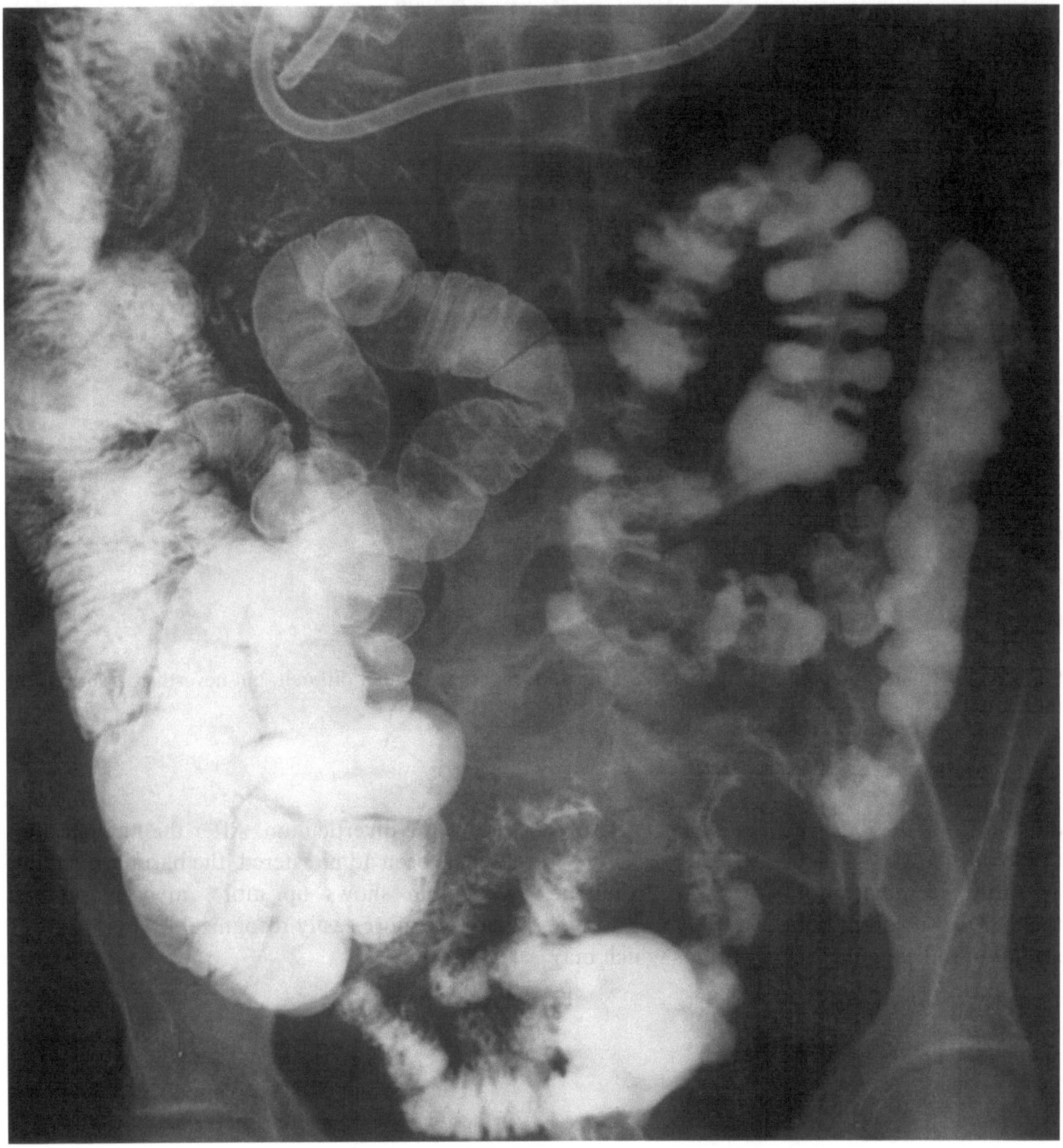

Fig. 5.6.-2. Nonrotation. Absence of the ascending duodenum and duodenojejunal junction (see course of tube). The descending part goes directly into the jejunum and ileum in the right abdomen. The terminal ileum coming from the right, is running into the cecum, which lies together with the remainder of the colon in the left abdomen. There is inadequate filling with local hyperperistalsis at the jejunoileal junction with some prestenotic dilatation of the jejunum due to adhesions after appendectomy

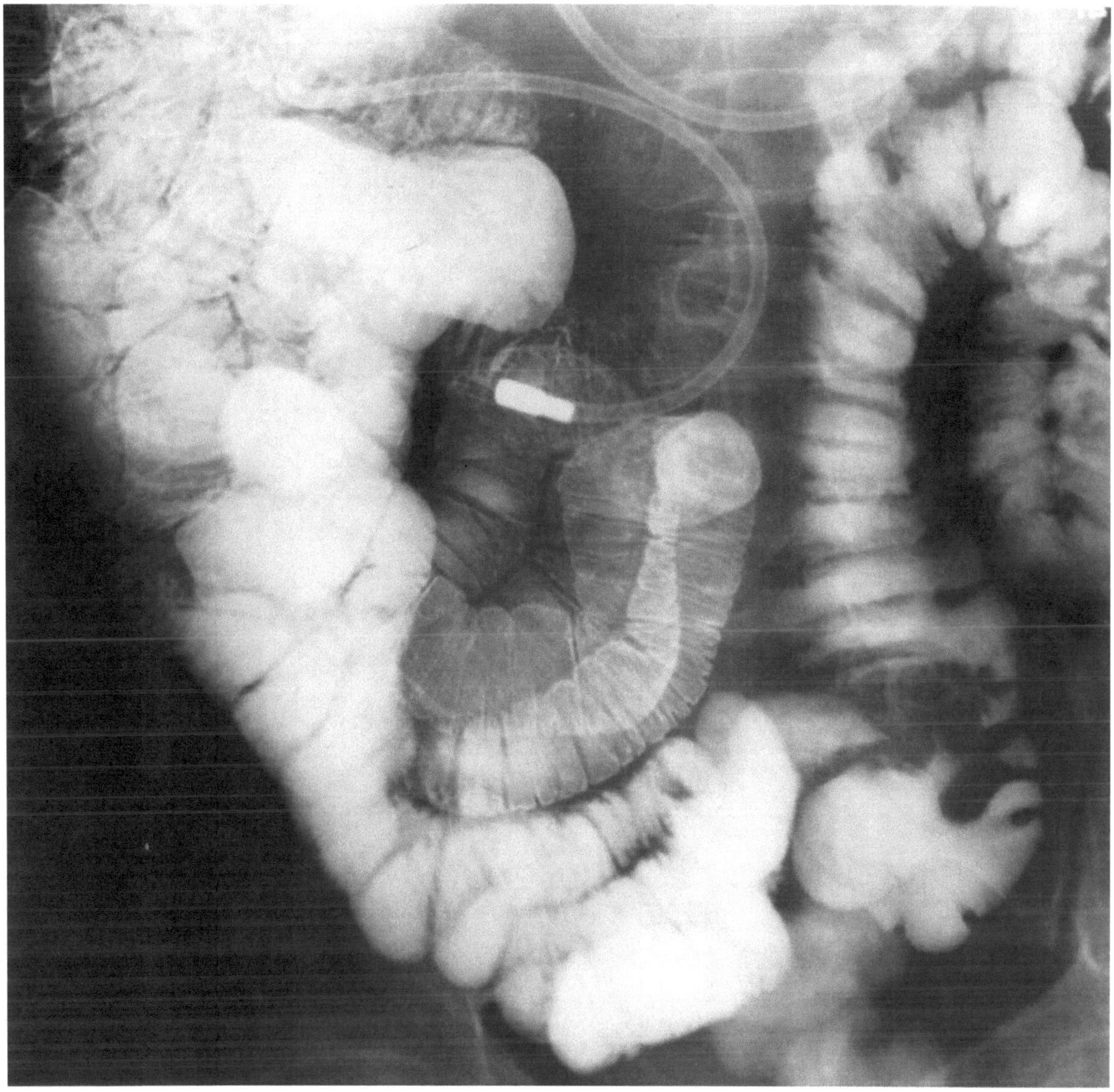

Fig. 5.6.-3. Nonrotation. The ascending duodenum is already partially developed, as can be seen by the course of the tube

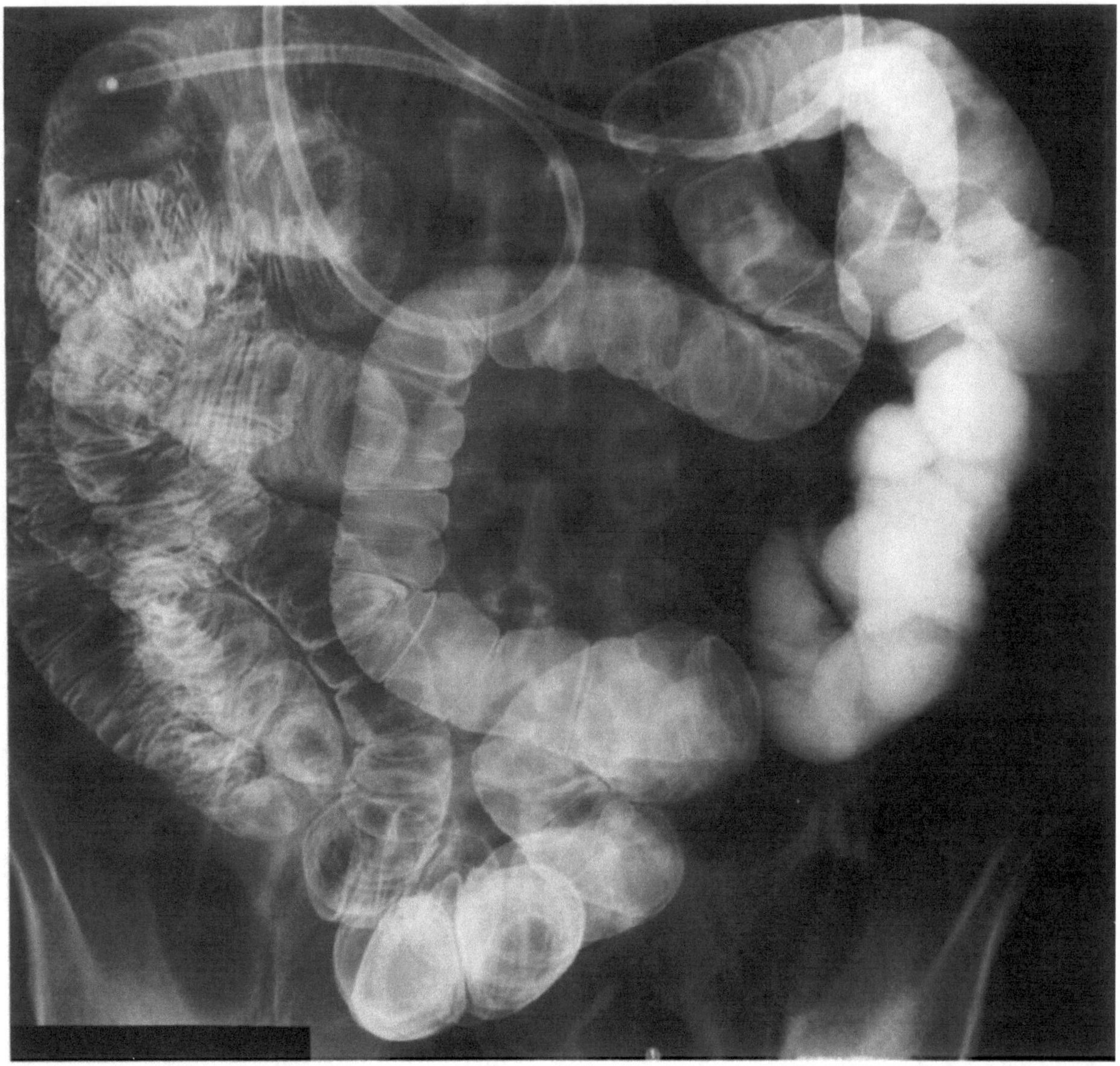

a

Fig. 5.6.-4a and b. Malrotation I. Same patient: In the first examination (**a**), the tube advances to the right after passing the duodenojejunal junction, positioned farther right than usual. The major part of the jejunum is situated on the right. In a control examination (**b**), the jejunal loops are placed more in the center and in the left upper quadrant. The cecum and the rest of the colon are correctly positioned. For about 10 years, the patient had complained of recurring midabdominal pain with gurgling, spurting gut sounds lasting for hours. This may be explained by temporary vessel torsion in an augmented movable mesentery or torsion of the intestine

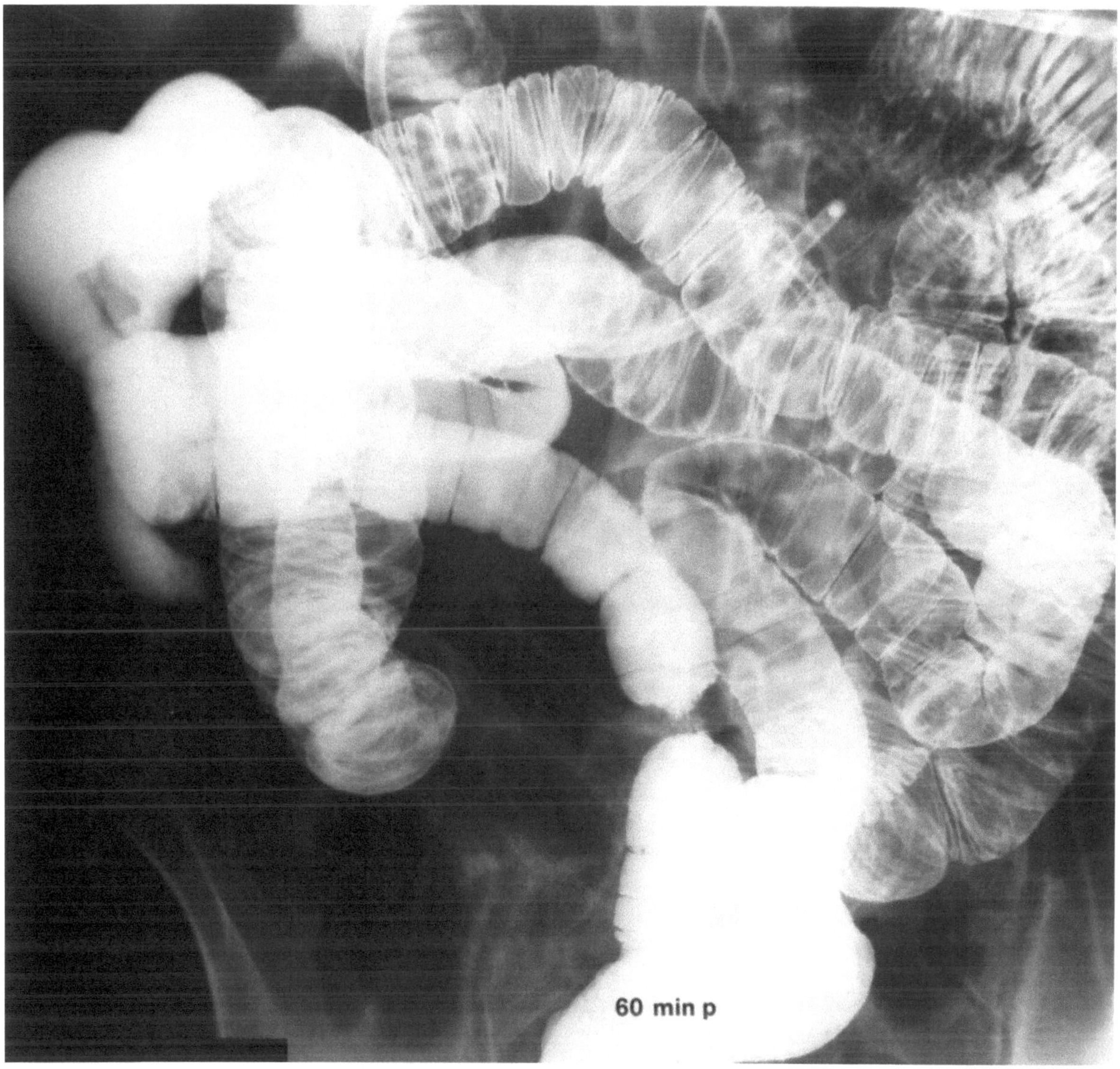

Fig. 5.6.-4b

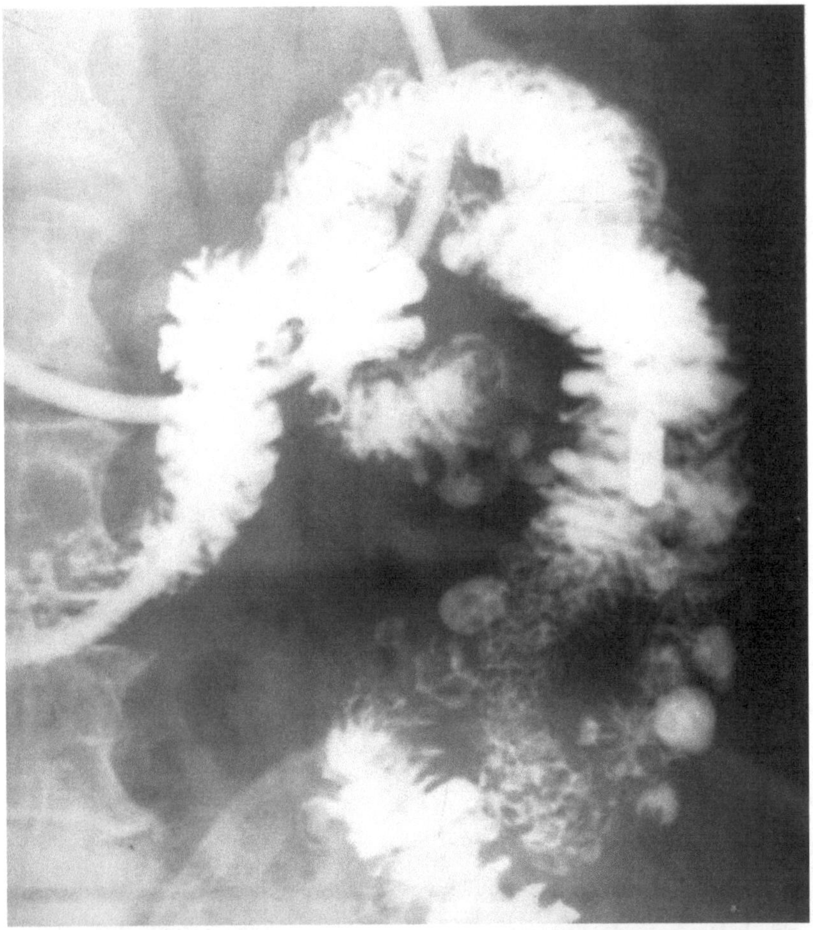

Fig. 5.6.-5. Diverticula. Multiple diverticula of varying size, found in the jejunum. Incidental finding

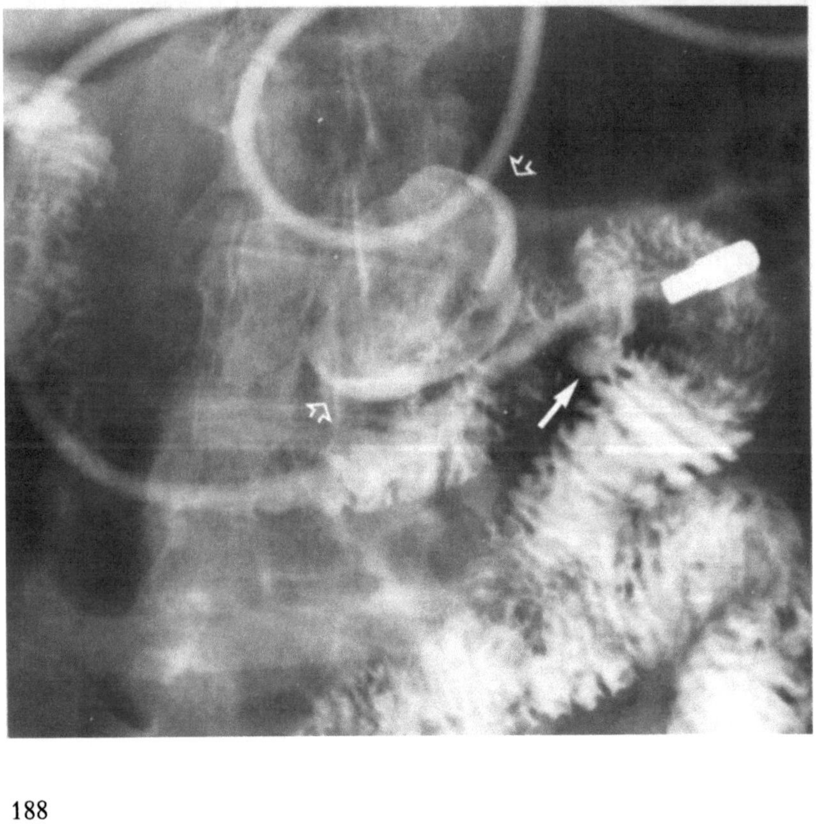

Fig. 5.6.-6. Diverticulum. Contrast medium around a trichobezoar in a large diverticulum (⇒) on the duodenojejunal junction. Additional small jejunal diverticulum (→). Incidental finding, confirmed endoscopically

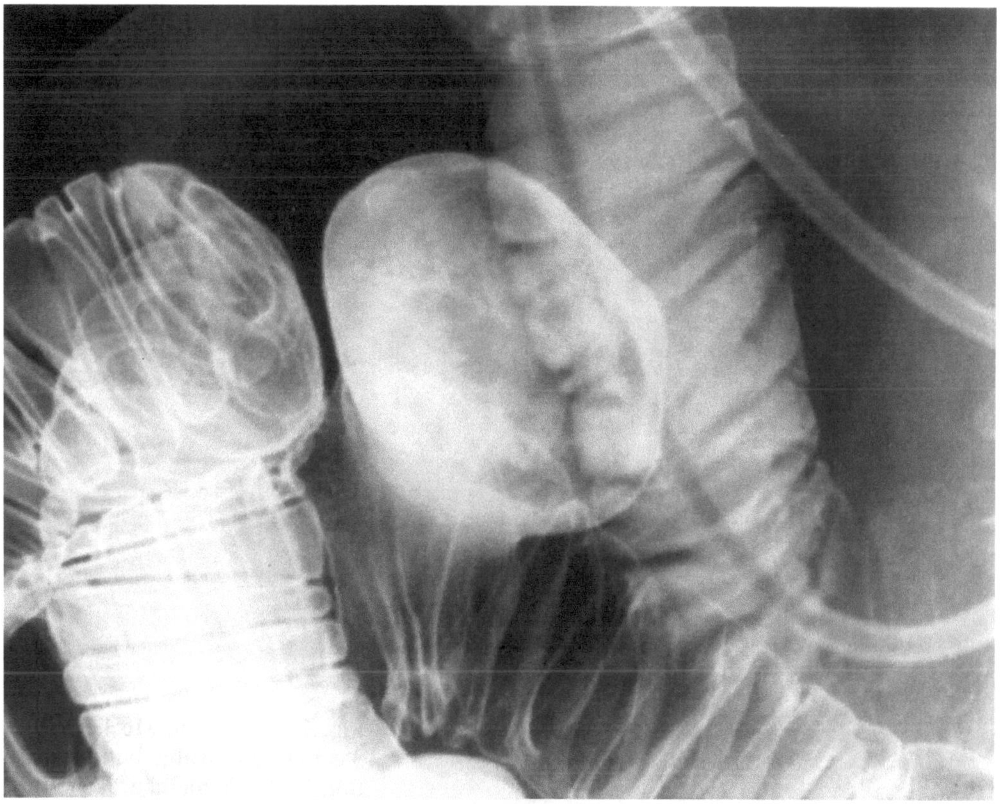

Fig. 5.6.-7. Diverticulum. Jejunal diverticulum causing gastrointestinal bleeding. Radiologically, there is no evident cause visible

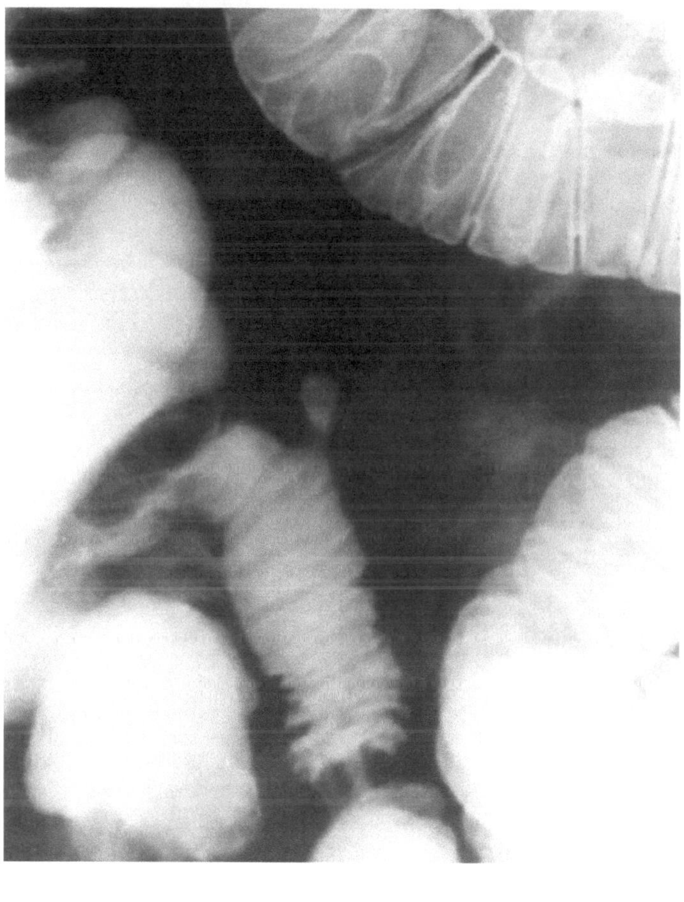

Fig. 5.6.-8. Diverticulum. Tiny, acquired diverticulum in the distal ileum on the mesenteric border in an asymptomatic patient. Incidental finding. Diverticula on the terminal ileum are rare

a

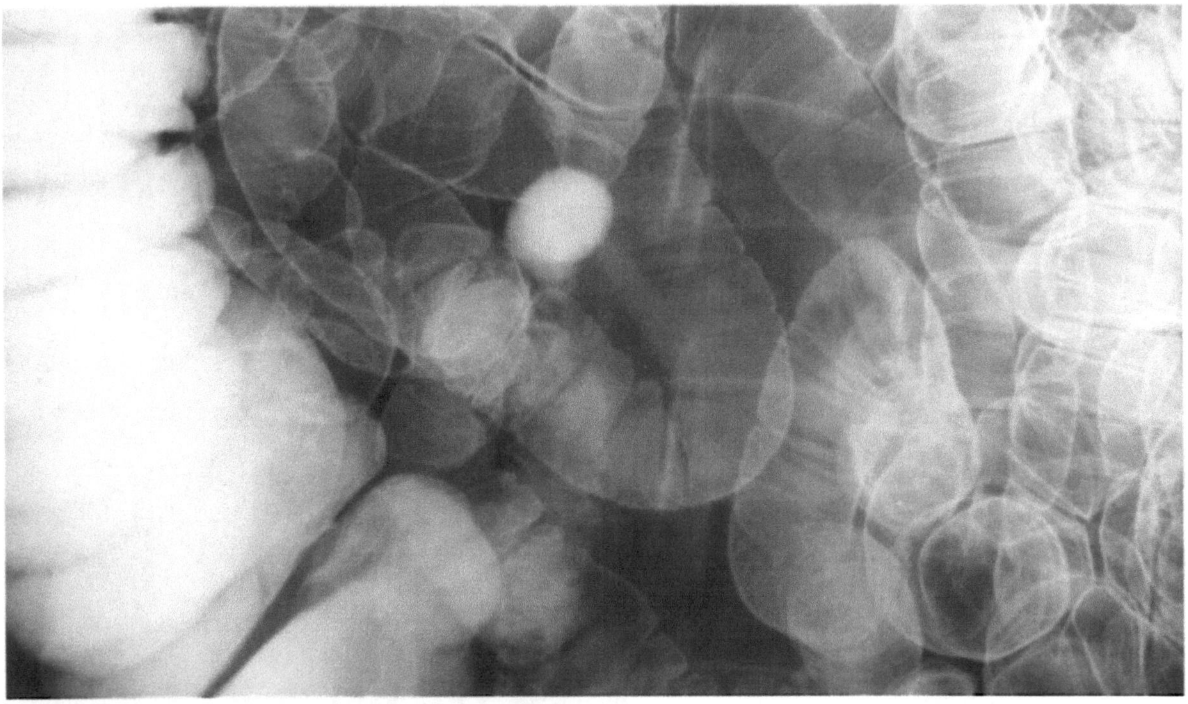

Fig. 5.6.-9a and b. Meckel's diverticulum. Ca. 3 cm large movable blind sack at a typical location in the ileum, characteristic of type A. The diverticulum is more easily recognizable in the early methylcellulose phase when it is still filled with barium (**a**) than later in pure double contrast (**b**). Incidental finding

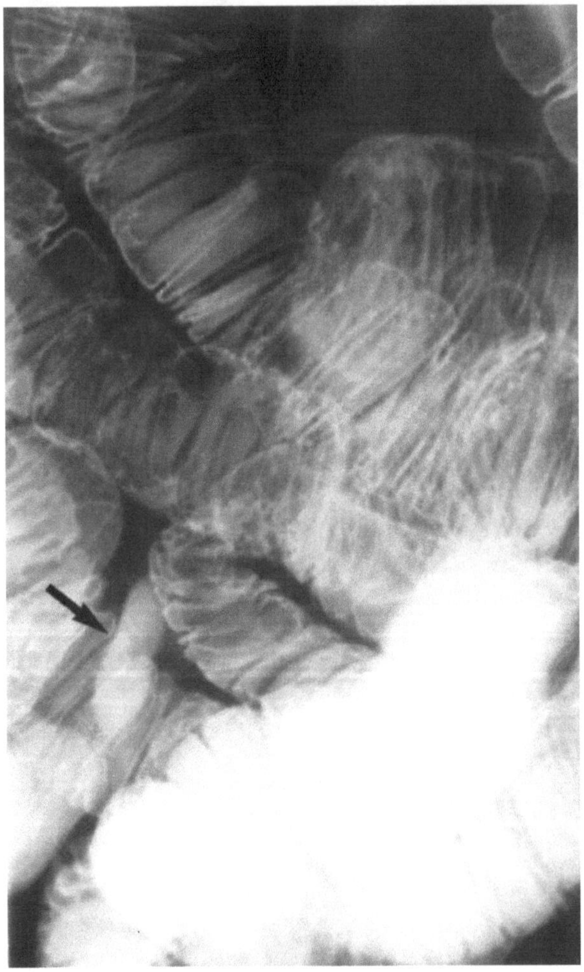

Fig. 5.6.-10. Meckel's diverticulum. Small longitudinal diverticulum which always projects on the same place, therefore characteristic of type B (→). The diverticulum is more easily recognized as long as it is adequately filled with barium. Patient had bled from this diverticulum

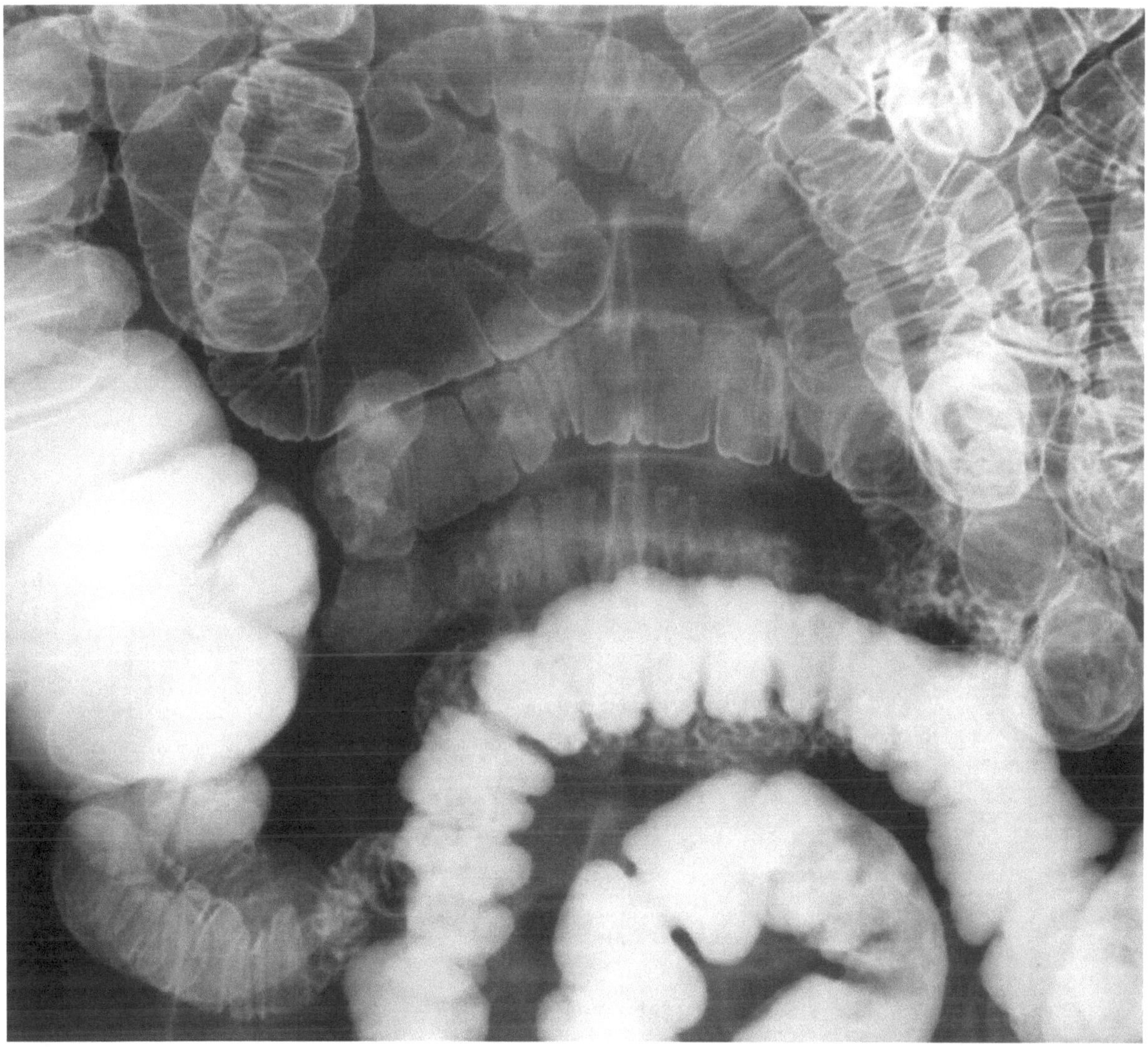

Fig. 5.6.-9b

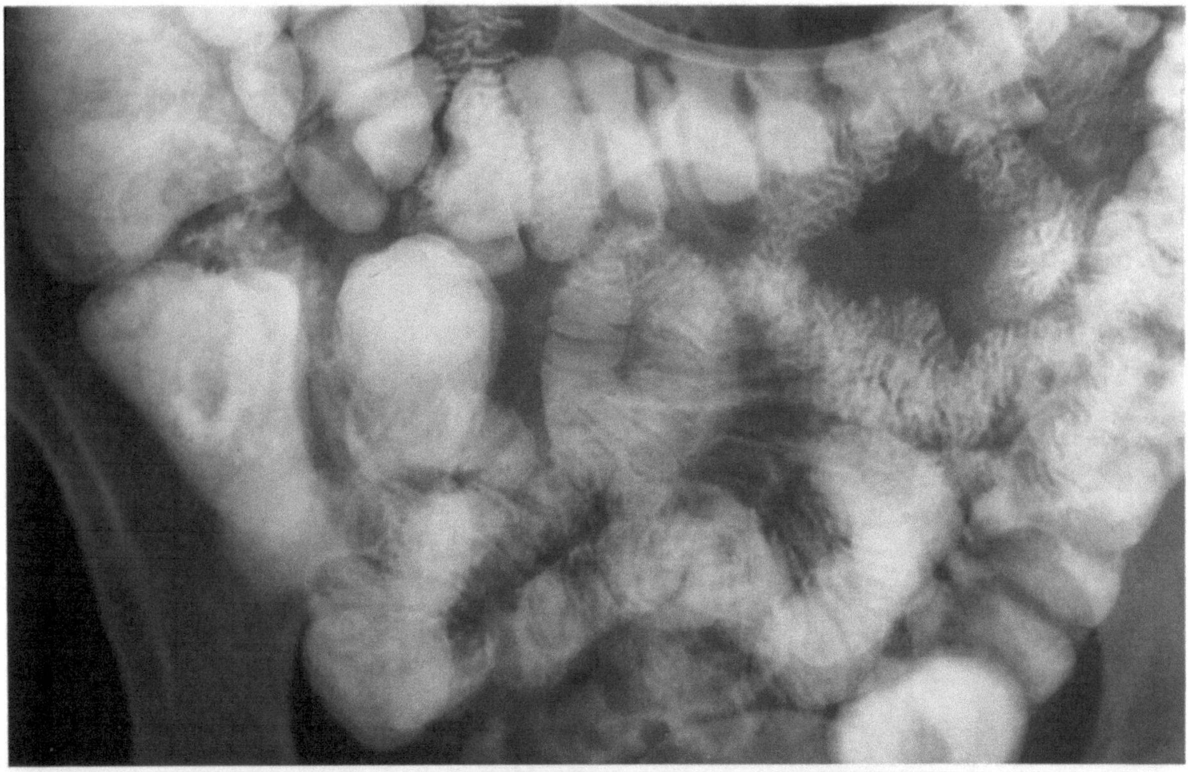

a

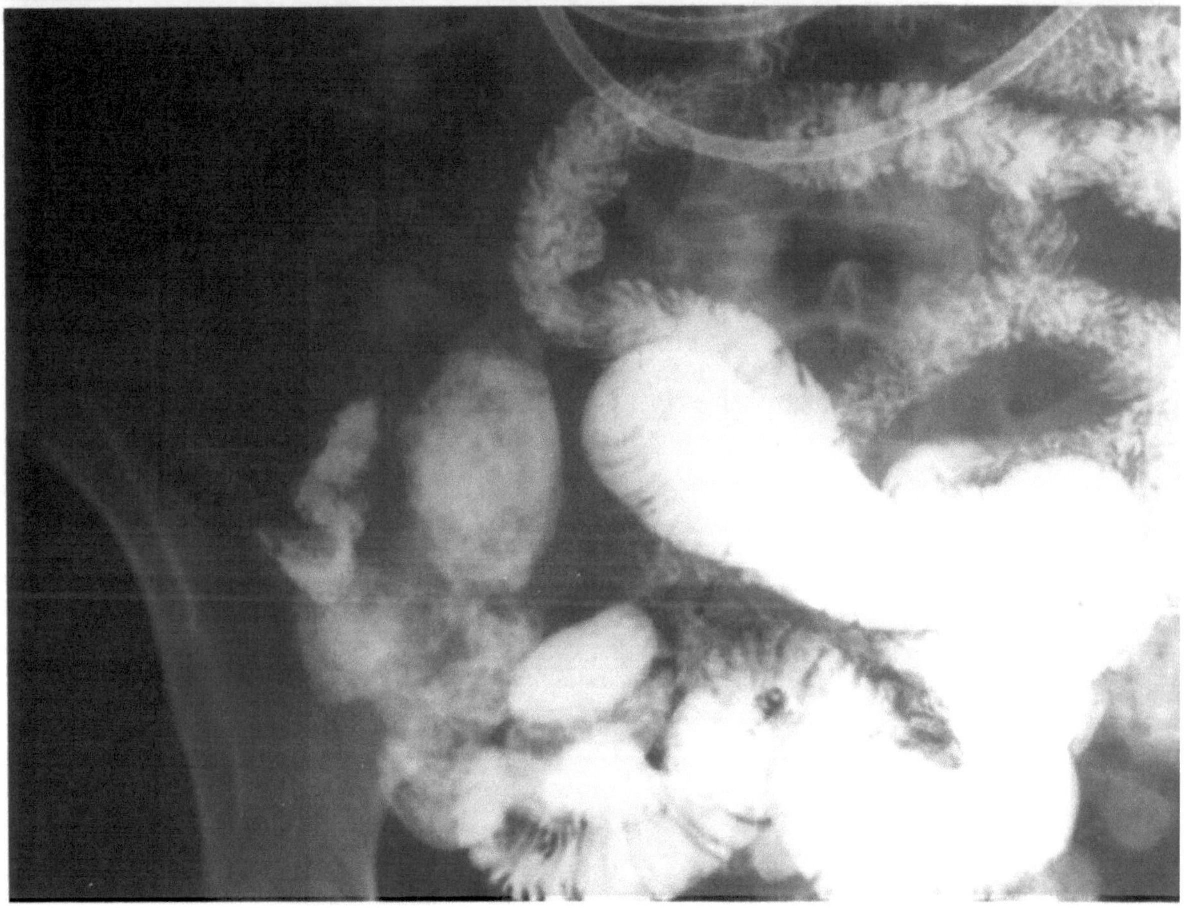

b

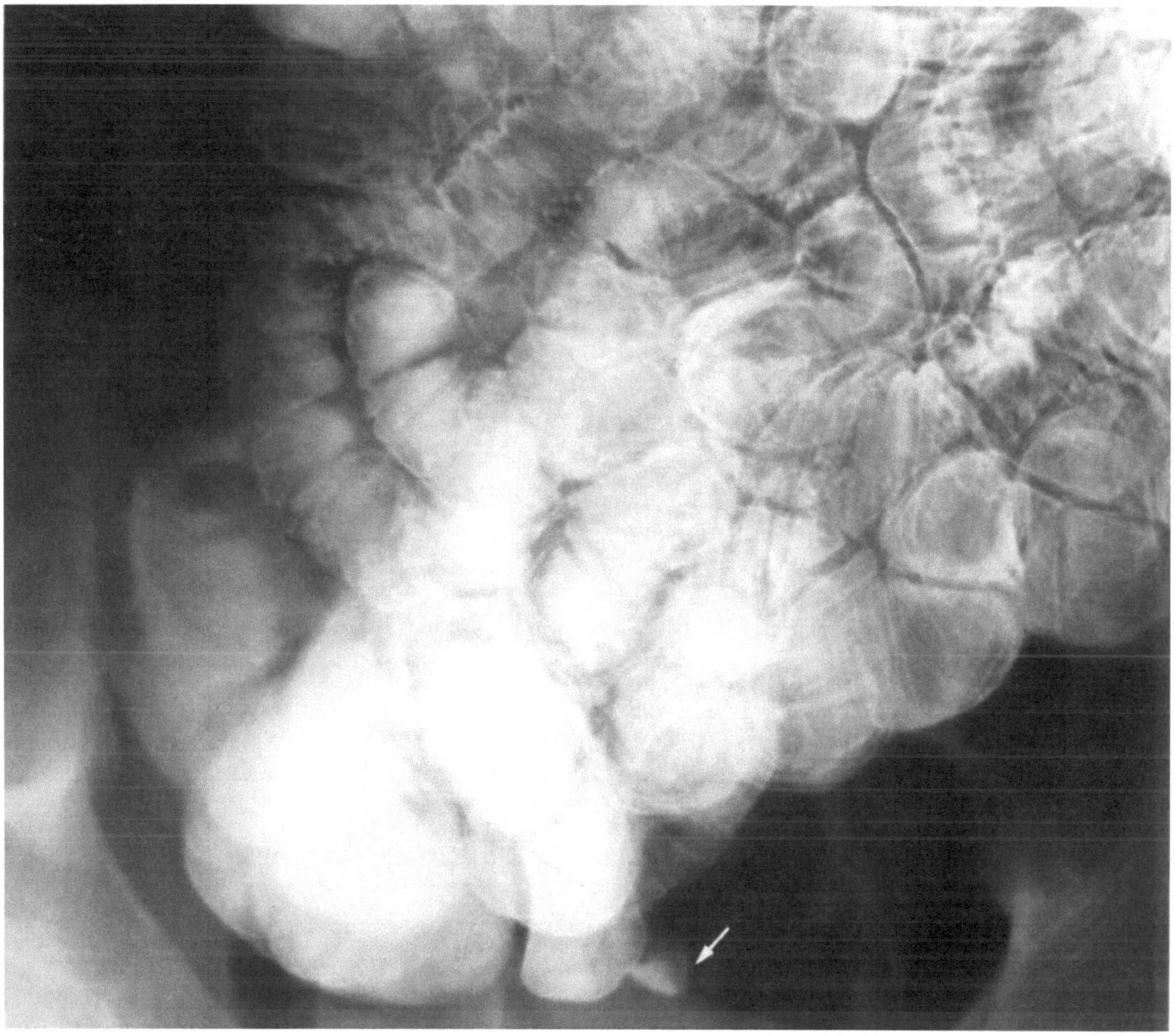

Fig. 5.6.-12. Meckel's diverticulum. Small diverticulum (→) always found at the same place (type B). Incidental finding in a patient with Crohn's disease

◀ **Fig. 5.6.-11 a and b.** Meckel's diverticulum. Medium size, ca. 6 cm long (**a**) representing type A. In the filling phase, the diverticulum is easily recognizable (**b**). The patient suffered gastrointestinal bleeding. No ectopic mucosa was found in the diverticulum

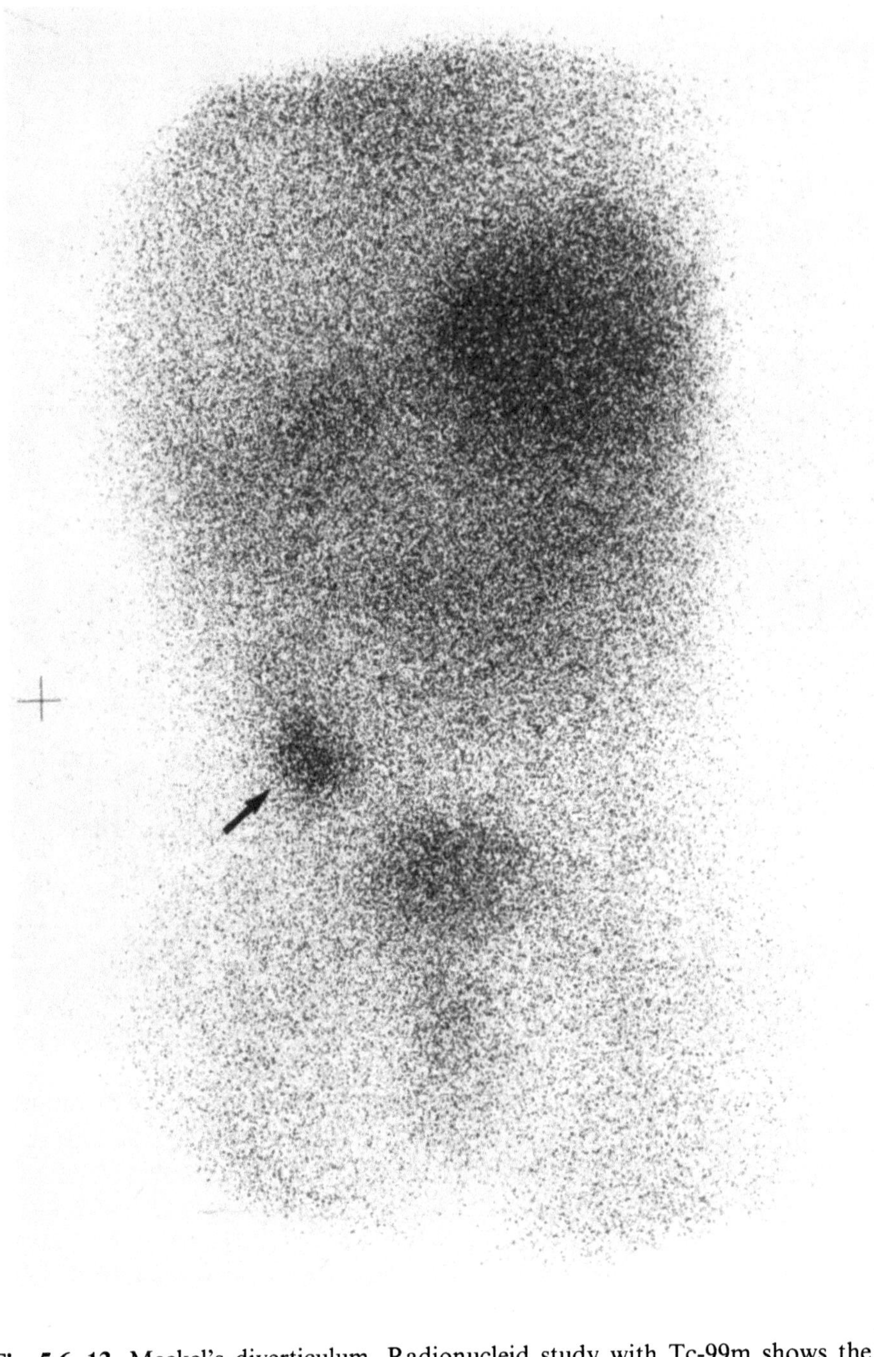

Fig. 5.6.-13. Meckel's diverticulum. Radionucleid study with Tc-99m shows the ectopic gastric mucosa in the diverticulum (→). 6-month-old baby with recurrent intestinal bleeding. Enteroclysis was negative

Bibliography

Chapter 1 "Introduction"

Antes G, Lissner J (1981) Die Doppelkontrastdarstellung des Dünndarms mit Barium und Methylcellulose. Fortschr Röntgenstr 134, 1:10–15

Antes G, Lissner J (1983) Double contrast small-bowel examination with barium and methylcellulose: Results in 300 cases. Radiology 148:37–40

Bilbao MK, Frische LH, Dotter ChT, Rösch J (1967) Hypotonic duodenography. Radiology 89:438–443

Einhorn M (1926) The Duodenal Tube and its Possibilities, 2nd edn. Davis, Philadelphia

Ekberg O (1977) Crohn's disease of the small bowel examined by double contrast technique. A comparison with oral technique. Gastrointest Radiol 1:355–359

Fleckenstein P, Pedersen G (1975) The value of the duodenal intubation method (Sellink modification) for the radiological visualization of the small bowel. Scand J Gastroenterol 10:423–425

Fried AM, Poulos A, Hatfield DR (1981) The effectiveness of the incidental small-bowel series. Radiology 140:45–46

Geiter B, Fuchs H-F (1977) Dünndarm-Kontrasteinlauf: Indikationen und Technik. Dtsch Ärztebl 43:2575

Gershon-Cohen J, Shay H (1939) Barium enteroclysis. Am J Roentgenol 42:456–458

Gianturco C (1967) Rapid fluoroscopic duodenal intubation. Radiology 88:1165

Gmünder U, Wirth W (1970) Dünndarmdoppelkontrastdarstellung. Schweiz Med Wochenschr 100:1236

Golden R (1959) Radiologic examination of the small intestine, 2nd edn. Lippincott, Philadelphia

Herlinger H (1978) A modified technique for the double contrast small-bowel enema. Gastrointest Radiol 3, 2:201–207

Herlinger H (1979) Small bowel. In: Laufer I (ed) Double Contrast Gastrointestinal Radiology. Saunders, Philadelphia

Lura A (1951) Enema of the small intestine with special emphasis on the diagnosis of tumours. Br J Radiol 24:264–271

Maglinte DDT, Burney BT, Miller RE (1982) Lesions missed on small-bowel follow-through: Analysis and recommendations. Radiology 144:737–739

Marshak RH, Lindner AE (1976) Radiology of the small intestine. Saunders, Philadelphia

Ott DJ, Yu Men Chen, Gelfand DW, van Swearingen F, Munitz HA (1985) Detailed per-oral small bowel examination vs. enteroclysis. Radiology 155:29–34

Pansdorf H (1937) Die fraktionierte Dünndarmfüllung und ihre klinische Bedeutung. Fortschr Röntgenstr 56:627–634

Pesquera GS (1929) A method for the direct visualization of lesions in the small intestine. Am J Roentgenol 22:254–257

Pribram BO, Kleiber N (1927) Ein neuer Weg zur röntgenologischen Darstellung des Duodenums (Pneumo-duodenum). Fortschr Geb Röntgenstr Nuklearmed 36:739

Pygott F, Street DF, Shellshear MF, Rhodes CJ (1960) Radiological investigation of the small intestine by small bowel enema technique. Gut 1:366–370

Rabe FE, Becker GJ, Besozzi MJ, Miller RE (1981) Efficacy study of the small-bowel examination. Radiology 140:47–50

Sanders DE, Ho CS (1976) The small bowel enema, experience with 150 examinations. Am J Roentgenol 127:743–751

Schatzki R (1943) Small intestinal enema. Am J Roentgenol 50:743–751

Scott-Harden WG, Hamilton HAR, McCall Smith S (1961) Radiological investigation of the small intestine. Gut 2:316–322

Sellink JL (1971) Examination of the Small Intestine by Means of Duodenal Intubation. Stenfert Kroese, Leiden

Sellink JL (1974) Radiologic examination of the small intestine by duodenal intubation. Acta Radiol 15:318–332

Sellink JL (1976) Radiological Atlas of Common Diseases of the Small Bowel. Stenfert Kroese, Leiden

Trickey SE, Halls J, Hodson CJ (1963) A further development of the small bowel enema. Proc R Soc Med 56:1070–1073

Vallance R (1980) An evaluation of the small bowel enema based on an analysis of 350 consecutive examinations. Clin Radiol 31:227–232

Chapter 2 "Examination Technique" and Chapter 4 "Basic Signs and Interpretation"

Abu-Yousef MM, Benson CA, Lu CH, Franken EA (1983) Enteroclysis aided by an electric pump. Radiology 147:268–269

Antes G, Eggemann F (1987) Problemlose Sondenlegung beim Dünndarmeinlauf (Enteroclysis). Röntgenpraxis (in press)

Antes G, Lissner J (1981) Die Doppelkontrastdarstellung des Dünndarms mit Barium und Methylcellulose. Fortschr Röntgenstr 134, 1:10–15

Antes G, Lissner J (1983) Double-contrast small-bowel examination with barium and methylcellulose. Results in 300 cases. Radiology 148:37–40

Bautz W, Schindler G (1983) Vergleichende Röntgenuntersuchung des Dünndarms mit Mono- und Doppelkontrast. Radiologe 23:295–303

Cohen M (1982) Prolonged Visualization of the Gastrointestinal Tract with Metrizamide. Radiology 143:327–328

Efsing HO, Lindroth B (1980) Small bowel examination after injection of Cholecystokinin. Clin Radiol 31:225–226

Ekberg O (1977) Double contrast examination of the small bowel. Gastrointest Radiol 1:349–353

Frimberger E, Kühner W, Eggemann F, Ottenjann R (1983) Koloskopischer Dünndarmeinlauf. Dtsch Med Wochenschr 108:1546–1548

Geiter B, Fuchs HF (1977) Dünndarm-Kontrasteinlauf: Indikationen und Technik. Dtsch Ärztebl 43:2575

Herlinger H (1979) Small bowel. In: Laufer I (ed) Double Contrast Gastrointestinal Radiology. Saunders, Philadelphia

Herlinger H, Maglinte DDT (1986) Jejunal Fold Separation in Adult Celiac Disease: Relevance of Enteroclysis. Radiology 158:605–611

Hirsch J, Ahrens E, Blankenhorn DH (1956) Measurement of the human intestinal length in vivo and some causes of variation. Gastroenterology 31:274–285

Kaufmann HJ, Langer R (1985) Anwendung nichtionischer Kontrastmittel in der Magen-Darm-Diagnostik von Neugeborenen und Säuglingen. In: Kaufmann HJ (Hrsg) Kontrastmittel in der Kinderradiologie. Karger, Basel

Maglinte DDT, Lappas JC, Chernish SM, Sellink JL (1986) Intubation Routes for Enteroclysis. Radiology 158:553–554

Meyers MA (1976) Clinical involvement of mesenteric and antimesenteric borders of small bowel loops. II. Radiological interpretation of pathologic alterations. Gastrointest Radiol 1:49–58

Miller RE (1965) Complete reflux small bowel examination. Radiology 84:457–463

Miller RE, Sellink JL (1979) Enteroclysis: the small bowel enema. How to succeed and how to fail. Gastrointest Radiol 4:269–283

Ott DJ, Yu Men Chen, Gelfand DW, van Swearingen F, Munitz HA (1985) Detailed per-oral small bowel examination vs. enteroclysis – part I: expeditures and radiation exposure. Radiology 155:29–34

Pansdorf H (1937) Die fraktionierte Dünndarmfüllung und ihre klinische Bedeutung. Fortschr Röntgenstr 56:627–634

Salomonowitz E, Czembirek H, Kletter K, Achter E (1980) Die Strahlenbelastung bei der modifizierten Doppelkontrastuntersuchung des Dünndarms. Fortschr Röntgenstr 133, 4:430–433

Salomonowitz E, Wittich G, Czembirek H (1983) Ergebnisse der Doppelkontrast-Untersuchung des Dünndarms. Radiologe 23:289–294

Sellink JL (1976) Radiological Atlas of Common Diseases of the Small Bowel. Stenfert Kroese, Leiden

Sellink JL, Rosenbusch G (1981) Moderne Untersuchungstechnik des Dünndarms oder Die zehn Gebote des Enteroclysma. Radiologe 21:366–376

Thompson WM, Amberg JR (1978) Use of the c-terminal octapeptide of Cholecystokinin in clinical radiology. II. The small bowel. Gastrointest Radiol 3:195–199

Treichel J (1981) Anforderungen an die röntgenologische Untersuchung des oberen Gastrointestinaltraktes und des Dünndarms. Röntgenpraxis 34:357–365

Trüber E, Fuchs HF (1981) Die neoplastischen und entzündlichen Dünndarmveränderungen im Röntgenbild. Radiologe 21:377–380

Underhill BML (1955) Intestinal length in man. Br Med J 4950:1243–1246

Vogel H, Löhr H (1978) Strahlenexposition und Strahlenrisiko bei Röntgenuntersuchungen des Dünndarms mit der Sonde. Radiol Diagn 6:812–817

Chapter 5.1 "Crohn's Disease"

Berridge FR (1971) Two unusual radiological signs of Crohn's disease of the colon. Clin Radiol 22: 444–451

Crohn BB, Ginzburg L, Oppenheimer GD (1932) Regional ileitis: a pathological-clinical entity. J Am Med Assoc 99:1323–1328

Ekberg O (1977) Crohn's Disease of the Small Bowel Examined by Double Contrast Technique: a Comparison with Oral Technique. Gastrointest Radiol 1:355–359

Ekberg O (1984) Barium/air double contrast examination of the small bowel in Crohn's disease. Fortschr Röntgenstr 140, 4:379–386

Ekberg O, Bååth L, Sjöström B, Lindhagen T (1984) Are Superficial Lesions of the Distal Part of the Ileum Early Indicators of Crohn's Disease in Adult Patients with Abdominal Pain? A Clinical and Radiologic Long Term Investigation. Gut 25:341–346

Ekberg O, Fork FT, Hildell J (1980) Predictive Value of Small Bowel Radiography for Recurrent Crohn Disease. Am J Radiol 135, 5:1051–1055

Ekberg O, Lindström C (1979) Superficial Lesions in Crohn's Disease of the Small Bowel. Gastrointest Radiol 4:389–393

Feczko PJ (1987) Malignancy Complicating Inflammatory Bowel Disease. Radiol Clin North Am 25, 1:157–174

Frick MP, Salomonowitz E, Gedgaudas E (1984) The Value of Computed Tomography in Crohn's Disease. Mt Sinai J Med 51, 4:368–371

Gelfand DW (1984) Gastrointestinal Radiology. Churchill Livingstone, Edinburgh London

Gelfand DW, Ott DJ (1981) Radiographic Demonstration of Small Intestinal Villi on Routine Clinical Studies. Gastrointest Radiol 6:21–27

Glick SN, Teplick SK (1985) Crohn Disease of the Small Intestine: Diffuse Mucosal Granularity. Radiology 154:313–317

Gürtler KF, Erbe W (1980) Röntgenuntersuchung des operierten Darmes bei Morbus Crohn. Röntgenblätter 33, 9:453–458

Herlinger H (1979) Small Bowel. In: Laufer I (ed) Double Contrast Gastrointestinal Radiology. Saunders, Philadelphia

Herlinger H (1982) The Small Bowel Enema and the Diagnosis of Crohn's Disease. Radiol Clin North Am 20, 4:721–742

Hildell J, Lindström C, Wenckert A (1980) Radiographic Appearances in Crohn's Disease. IV. The New Distal Ileum after Surgery. Acta Radiol 21: 221–229

Kerber GW, Frank PH (1984) Carcinoma of the Small Intestine and Colon as a Complication of Crohn Disease. Radiologic Manifestations. Radiology 150:639–645

Kirsner JB, Shorter RG (1982) Recent Developments in "Non-specific" Inflammatory Bowel Disease. N Engl J Med 306, 13:775–785

Korelitz BI (1984) The Ileorectal and Ileosigmoidal Fistula in Crohn's Disease: A Clinical-Radiological Correlation. Mt Sinai J Med 51, 4:341–346

Marshak RH (1975) Granulomatous disease of the intestinal tract (Crohn's disease). Radiology 114:3

Morson BC (1964) Pathologisch-anatomische Veränderungen des Dickdarmes und der Analregion bei Crohn'scher Erkrankung. Z Gastroenterol 2:255–268

Morson BC, Dawson J (1979) Gastrointestinal Pathology. Blackwell Scientific Publications, Oxford

Nolan DJ, Piris J (1980) Crohn's Disease of the Small Intestine: a Comparative Study of the Radiological and Pathological Appearances. Clin Radiol 31, 5:591–596

Sartoris DJ, Harell GS, Anderson MF, Zboralske FF (1984) Small-Bowel Lymphoma and Regional Enteritis: Radiographic Similarities. Radiology 152: 291–296

Sellink JL, Miller RE (1982) Radiology of the Small Bowel. Martinus Nijhoff, The Hague

Chapter 5.2 "Inflammatory Diseases apart from Crohn's Disease"

Ament ME, Rubin CE (1972) Relation of Giardiasis to abnormal intestinal structure and function in gastrointestinal immunodeficiency syndroms. Gastroenterology 62:216–226

Antes G, Kruis W (1982) Whipple's Disease demonstrated by double contrast small bowel enema with barium and methylcellulose. Eur J Radiol 2: 238–241

Antes G, Lissner J (1983) Double-contrast small-bowel examination with barium and methylcellulose. Results in 300 cases. Radiology 148, 1:37–40

Brombart MM (1980) Radiologie des Verdauungstraktes. Thieme, Stuttgart

Bruneton JN, Faure X, Bourry J, Chauvel P, Abbes M, Lecomte P, Delmont J (1982) A radiologic study of chronic radiation-induced injury of the small intestine and colon. Fortschr Röntgenstr 136, 2:129–132

Chau PM, Fletcher GH, Rutledge FN, Dodd jr GD (1962) Complications in high dose whole pelvis irradiation in female pelvic cancer. Am J Roentgenol 87:22–40

De Cosse JJ, Rhodes RS, Wentz WB, Reagan JW, Dworken HJ, Holden WD (1969) The natural history and management of radiation induced injury of the gastrointestinal tract. Ann Surg 170:369–384

Crohn BB, Ginzburg L, Oppenheimer GD (1932) Regional ileitis: a pathological-clinical entity. J Am Med Assoc 99:1323–1328

Evert JA, Black BM, Dockerty MB (1948) Primary nonspecific ulcers of the small intestine. Surgery 23:185

Golden R (1945) Radiologic examination of the small intestine. Lippincott, Philadelphia

Graham JB, Villalba RJ (1963) Damage to small intestine by radiotherapy. Surg Gynecol Obstet 116:665

Graundins J (1969) Über Strahlenspätschäden am Dünndarm. Langenbecks Arch Klin Chir 324:120–130

Herlinger H (1969) Small bowel: In: Laufer I (ed) Double Contrast Gastrointestinal Radiology. Saunders, Philadelphia, p 484

Hermans PE, Huizenga KA, Hoffman HN, et al. (1966) Dysgammaglobulinemia associated with nodular lymphoid hyperplasia of small intestine. Am J Med 40:78

Joelsson I, Raf L, Soderberg G (1971) Stenosis of the small bowel as a complication in radiation therapy of carcinoma of the uterine cervix. Acta Radiol [Ther] (Stockh) 10:593–604

Lasserich MA (1953) Röntgenologische Studien an der terminalen Ileumschlinge bei gesunden Kindern. Z Kinderheilkunde 74:77–84

Marshak RH, Hazzi C, Lindner AE, et al. (1974) Small bowel in immunoglobulin deficiency syndroms. Am J Roentgenol 122:227

Mason GR, Dietrich P, Friedland GW, Hankes GE (1970) The radiological findings in radiation induced enteritis and colitis. Clin Radiol 21:232–247

Neumeister K, Pfeiffer J (1966) Klinische Analyse der akuten intestinalen Strahlenreaktionen bei Röntgen-Radium- und Telekobaltbestrahlungen. Strahlentherapie 129:512–519

Prévôt R (1950) Röntgendiagnose der entzündlichen Darmerkrankungen. Fortschr Röntgenstr 72:547–563

Rogers LF, Goldstein HM (1977) Roentgen manifestations of radiation injury to the gastrointestinal tract. Gastrointest Radiol 2:281–291

Rubin P, Casarett GW (1968) Clinical Radiation Pathology. Saunders, Philadelphia

Ruppin H (1980) Unspezifische Enteritis. Dtsch Ärztebl 50:2959–2969

Strockbine MF, Hancock JE, Fletcher GH (1970) Complications in 831 patients with squamous cell carcinoma of the intact uterine cervix treated with 3000 rads or more whole pelvis irradiation. Am J Roentgenol Radium Ther Nucl Med 108:293–304

Sturges HF, Krone ChL (1973) Ulceration and structure of the jejunum in a patient on long-term Indomethacin therapy. Am J Gastroenterol 59:162

Wells J (1948) The mucosal pattern of the terminal ileum in children. Radiology 51:305–309

Chapter 5.3 "Tumors"

Bancks NH, Goldstein HM, Dodd GD (1975) The Roentgenologic Spectrum of Small Intestinal Carcinoid Tumors. Am J Roentgenol 123:274–280

Barclay THC, Schapira DV (1983) Malignant Tumors of the Small Intestine. Cancer 51:878–881

Boijsen E, Kaude J, Tylén U (1974) Radiologic Diagnosis of Ileal Carcinoid Tumours. Acta Radiol [Diagn] (Stockh) 15:65–80

Bruneton J-N, Drouillard J, Roux P, Lecomte P, Tavernier J (1981) Leiomyoma and Leiomyosarcoma of the Digestive Tract – A Report of 45 cases and Review of the Literature. Eur J Radiol 1:291–300

Castellino RA (1986) Hodgkin Disease: Practical Concepts for the Diagnostic Radiologist. Radiology 159:305–310

Clements jr JL, Hixson GL, Berk RN, Dodds WL, Goldstein H (1984) Gastrointestinal Carcinoid Tumours: An Analysis of 104 Cases. Mt Sinai J Med 51, 4:351–359

Ekberg O, Ekholm S (1980) Radiography in Primary Tumors of the Small Bowel. Acta Radiol [Diagn] (Stockh) 21:79–84

Ekberg O, Ekholm S (1980) Radiology of Primary Small Bowel Adenocarcinoma. Gastrointest Radiol 5:49–53

Lennert K (1981) Histopathologie der Non-Hodgkin-Lymphome. Springer, Berlin Heidelberg New York

Marshak RH, Lindner AE (1976) Radiology of the Small Intestine, 2nd edn. Saunders, Philadelphia

Meschan I (1984) An Overview and Summary of Roentgen Signs of Diseases of the Small Intestine. Mt Sinai J Med 51, 4:319–336

Morson BC (ed) (1976) International Histological Classification of Tumors: Histological Typing of Intestinal Tumours. WHO

Morson BC, Dawson J (1979) Gastrointestinal Pathology. Blackwell Scientific Publications, Oxford

Sartoris DJ, Harell GS, Anderson MF, Zboralske FF (1984) Small-Bowel Lymphoma and Regional Enteritis: Radiographic Similarities. Radiology 152: 291–296

Sellink JL, Miller RE (1982) Radiology of the Small Bowel. Martinus Nijhoff, The Hague

Smith SJ, Carlson HC, Gisvold JJ (1977) Secondary Neoplasmus of the Small Bowel. Radiology 125: 25–33

Chapter 5.4 "Motility Disorders"

Cornell AM (guest editor) (1982) Motility and its disturbances. In: Clinics in Gastroenterology, vol 11, no 3. Saunders, Philadelphia

Erckenbrecht J, Wienbeck M (1984) Störungen der Dünndarmmotilität. In: Wienbeck M, Siewert JR (Hrsg) Therapie gastrointestinaler Motilitätsstörungen. Edition Medizin, Weinheim, pp 47–58

Franken jr EA, Smith WL, Smith JA (1980) Paralysis of the small bowel resembling mechanical intestinal obstruction. Gastrointest Radiol 5:161–167

Gupta A (1984) Radiological lactase deficiency – a population survey. In: Capesius P (ed) Proceedings of the XVth International Congress of Radiology, Brussels 1981. Abdomen and Gastrointestinal Tract. Interimages, Luxembourg, pp 514–518

Herlinger H, Maglinte DDT (1986) Jejunal Fold Separation in Adult Celiac Disease: Relevance of Enteroclysis. Radiology 158:605–611

Horowitz AL, Meyers MA (1973) The "hide-bound" small bowel of scleroderma. Am J Roentgenol 119: 332–334

Naish JM, Capper WM, Brown NJ (1960) Intestinal pseudo-obstruction with steatorrhoea. Gut 1: 62–66

Olmsted WW, Madewell JE (1976) The esophageal and small-bowel manifestation of progressive systemic sclerosis. Gastrointest Radiol 1:33–36

Sellink JL (1976) Radiological Atlas of Common Diseases of the Small Bowel. Stenfert Kroese, Leiden

Shimkin PM, Waldmann TA, Krugman RL (1970) Intestinal lymphangiectasia. Am J Roentgenol 110: 827

Shermling DH, Leisinger P, Prader A (1972) On the familial occurrence of coeliac disease. Acta Paediatr Scand 61:501

Wienbeck M (1980) Normale and pathologische Motilitätsmuster im Dünndarm. In: Symposion über Motilitätsstörungen, XI. Internationaler Kongreß für Gastroenterologie, Hamburg 1980. Pharmazeutische Verlagsgesellschaft, Hamburg

Wienbeck M, Erckenbrecht J (1983) Funktionelle Störungen des Dünndarms. In: Caspary WF (Hrsg) Dünndarm. Handbuch der Inneren Medizin, 3. Band, 3. Teil, B. Springer, Berlin Heidelberg New York Tokyo, pp 631–639

Chapter 5.5 "Obstructions"

Bizer LS, Liebling RW, Delany HM, Gliedman ML (1981) Small Bowel Obstruction. Surgery 89: 407–413

Caroline DF, Herlinger H, Laufer I, Kressel HY, Levine MS (1984) Small Bowel Enema in the Diagnosis of Adhesive Obstructions. Am J Roentgenol 142:1133–1139

Maglinte DDT, Miller RE (1984) Intubation Infusion Method: Reliability in Diagnosis of Mechanical Partial Small-Bowel Obstruction. Mt Sinai J Med 51:372–377

Maglinte DDT, Miller RE, Lappas JC (1984) Radiologic Diagnosis of Occult Incisional Hernias of the Small Intestine. Am J Roentgenol 142:931–932

Maglinte DDT, Peterson LA, Vahey TN, Miller RE, Chernish SM (1984) Enteroclysis in Partial Small Bowel Obstruction. Am J Surg 147:325–329

Ott DJ, Yu Men Chen, Gelfand DW, van Swearingen F, Munitz HA (1985) Detailed per-oral small bowel examination vs. enteroclysis. Radiology 155:29–34

Chapter 5.6 "Malformations"

Aldrich EM, Morton CB, Baker JP (1955) Intestinal obstruction resulting from malrotation of the intestine. Ann Surg 141:765–777

Altschul W (1924) Mesenterium commune. Fortschr Röntgenstr 32:580–585

Arey LB (1947) Developmental Anatomy. A textbook and laboratory manual of embryology. Saunders, Philadelphia

Berne AS (1959) Meckel's diverticulum. X-ray diagnosis. N Engl J Med 260:690–696

Berquist HT, Nolan NG, Adson MA, Schutt AJ (1973) Diagnosis of Meckel's diverticulum by radioisotope scanning. Mayo Clin Proc 48:98–102

Christie A (1931) Meckel's diverticulum. Am J Dis Child 42:544–553

Duszynski DO, Jewett TC, Allen JE (1971) Tc 99m-Na pertechnetate scanning of the abdomen with particular reference to small bowel pathology. Am J Roentgenol 113:258

Ferner H (1964) Grundriß der Entwicklungsgeschichte des Menschen, 8. Auflage. Einhardt, München Basel

Gardner jr CE, Hart D (1934) Anomalies of intestinal rotation as a cause of intestinal obstructions. Review of hundred and three reported cases. Arch Surg 29:942–981

Grob M (1953) Über Lageanomalien des Magendarmtractes infolge Störungen der fetalen Darmdrehung. Schwabe, Basel

Gross RE, Holcomb GW, Farber S (1952) Duplications of the alimentary tract. Pediatrics 9:449–468

Ladd WE (1942) Meckel's diverticulum. In: Christopher F (ed) Textbook of Surgery, 3rd edn. Saunders, Philadelphia, p 1163

Maglinte DDT, Elmore MF, Isenberg M, Dolan PA (1980) Meckel diverticulum: Radiologic demonstration by enteroclysis. Am J Roentgenol 134: 925–932

Moore TC, Battersby JS (1952) Congenital duplications of the small intestine. Surg Gynecol Obstet 95:557–567

Parsons B (1953) Paraduodenal hernias. Am J Roentgenol 69:563

Prévôt R (1968) Erkrankungen des Dünndarms. Handbuch der Medizinischen Radiologie, Band XI, Teil 2. Springer, Berlin Heidelberg, p 19

Rösch W (1978) Divertikel am Verdauungstrakt. Dtsch Ärztebl 44:2569–2573

Rosenthal L, Henry JN, Freeman LM (1972) Radiopertechnetate imaging of the Meckel's diverticulum. Radiology 105:371–373

Sandera R (1931) Duodenum mobile im Röntgenbilde. Fortschr Röntgenstr 44:574–599

Sellink JL (1976) Radiological Atlas of Common Diseases of the Small Bowel. Stenfert Kroese, Leiden, p 333

Smith JR (1960) Accessory enteric formations – a classification and nomenclature. Arch Dis Child 35:87–89

Stein GN, Bennet HH, Finkelstein A (1958) The preoperative roentgen diagnosis of Meckel's diverticulum in adults. Am J Roentgenol 79:815–822

Index

MIX
Papier aus verantwortungsvollen Quellen
Paper from responsible sources
FSC® C105338

If you have any concerns about our products,
you can contact us on
ProductSafety@springernature.com

In case Publisher is established outside the EU,
the EU authorized representative is:
Springer Nature Customer Service Center GmbH
Europaplatz 3, 69115 Heidelberg, Germany

Printed by Libri Plureos GmbH
in Hamburg, Germany